Of Medicine and Men

Of Medicine and Men

Biographies and Ideas in European Social Medicine between the World Wars

Edited by Iris Borowy
and Anne Hardy

PETER LANG
Frankfurt am Main · Berlin · Bern · Bruxelles · New York · Oxford · Wien

Bibliographic Information published by the Deutsche Nationalbibliothek
The Deutsche Nationalbibliothek lists this publication in the Deutsche Nationalbibliografie; detailed bibliographic data is available in the internet at <http://www.d-nb.de>.

Cover illustration:
© United Nations Office at Geneva,
United Nations Library,
League of Nations Archive

ISBN 978-3-631-58044-8

www.peterlang.de

Table of Contents

Of Medicine and Men – Introduction

Iris Borowy

Biography is a popular genre. We like stories about people, whose courses through life we can follow and understand. In reassuring ways the lives of even the most extraordinary persons, the heroes, the saviours and the monsters, unfold in categories we can relate to: hopes and ambitions, successes and failures, friendship, trust, deceit, love and hate. Biographies on Hitler, Stalin or the Soong siblings sell very well and are widely read. They have a prominent place in historiography, and justifiably so. Since by history we axiomatically assume the history of humans at its simplest level, all history is biography: an account of how people have experienced their environments, how they have reacted to them, what decisions they have taken and how these decisions have influenced the people and the world around them. Even mass phenomena consist of the aggregate individual fates: famine means many people suffering hunger, demographic growth means many people having three and more surviving children and living long lives, industrial revolution means many people making inventions, working in factories and living in an increasingly urban and technological environment. While we need statistics to grasp the quantitative component of reality, we need an understanding of individual fates to make sense of the numbers.

However, the dangers of biographies are equally obvious and well known: an overgeneralization of individual experiences i.e. accepting a few cases with their idiosyncratic aspects as representative of the large picture, overrating the impact of specific individuals in relation to cultural and political development beyond their control, the danger of filling in gaps of people's lives by speculations or imagination, concentration on seemingly important people and an uncritical or unbalanced assessment of their achievements, in short, neglecting analysis for the sheer story. Besides, the very popularity of biography presents a problem for scholarly analysis. In Austria, the issue has been considered sufficiently important in 2005 to establish an institute for the history and theory of biography, which justifies its existence by the fact that its genre has long been underestimated by professional scholars because of its murky place between fact and fiction. It defines its object of study as: 'Biography forms an intersection point between academia, art and entertainment.'[1] Today, biography can hardly be considered a neglected area. Several other institutes between the Netherlands and Australia devote all or part of their resources to the study of biography,[2] and at least seven journals focus on biography.[3] They can rely on and will no doubt add to an already impressive body of books relating to science/art and craft of writing biography.[4]

In fact, the genre is sufficiently extensive to allow the medical biography as a sub-field, including its own Journal of Medical Biography, dedicated to the study of 'lives of people in or associated with medicine...'[5] However, medical biography offers particular difficulties, derived from generations of historiographic baggage. Traditionally, the history of medicine has been perceived as the history of discoveries of physicians and scientists. Indeed, it is difficult to imagine how any history of medicine or health could possibly be written without mentioning personalities like Edward Jenner, Louis Pasteur or Robert Koch, not to mention Hippocrates. Thus, biographical data inevitably must be considered for the interpretation of past conceptualizations of disease, therapeutic traditions, the social repercussions of health and disease and a host of other facets, and justifiably, collections of doctors' biographies are considered important projects in the history of medicine.[6] But the very attention historiography grants them, and has to grant them as essential players in all matters regarding medicine and health, risks overrating them. For too long classic narratives granted medical men the role of heroes as selfless helpers of the sick and infirm or as similarly selfless researchers, who put their genius to the use of science for the benefit of mankind, as 'medical history ... seemed to celebrate medical science, glorify the role of physicians, and project a positivist view of scientific progress...'.[7] Such a view is no longer tenable, as revisionist analysis has revealed the profound involvement of physicians and science in general in all phenomena that have accompanied human history, the good, the bad and the ugly, including imperialism, colonialism, racism and genocide.[8] Also, at least since Thomas McKeown demonstrated that falling mortality rates in Europe pre-dated therapeutic competence, the relative importance of physicians for public health has had to be viewed critically.[9] Not surprisingly, a growing amount of scholarship addresses the particular problems surrounding biographies of scientists, trying to identify strategies that do justice to the ambivalence of the genre.[10] But at the moment, this theoretical interest is not borne out by successful practice. As Thomas Söderqvist shows in his recent overview, scientific biography merely represents a pointed version of biography in general: a large number of scientific lives face a dearth of scholarly treatments.[11]

Patrick Zylberman's paper in this volume is one attempt to bridge this gap by reconciling the complex historical baggage of professional ritual within the science community with a modern scholarly view. As his analysis makes clear, medical biographies have long existed in a multifaceted cultural context and have carried a variety of subtle meanings, which are near impossible to detach from present-day perspectives. Inevitably, the legacy of this context colours all subsequent memory of individuals, including the choice of who is remembered favourably, often, or even at all. Bearing these cautions in mind, this book aims to understand the health experience of a period through a small group of physician-scientists. For a number of reasons, the early twentieth century is a particularly rich period for biographical analysis. The important role medicine played in Nazi Germany has served to direct attention to doctors' interaction with National Socialism.[12] In other countries, important developments such as the introduction of the welfare state and the evolution of social hygiene have sparked interest in prominent proponents.[13] But as medicine and public health became international, one of the main themes of this volume, an increasing number of people have been perceived as international personae. Thus, a number of personalities that marked the international health scene have already been the object of publications. In recent years Heinrich Zeiss has attracted substantial attention for the clear political repercussions of his position between Weimar Germany, Soviet Russia and Nazi ideology and his ambivalent concept of 'geomedicine.'[14] Maxime Kuczinsky-Godard's activities in several continents have been examined exhaustively.[15] Similarly, with Alan Gregg, Jacques Parisot and René Sand, some of the influential men of the international public health scene of the period have been described.[16]

So what has determined the selection of men in this volume? Zylberman's sharp analysis makes it impossible to ignore the extent to which the framework of organisational structure and memory context has also affected the preparation of this volume. Thus, the selection of personalities was partly dictated by institutional affiliation to the League of Nations Health Organisation (LNHO), arguably the centre of international health in Europe at the time.[17] It was also the only international health organization to develop a clear social hygienic approach to public health and to forge ties between scientists along those lines. While the Rockefeller Foundation, which likewise plays a significant role in the story of this volume, remained committed to a vertical, disease-centred view of public health, and the *Office International d'Hygiène Publique* focused on an older epidemiological paradigm, the LNHO organized comprehensive projects regarding the social determinants of health and thus became the natural point of reference for work of social medicine at the time.[18] This context connected a social and political to the medical-scientific agenda of the people involved. Social medicine was then a major conceptual framework of health. It derived from a growing awareness of the detrimental repercussions of industrialisation on the health of the worker population, often overworked and underfed and crammed into dismal housing.[19] An increasing realization of the serious health effects of such conditions gave rise to an international movement of health experts, who never organised into a coordinated pressure group, but who were vaguely united in 'a critical approach to health care that stressed the social determinants of disease.'[20] These determinants included working and living conditions and their contexts. A social medical approach to public health typically was horizontal, addressing not specific diseases but the general measures needed to prevent the outbreak of an array of diseases. Thereby, social medicine combined descriptive and normative components: the former sought to determine the conditions that led to specific diseases or increased morbidity among special risk groups, a process that necessitated comprehensive statistical evidence, while the latter aimed at identifying structures that would prevent these diseases and result in good health among all parts of society, notably the underprivileged. Increasingly, it formed part of the mainstream of medical and societal discourse. While the exact meaning of social medicine remained vague and adaptable to local circumstances, the central idea informed crucial welfare legislation as well as contemporary understanding of public health.[21] Originally, the focus on the need for social reform as a prerequisite of improving public health identified social medicine with left-wing, socialist positions. However, ideological lines were not that clearly defined. The preventive element of social hygiene could be interpreted as a prevention of disease in future generations, forming connections to eugenics and racial hygiene.[22]

By the 1930s, a social medical approach to public health had found forceful institutional endorsement in the League of Nations Health Organisation (LNHO). The impact of the LNHO on the international discourse can hardly be overestimated. It attracted international cooperation because it offered funds, professional expertise, a safe framework for open discussion and, to many, a promise of modernity. In several fields of work, it elicited the enthusiastic cooperation of some of the best minds of the time.[23] In some way our subjects were all connected with it, though Selskar Gunn never belonged to it or cooperated in LNHO projects. But his unwavering support for the institution within the Rockefeller Foundation was of substantial support. The importance of the interconnection of people affiliated with the LNHO has been pointed out before. Martin Dubin coined the expression of a 'biomedical/public health episteme' that characterised international cooperation among a group of medical and public health experts, who framed the discourse from within various international organisations.[24] A similar point has been made by Bridget Towers.[25] As both emphasise, strong, determined and sometimes brilliant individuals were the driving forces of the interwar health scene, but they gained their impact only through an informal yet effective network of colleagues. In some instances, as for Andrija Štampar or Franz Goldmann during World War II, this network may have been life-saving. Of the people in this volume, Andrija Štampar is probably the best known internationally. He and Selskar Gunn have been described in the English language.[26] Bela Johan has attracted substantial and controversial attention in his native Hungary. Franz Goldmann and Fritz Rott have both been the object of lengthy biographies but are otherwise little known outside of, or even in, Germany. Gustavo Pittaluga, Thorvald Madsen, Melville Mackenzie, Emil Roesle and Otto Olsen have received little attention before, and in some cases unearthing sufficient information about them has proved difficult. The story of many men who made up the vibrant international public health scene during the formative period after World War I is still untold, among them Oscar Velghe (Belgium), Alberto Lutrario (Italy), Hugh Cumming (USA), Antoine Lasnet (France), and Witold Chodzko (Poland). Regrettably it was not possible to include them in this volume because material or authors or both could not be found. The full story of international social medicine during the early twentieth century is still to be written. This book is meant to be one contribution to it.

At first sight, the men of this volume appear to be experts in different fields with only limited overlap. Pittaluga was by training a malarialogist, Johan a pathologist, Gunn a biologist, Štampar a social hygienist, Goldmann a public health expert, Mackenzie a general practitioner, Madsen a serologist, Olsen a clinician, Rott a paediatrician and Roesle a statistician. But a closer look reveals that they had more in common than seems immediately obvious. All devoted all or part of their attention to the conditions that determined the health of groups of people; all were active in the field of public health structures, often with a focus on rural areas. They were also all interdisciplinarians, combining two or more fields of work by mixing medical practice, scientific research, academic teaching and public health administration. The degrees to which they engaged in these respective duties differed. Some were primarily scientists (Roesle, Pittaluga, Madsen), others were more prominently public health officials (Johan, Štampar, Gunn), some spent prolonged periods as practicing physicians (Mackenzie, Pittaluga, Štampar) and others were long-time lecturers (Goldmann, Roesle). Several made significant contributions to conceptual developments in public health (Štampar, Johan, Goldmann, Rott), others contributed to it through diplomacy (Madsen, Gunn, Mackenzie). But all of them mixed duties, and it is remarkable how much they saw the various facets as complementary. To them, experience with patients inter-acted with theoretical knowledge (requiring as much as generating it), the collective experience with individuals needed to be enriched by laboratory findings and transformed into statistical evidence, and the understanding thus gained should feed back into health benefits via public health arrangements and training for new generations of doctors. Thus, they clearly agreed on several key issues:

- that individual health depended on public health policies and therefore there was a need for an active public health agenda,
- that prevention was at least as important as therapy,
- that in the interest of the general good some parts of society, notably children and rural populations, needed special attention;
- that effective efforts needed to be rational, holistic and science-driven, incorporating bacteriology and social hygiene,
- that public health was a collective responsibility of many, including governments, insurance funds, scientists and physicians, whose respective input required cooperation and coordination,
- that all progress depended on the international exchange of information.

The internationalism of this group was a formative component of their activities, and, by the same token, their and their colleagues' activities shaped the nature of international medico-scientific discourse at the time. For some of them, internationalism came naturally. Olsen's origins in the Danish minority in northern Germany automatically provided him with a bi-national background, and Pittaluga entered a transnational sphere when he left his native Italy for life and work in Spain. Several worked in foreign countries (Štampar, Mackenzie, Gunn, Madsen, Goldmann) or at least considered it (Johan). Such personal factors spurred these men's international outlook, but even those, whose work remained inside their native country (Rott, Roesle) appreciated the value of experience beyond its borders. This exchange was noteworthy because it was not limited to science, whose flow is inevitably international, even if and when scientists and governments try to put it to nationalist use. To an unprecedented degree, these people exchanged ideas about what constituted health and how societies could and should be organised to safeguard it. Collectively, they made use of this small window of opportunity where the breakdown of an old world order encouraged social experimentation before the advent of World War II, and subsequently the Cold War, froze a free flow of ideas. Although the interwar era was certainly rich in contradictory ideology, these ideological rifts did not divide public health theory into distinct and neatly packaged concepts.

The significance of the LNHO in the lives of these men has been noted. But there were other avenues of contact, both organizational and geographical. While they were most likely physically to meet in Geneva at meetings of LNHO committees many of them depended, financially and professionally, on the support of the Rockefeller Foundation (RF) for at least part of their careers. RF fellow Gunn helped negotiate the terms under which the RF underwrote some of the health reforms undertaken by Štampar in Yugoslavia and Johan in Hungary. Pittaluga likewise profited from RF funds, though to a lesser extent. Geographically, first Russia and then China turned out to be formative locales for interwar public health. Even before the First World War, Russia provided a key experience for Madsen. His observations during the 1908 cholera epidemic shocked him for the intensity of helpless misery that an infectious disease could still cause in a European country at the time, and it opened his eyes to the need for international cooperation in science as well as in issues of public health. Years later Mackenzie would undergo a very similar experience when acting as the only foreign doctor in a Russian province. While Russia acted as a catalyst for international public health efforts, it also provided illustration of the effects of the first – and only – communist administration, its radical break with conventional social policies and the effects on public health. As always, people's conclusions tended to reflect individual perspectives. While Mackenzie was appalled by what he perceived to be blatant abuse of healthcare in the interest of inhumane politics, Roesle was fascinated and Štampar clearly impressed. Only a few years later, the new National Government of China offered a second testing ground for the creation of a new public health system. But this time, there was no question of learning from Chinese experiments. Western health experts, who had invested considerable efforts in improving clearly inadequate health structures in their own countries, now turned to China with missionary zeal. While Gunn and Mackenzie undertook the coordination of modernization efforts for their respective institutions, Johan and Štampar provided conceptual cues, and after his forced departure from Croatia, Štampar strove to implement his ideas in China. Even Goldmann, desperate for a new professional home after German politics had made him a refugee, tried to save his own livelihood by working for China. The importance of these two countries was hardly coincidental. The nascent Soviet Union and China naturally attracted international physicians: as places of turmoil and the extensive prevalence of epidemic diseases with a clear need for medical help, but also as countries that were establishing new health systems in processes that offered both demonstration material and jobs. With their mixture of hygienic misery and promise, these two countries epitomized the feeling within medical circles of the time.

The world of international health was small, allowing for paths to cross frequently. Already in 1910-11 Štampar was impressed by the lectures of Ludwig Teleky in Vienna, some fifteen years before the latter would argue with Emil Roesle about the correct use of medical statistics.[27] Later in Croatia, Štampar used references by Alfred Grotjahn, who was also a formative influence on the careers of Franz Goldmann and Fritz Rott in Germany. Madsen was the driving force behind the connection of Germany to the LNHO and possibly both he and Grotjahn were directly involved in the employment of Otto Olsen at the LNHO Health Section in Geneva. Meanwhile, Štampar was one of the important contacts for Gunn during the latter's stay in Europe, another being Bela Johan in Hungary. In 1936, Štampar toured Europe with Pittaluga and in the same year he met Charles Winslow during a mission to the USSR. Winslow was then instrumental in opening doors to employment for Goldmann, who had taken refuge from Nazi Germany in the United States.

These contacts were facilitated by the characteristics they had in common. They came from comfortable, middle to upper middle class backgrounds, with Štampar, whose father was a village teacher, occupying the relatively lowest rank of the social ladder. Born between 1870 and 1895, they came of age before World War I. They were old enough to have experienced the world of the long nineteenth century with its scientific and social progressivism and its political conservatism. They had qualified as doctors and had gained various degrees of work experience when they witnessed the breakdown of the political order, often that of their own countries, notably the Habsburg Empire (Štampar, Johan) and the German monarchy (Goldmann, Rott, Roesle, Olsen). And even for those, who came from relatively stable societies in Denmark or the USA (Madsen, Gunn) World War I proved the pivotal event that radically transformed the conceptual conditions of their work. But they were also young enough to appreciate the opportunities inherent in the post-war crises. For them, the combination of reformist currents in science and social theory, medical needs and political options translated into tangible efforts towards new, improved health systems.

In retrospect, it is the ambivalent relation to politics which is most intriguing about the intertwined careers, portrayed in this volume. At all times, medicine and public health are political issues. As numerous publications have amply demonstrated in recent years, a plethora of decisions about the social construction of patients and diseases, about sanitary measures, and access to measures of prevention and cure are distinctly political.[28] None of these men could have been unaware of the close nexus between political decisions and public health output, since they were subjected to evidence of the process on a daily basis. Few countries enjoyed political stability. Madsen, Gunn and Mackenzie were among the lucky few, whose lives were based in countries with stable political regimes. But Pittaluga, Johan, Štampar and, obviously, their German colleagues experienced changes not only of government but of political system which threw into question the entire fabric of the social order. They knew that politics could overnight wipe out structures that had been built up over years.

Above all, the catastrophic First World War affected public health, both data and discourse, in all European countries, and in this context medical science entered political conceptualisations to a degree unknown before.[29] The war left scars everywhere, but it proved traumatic for the defeated. In Hungary, resentment over the treaty of Trianon gave birth to a psychological need to demonstrate Hungarian cultural superiority, a mindset that Bela Johan duly took into account when he portrayed public health work as part of a national-conservative policy for cultural assertion and when he made sure to stress real or imagined Hungarian origins of his plan for a major health reform. In Germany, widespread indignation about the treaty of Versailles restricted the possibilities of cooperation with the LNHO. And, similar to Hungary but with more devastating results, defeat was compensated by a search for perceived racial superiority. Scientific racism was hardly new, but it gained deadly strength in a climate in which the society eagerly sought this chance to repair their sense of victimization, and in which doctors eagerly sought this chance to improve both social standing and job opportunities.[30] In Spain, the experience of defeat in the 1898 Spanish-American War led not to introspection but, on the contrary, to an opening up to 'Europe," an imagined place of modernity and reform, which would allow the country to regain its rightful place in the international arena. Thus, while Johan, Goldmann, Roesle or Rott sometimes had to find ingenious ways to connect their work to outside influences, Pittaluga, by seeking international contact, merely met widespread expectations about his role as scientist – at least until civil war and the fascist rise to power turned political coordinates upside down. Meanwhile, Madsen, Mackenzie and Gunn enjoyed the luxury of stable systems that weathered the challenges of economic crisis and international political crisis through democratic changes of government within democratic order. In a sense, they even benefited from the war, which broadened their bio-political horizon and opened up new career opportunities to them. Madsen, while not having sought this path, gained international stature as a shrewd businessman, who combined economic opportunity with impartial – and life-saving – help to combatant troops, and as a diplomat in humanitarian mission. Mackenzie positively enjoyed his war experience, which he spent far away from frontline bloodshed and which introduced him to another life than that of a provincial GP. In dealing with people and administrations in turbulent places, these men could hardly afford to ignore political sensitivities. Gunn, as mediator between American and European public health efforts, and Mackenzie, temporarily responsible for public health decisions in Liberia and China, had to take cognizance of the politics of these countries in their charge. Thus, the lives of the people in this volume serve as illustrations of how interwar political thinking diffused into scientific work. Only Madsen seemed able to switch effortlessly between the complicated politics of his international engagement at the LNHO and the scientific retreat of his serological institute in peaceful Denmark. The neutral status of his country doubtlessly helped, but so supposedly did his calm bearing. Even so, politics caught up with him after the outbreak of World War II. Unlike most in the international scene, he apparently translated his loyalty to his German colleagues into pro-Axis sentiments, or so at least it seemed to French observers.[31]

The issue of Germany and German politics eventually forced the deepest rifts within the group. In some cases, the World War II position was a continuation of long-term ideological development, in which medical beliefs constituted a formative component. Thus, Fritz Rott began his career as a conservative side and inexorably veered further to the extreme right. His views on child welfare – perfectly in line with LNHO work during the 1920s – increasingly took on eugenic overtones. After 1933, Rott embraced racial hygiene and continued a successful career in National-Socialist Germany. For others, living with National Socialism appeared a matter of political compromise without conceptual connection to their bio-medical agenda. Faced with the demands of dictatorships Bela Johan and Otto Olsen tried to manoeuvre their way through difficult times in ways that evade simple moral judgment. Such ambivalence was not open to all. Jewish Franz Goldmann was forced to leave Germany because staying was tantamount to a death sentence. Štampar's life was no less in jeopardy. After losing his position due to nationalist intrigue in his country and spending several years on temporary assignments, he was imprisoned by German occupation forces and forced into an internment camp. He probably survived only because of the intervention of a 'German professor,' whose identity remains obscure. Not all men endured such a dramatic, life-threatening turn of events, but several experienced political difficulties of varying degrees. Pittaluga had to leave Spain when a workers' committee removed him from his office, and he then found himself dismissed twice, first by the Republican and later again by the Francoist government. Johan was detained for a few days by Communist authorities in 1950, probably under suspicion of overly close contact with Western scientific circles. He was released unharmed, but worked for the rest of his life in pharmaceutical research, outside the field of public health administration. Roesle probably owed his relative safety during National Socialism to the usefulness of his expertise, despite his pro-Soviet sympathies. Attitudes to the Soviet Union divided the group almost as much as those to Germany. Štampar was dismayed by the growing tide of fascism he witnessed in Europe and found reason to admire developments in Communist Russia, apparently blind to the genocidal starvation its policies caused in the Ukraine (and elsewhere). By contrast Mackenzie, while never in danger of turning fascist, was repelled by his experience with Communism in the Soviet Union and retained a conservative outlook that effortlessly reconciled internationalism with loyalty to the British Empire. The group's views on the US health system were correspondingly diverse. While Johan looked towards the USA as a model to learn from, Štampar considered it backward and in need of progressive reform. Gunn tried to distance himself from the tendency of the Rockefeller Foundation to export its American system throughout the world but never doubted that it was a model worth exporting when adapted to local circumstances.

Between them, these men represent the entire range of politics on offer during the period. Inevitably, these differences placed them on different sides of the political divides, defined by those in power in their countries during and after World War II. Johan, Rott and to some extent Olsen were on the 'right' side of power during the war and unable to cleanse themselves of the political stain afterwards. Štampar, Goldmann and, though in a different way, Roesle were on 'wrong' side before or during the war, but exonerated afterwards. Those who were blessed by the absence of dictatorship, Gunn, Mackenzie and Madsen, were consistently on the 'right" side or, in the case of Madsen, at least escaped further scrutiny of his wartime attitude. Relatively the saddest case may be Pittaluga, who never managed to establish himself in a place with whose politics he was fully in harmony. He was survived by dictatorship.

There remains the paradox that people with such contrasting political beliefs could, at one time, work together within a framework of organised international cooperation and could hold very similar bio-medical views. Part of the explanation may be that to a substantial extent they acted under the express credo of the apolitical character of health. Indeed, several of them flatly denied the political nature of their work. Pittaluga tried to organise malaria commissions in ways that kept them independent from government influence. Both Štampar and Mackenzie ostensibly aimed at keeping their health work separated from 'politics.' This attitude is non-sensical not only because of the evident political component of public health concepts and strategies, but because several of the men themselves were active in politics. Johan was political secretary in the Ministry of the Interior from summer 1935 until October 1944. Štampar was chairman of the Department of Racial, Public and Social Hygiene in the newly founded Ministry of Public Health. Rott was deputy director of the new Imperial Centre for Health Matters, and Goldmann worked at the Imperial Health Bureau. Pittaluga joined the newly founded Reformist party and won a seat in the last democratically elected parliament before the military dictatorship of Primo de Rivera, and later he held several public service positions under the short-lived Second Republic. Ironically, the person who most emphatically rejected a political component of medicine, Mackenzie, accepted the most clearly political twist in his career. On behalf of the League he repeatedly engaged in missions, which had only scant connection to medical affairs, such as his missions to Liberia or his responsibility for League work in China. Still, although these people's lives in themselves belied the idea of non-political health, the concept nevertheless held true in the understanding of a basic humanity, common to all people, which transcended political considerations. And, as Zoe Sprigings points out, this belief was certainly held dear by some experts in ways that were self-delusive as much as they were idealistic. And without doubt it paved the way for their direct or indirect cooperation across ideological divides.

On a practical level, however, cooperation was often less complicated than ideological differences might suggest. As indicated above, many ideas about best practice in public health were shared across belief barriers, which only later became ideologically prohibitive. At the time, numerous measures (mass screenings and mass vaccinations, health propaganda, the control of water quality and the establishment of a rational infrastructure of health institutions) were compatible with fascism, communism or liberalism. In a remarkable congruence of thought the health centre epitomizes this shared pool of ideas. Virtually all the men portrayed in this volume endorsed, recommended, established or worked in a health centre type of institution at some point or other. The concept clearly had broad appeal, possibly for a combination of elements: the idea a central place of reference for health matters, mainly but not exclusively preventive, where people from different disciplines cooperated or its embeddedness in the social fabric of a people. Not surprisingly, they made common enemies among practicing physicians, who defended their status as a liberal profession, the group whose status was most threatened by broad based public health activities.

As individuals, all these men had periods of success and failure, but in the end their fates took distinctly different turns. Madsen, Mackenzie and Štampar ended their lives as highly respected personalities, whose expertise was sought and whose contribution to the international health scene was valued at renowned research institutes or at the World Health Organization. By contrast, Pittaluga spent his last years in exile in Cuba with most of his work destroyed by the dictatorship that prevented his return. Several continued their careers in unspectacular ways. Roesle and Madsen, the two oldest of the group, approached retirement in their professional environment. Goldmann had a prestigious position at Harvard but suffered from seeing his ideas ignored. Those who were tainted with Nazi collaboration continued on a more subdued level. Johan was discredited through his temporary connection with the occupation forces, but he was nevertheless able to gain a scientific foothold in pharmaceutical production. Rott evaded scrutiny of his role in the Nazi administration through an unglamorous but solid private practice, and Olsen apparently remained loosely connected with the general field of public health without, however, being able to regain secure employment.

The result of their work is difficult to define, both collectively and individually, and assessment invariably depends on whether one chooses a short- or long-term perspective. As the controversy around Bela Johan in Hungary proves, evaluation also depends on political circumstances and is far from over. But some people's legacy seems comparatively clear. Štampar's significance as a formative figure in the establishment of public health structures in Yugoslavia and as co-founder of the WHO is uncontested. Madsen is justifiably remembered as a long-time Director of the Danish State Serum Institute and a central personality in serological standardization. Roesle's contribution to medical statistics is recognised among statisticians. The achievements of Pittaluga, Gunn, Goldmann, Rott, Olsen and Mackenzie are known only to a small group of specialists, and clearly their significance is limited. Gunn, Olsen and Mackenzie were mainly organisers, important in their times for the functioning of international cooperation but with little conceptual input into the overall discourse to leave as legacy. Goldmann's ideas still have their place in today's discussions of modern public health systems, while Rott's writings have dated and are to a large extent discredited by his Nazi connection. Pittaluga has left his mark on the development of public health in democratic Spain and on malariology.

In the end, the collective significance of these men is more than the sum of their individual successes and failings. They were influential – though not the only – pioneers of a culture of international, interdisciplinary and holistic commitment to public health. Their cooperation was made possible by the existence of international organisation, above all the LNHO, but by the same token these organisations existed only through their activities. They were the first generation of bio-medical experts who perceived health issues in their medical, scientific and social shape as challenges for international engagement, to which they contributed and from which they drew support. With their visions, their differences among themselves and also their shortcomings, they drove a process towards an approach to global health which now appears natural, almost self-evident, to us. Though their immediate goals were usually much more modest, and often more self-serving, together they were essential contributors to the efforts of humanity towards a global civil society.

Acknowledgments
I would like to thank Esteban Rodríguez-Ocaña, Erik Ingebrigsten, and Anne Hardy for helpful comments on the paper.

---

1 Ludwik Boltzmann Institut. Geschichte und Theorie der Biographie. Quoted at: http://gtb.lbg.ac.at/index.php?pId=k4536bm15819gvg200526&mediaId=1, viewed 1 Feb 2008.

2 Including the Biografie Instituut at the University of Groningen; The Center for Biographical Research at the University of Hawaii, the Biography Institute at the Humanities Research Centre of the Australian National University.

3 a/b: Auto/Biography Studies; Auto/Biography; Biography, BIOS, Journal of Historical Biography, Life Writing and Life Writing Annual.

4 See for instance L.E. Ambrosius (ed.), *Writing Biography: Historians and Their Craft* (Lincoln: University of Nebraska Press, 2004); H.E. Bödeker (ed.), *Biographie schreiben* (Göttingen: Wallstein Verlag, 2003); W. Fuchs-Heinritz, *Biographische Forschung. Eine Einführung in Praxis und Methoden* (Wiesbaden: Verlag für Sozialwissenschaft, 2002); M. Holroyd, *Works on Paper: The Craft of Biography and Autobiography* (London: Little Brown, 2002); C.N. Parke, *Biography: Writing Lives* (New York: Routledge, 2002).

5 Journal of Medical Biography, http://www.rsmpress.co.uk/jmb.htm, seen 7 July 2008.

6 W. Eckart and C. Gradmann (eds.), *Ärzte-Lexikon, Von der Antike bis zur Gegenwart* (Berlin: Springer Verlag, 2006).

7 See E. Fee, 'Public Health, past and present: A shared social vision', Introduction to George Rosen, *A History of Public Health* (Baltimore: Johns Hopkins University Press, 1993), x.

8 P. Weindling, *Epidemics and Genocide in Eastern Europe, 1890-1945* (Oxford: OUP, 1999).

9 For a review of McKeown's thesis and arguments of his critics, see B. Harris, 'Public Health, Nutrition, and the Decline of Mortality: The McKeown Thesis Revisited', *Social History of Medicine*, 17:3 (2004), 379-407.

10 M. Greene, 'Writing Scientific Biography', *Journal of the history of biology*, 40:4 (2007), 727-760; C. Carson and S. Schweber, 'Recent biographical studies in the physical sciences', *Isis* 85 (1994), 284-292; T.L. Hankins, 'In Defence of Biography. The Use of Biography in the History of Science', *History of Science* 17 (1979), 1-16; M. Shortland and R. Yeo (eds.), *Telling Lives in Science. Essays on Scientific Biography* (Cambridge: Cambridge University Press, 1996).

11 T. Söderqvist, 'A New Look at the Genre of Scientific Biography', in T. Söderqvist (ed.), *The History and Poetics of Scientific Biography* (London: Ashgate, 2007), 1-15.

12 R.J. Lifton, *The Nazi doctors: medical killing and the psychology of genocide* (New York: Basic Books, 1986); A. Ebbinghaus and K. Dörner (eds.), *Vernichten und Heilen* (Berlin: Aufbau Taschenbuch Verlag, 2001); E. Klee, *Deutsche Medizin im Dritten Reich. Karrieren vor und nach 1945* (Frankfurt a.M.: S. Fischer Verlag, 2001); R. Proctor, *Racial Hygiene: medicine under the Nazis, Cambridge* (Harvard: HUP, 2000).

13 E. Bendiner, 'Sara Josephine Baker: A Crusader for Women and Children's Health', *Hospital Practice* 30:9 (1995), 68-77; N. Goodman, *Wilson Jameson. Architect of National Health* (London: George Allen and Unwin Ltd., 1970); Jose Harris, *William Beveridge* (Oxford: Clarendon Press, 1997).

14 P. Weindling, 'Heinrich Zeiss, Hygiene and Holocaust,' in D. Porter and R. Porter (eds.), *Doctors, politics and society: historical essays* (Amsterdam: Rodopi, 1993), 174-

187; W. Eckart, 'Creating Confidence': Heinz Zeiss as a Traveller in the Soviet Union, 1922-1932', in S. Gross Solomon (ed.), *Doing Medicine Together: Germany and Russia between the Wars* (Toronto: University of Toronto Press, 2006), 199-239; S. Gross Solomon, 'Infertile Soil: Heinz Zeiss and the Import of Medical Geography to Russia, 1922-1930', ibid., 240-290; S. Schleiermacher, 'The Scientist as Lobbyist: Zeiss and *Auslandsdeutschtum'*, ibid., *291-324;* S. Schleiermacher, 'Der Hygieniker Heinz Zeiss und sein Konzept der 'Geomedizin des Ostraums",' in R. vom Bruch and C. Jahr (eds.), *Die Berliner Universität in der NS-Zeit*, (Stuttgart: Steiner, 2005), 17-34.

15 M. Cueto, 'Social Medicine and 'Leprosy" in the Peruvian Amazon', *The Americas* 61:1 (2004), 61; B.A. Zuno, 'Maxime Kuczynski-Godard, un pionero de la salud pública', *Rev. perú. med. ex salud publica* 20:4 (2003), 231; M. Knipper and M. Cueto (eds.), *Social medicine, medical geography and health care for indigenous peoples: 'Ethnic Pathology'in Germany, Russia, Latin America and beyond*, (forthcoming).

16 P. Zylberman, 'Fewer Parallels than Antitheses: René Sand and Andrija Štampar on Social Medicine, 1919-1955', *Social History of Medicine*, 17:1 (2004), 77-92; Lion Murard, 'Health Policy between the International and the Local: Jacques Parisot in Nancy and Geneva', in I. Borowy and W.D. Gruner, *Facing Illness in Troubled Times* (Berlin: Peter Lang Verlag, 2005), 207-245; A. Anciaux, *Le docteur René Sand ou la culture des valeurs humaines* (Bruxelles: Conseil International de l'action social, 1988); W. Schneider, 'The Model American Foundation Officer: Alan Gregg and the Rockefeller Foundation Medical Divisions', *Minerva* 41:2 (2003), 155-166.

17 See I. Borowy, *Coming to Terms with World Health, The League of Nations Health Organisation,* Rochester University Press, (forthcoming).

18 I. Borowy, 'Social Medicine between the Wars. Positioning a Volatile Concept', *Hygiea Internationalis,* 6:2 (2007), 13–35.

19 About social medicine see also: M. R. Anderson, L. Smith, and V.W. Sidel, 'What is Social Medicine?', *Monthly Review*, 56:8 (2005), 27-34; G. Moser and J. Fleischhacker, 'People's health and Nation's body. The modernisations of statistics, demography and social hygiene in the Weimar Republic', in E. Rodríguez-Ocaña (ed.), *The Politics of the Healthy Life, an International Perspective* (Sheffield: EAHMH, 2002), 151-179; L. Murard and P. Zylberman, 'French social medicine on the international public health map in the 1930s', ibid., 197-218; D. Porter and R. Porter, 'What was Social Medicine? An Historiographical Essay', *Journal of Historical Sociology,* 1 (1989), 90-106.

20 E. T. Morman, 'George Rosen, Public Health and History', in George Rosen, *A History of Public Health* (Baltimore: John Hopkins University Press, 1993), lxix.

21 See E. Fee and Roy Acheson (eds.), *A History of Education in Public Health* (Oxford: OUP, 1991), and for a contemporary perspective R. Wilkinson and M. Marmot (eds.), *The Social Determinants of Health* (Oxford: OUP, 1999).

22 See A. Labisch, ‚Die „hygienische Revolution" im medizinischen Denken. Medizini--sches Wissen und ärztliches Handeln,' in A. Ebbinghaus and K. Dörner (eds.), *Vernichten und Heilen* (Berlin: Aufbau Taschenbuch Verlag, 2001), 68-89.

23 See I. Borowy, 'International Social Medicine Between the Wars. Positioning a Volatile Concept,' *Hygiea Internationalis*, 6:2 (2007), 13–35.

24 M. Dubin, 'The League of Nations Health Organisation', in P. Weindling (ed.), *International health organisations and movements, 1918-39* (Cambridge: CUP, 1995), 56-80.

25 B.A Towers, *The Politics of Tuberculosis in Western Europe 1914-40. A Study in the Sociology of Policymaking,* Ph.D. thesis, London University, 1987.

26 S. Litsios, 'Selskar Gunn and China: The Rockefeller Foundation's 'Other" Approach to Public Health', *Bulletin of the history of medicine,* 79:2 (2005), 295-318; P. Zylberman,,'Fewer Parallels than Antitheses: René Sand and Andrija Štampar on Social Medicine, 1919-1955', *Social History of Medicine*, 17: 1 (2004), 77-92; T.M. Brown, 'Andrija Stampar: Charismatic Leader of Social Medicine and International Health', *American Journal of Public Health,* 96:8 (2006), 1383-1385.

27 I. Borowy, 'Counting Death and Disease - Classification of Death and Disease in the Interwar Years, 1919 – 1939', *Continuity and Change,* 18:3 (2003), 457 - 481.

28 See e.g. A.T. Price-Smith, *The Health of Nations* (Cambridge, Mass.: MIT Press, 2002); R. Cooter and J. Pickstone (eds.), *Companion to Medicine in the Twentieth Century* (London and New York: Routledge, 2003); E. Rodríguez-Ocaña (ed.), *The Politics of the Healthy Life* (Sheffield: EAHMH Publications, 2002); R.B. Proctor, *The Nazi War on Cancer* (Princeton: Princeton University Press, 1999).

29 See chapter three in Mark Mazower, *Dark Continent: Europe's twentieth Century* (London: Penguin Books, 1998).

30 See P. Weindling, *Health race and German politics between national unification and Nazism, 1870-1945* (Cambridge: Cambridge University Press), 1993.

31 Ministre des Affaires Etrangères to Ministre de la Guerre, stamped 26 October 1939, and response, AMAE, Serie SDN. IL – Hygiene. Nr. 1562. Composition du Comite d'Hygiene; Report, untitled, unsigned and undated, AMAE, SDN, IL-Hygiène, 1561, 193-6. The description of Madsen is credible in as much as he did, indeed, have close personal ties to Germany. It is, however, strange to imagine him turning against Poland, the home of his long-time friend and LNHO partner, Rajchman.

Selskar 'Mike' Gunn and Public Health Reform in Europe

Socrates Litsios

Introduction

Selskar 'Mike' Gunn is the only person included in this volume whose responsibilities were not primarily national in character. Instead, in his capacity as Director of the Rockefeller Foundation's Paris Office (1922-1932), he interacted with many, if not all, the 'big names' of this book, and others, to help shape the support provided by the Foundation to national public health systems throughout Europe. This chapter examines Gunn's growing frustration with what he perceived as serious weaknesses in the Foundation's strategy concerning the training of medical doctors in public health, both undergraduate students in medicine and health officers already employed. In documenting Gunn's failure to alter the approach of the Foundation in Europe, I hope to shed more light on issues that are of importance today, in particular the problem of developing a productive relationship between medical interests and those of public health. This history suggests that the Rockefeller Foundation had other options in Europe that might have proved more productive than the ones they chose to follow.

Background

Concerned with the debilitating impact of hookworm on education, the Rockefeller family established the Rockefeller Sanitary Commission in late 1909 with Wickliffe Rose, an educator, in charge. In the course of the effort to control this disease in several Southern US States, it became evident to Rose that the lack of a public health infrastructure prevented the achievement of permanent gains. The best that could be done was to demonstrate what methods worked, in the hope that local governments would incorporate them into their health programmes. Such demonstrations would serve as 'an entering wedge, a method by which states and nations could be induced to build up permanent machinery to take care of the whole problem of public health'.[1] They were also educational, with the public as 'first priority', [2] and it was they that would lead to 'a consideration of the whole question of medical education, the organization of systems of public health, and the training of men for the public health service'.[3] In 1913 an International Health Commission (IHC) was established with Rose as Director to extend the hookworm campaign around the world. Rose's travels abroad convinced him that 'there was a general need for public health workers at all levels'.[4] To achieve this he envisioned a system for public health similar to the teacher training system used in the Southern United States. In 1914 he prepared a report on Training for Public Health Service for America which embodied the notion of such a system. This report led to studies which in time led to the establishment of the Johns Hopkins School of Hygiene and Public Health. Although Rose worked with William Welch, professor of pathology at the Johns Hopkins Medical School, in determining what kind of public health school was needed, it was Welch who ended up having the last word, in a process that has been extensively described by historians.[5] Welch believed that public health leaders should have medical degrees. Contrary to the wishes of Rose and senior public health specialists who participated in the discussions which led to the establishment of the Johns Hopkins School, the Hopkins curriculum gave preference to advanced education, giving priority to research and research methods. None of the faculty of the new school 'had ever been a public health officer or had any direct experience of public health practice'.[6] Welch went so far as to indicate that the school need not 'meet the immediate needs of the public health service'.[7] This helps explain why he saw no place for Gunn in his school in 1917, when George Vincent, the newly designated president of the Rockefeller Foundation, proposed that Welch hire him. At the time Gunn was editor of the *American Journal of Public Health*, and had already shown an aptitude in the development of educational campaigns in his capacity as part-time director of the Massachusetts's Division of Hygiene.[8] Welch did not want his faculty to be disturbed 'by having to do popular work or by being part of a large organization part of which [was] meant to do popular work'.[9] Instead, Gunn was engaged by the Foundation as associate director of the Foundation's Commission for the Prevention of Tuberculosis in France.[10]

Rose's early vision for America was a network of public health schools spread out across the country with one or more institutes at the centre. The role of the central institutes would be to produce knowledge needed in public health and to guide smaller schools, which would be responsible for educating local health officers. In 1919 he extended this vision to the whole world: 'a series of schools of hygiene at strategic places all over the world, with relations of interchange, and including the building up of public health organization, statistics and public health laboratory services, and demonstrations in the control of [certain key diseases]'.[11] Vincent organized a conference of Foundation officers and advisors in 1920 to consider the question of training centres in public health for America. Although Rose was not present, his vision of a hierarchical network of schools was still in place, as can be judged by the three types of educational centres that Vincent proposed for discussion: (a) 'scientific study, research and inspiration, which will extend fundamental sciences of public health'; (b) 'sound training school which will stress preparation of health officers and technicians'; and (c) 'short, practical field training courses in connection with State Boards of Health'.[12] Johns Hopkins was given as an example of the first centre, the Harvard-MIT school for health officers of the second, and New York State and Ohio of the third. The idea that the Hopkins school 'would be a kind of foster mother to all, furnishing teachers, leaders, etc...,' still prevailed. Welch, who was present, thought it would be 'unfortunate' to differentiate between the types of training planned at Hopkins and Harvard. Each place should combine scientific research and professional training, adding that research was a 'necessary feature of a first class institution'. Vincent suggested the possibility of forming departments of public health in several medical schools 'rather than of forming additional separate schools'. For that, all that was needed, according to Welch, was a 'bacteriologist, a parasitologist, and a general hygienist, with their laboratories and equipment'. This would 'effect medical education and influence medical students, thus bringing physicians generally into sympathetic touch and cooperation' with the public health movement as well as 'develop the field on a nation-wide basis'.[13]

Although the word 'inspiration' was associated with the Hopkins school, by all accounts, William Sedgwick, the founder of the MIT School of Biology and one of the co-founders of the Harvard-MIT school, was considered by many to be the most inspirational teacher of public health at the time.[i] It was after hearing Sedgwick lecture at the end of 1901, his first year at MIT, that Gunn decided to shift from Electrical Engineering to biology.[14] Sedgwick was also associated with the idea that a medical degree was not a necessary prerequisite for public health. What Gunn's views were on the subject is not clear; nevertheless, when Marshall Balfour, who studied under Gunn while at MIT, asked for career advice in late 1921, Gunn replied 'take a medical course if [you want] to get into public health'.[15] Thus, while clearly inspired by Sedgwick, Gunn was not attempting to resurrect Sedgwick's idea of a public health career independent from that of medicine. Instead, Gunn's preoccupation was precisely with the second line of educational facility, one that aimed at preparing health officers and technicians. This helps explain why he examined first-hand the relationship between Harvard and MIT on almost each of his visits to the States during this period. The relationship between the two schools was altered by the establishment of the Harvard School of Public Health in 1921. With Sedgwick's agreement, and Rose's belief that the lack of interest in public health among the participating professors 'could be remedied', the new school of public health was located near the medical school.[16] David Edsall, at the time dean of both the Harvard School of Public Health and the Medical School, believed that medical students' attitudes would not change 'until we can change the attitude of the medical faculties'.[17] Unfortunately, Sedgwick died in early 1921 when he was actively working on the design of the new school in which MIT was expected to play an integral role. This perhaps explains why when Gunn visited the area in

---

i Allen Freeman, who taught public health at Hopkins in the 1920s, judged Sedgwick to be 'greatest teacher of the subject [public health] at the time'. (A. Freeman, '*Five Million Patients: The Professional Life of a Health Officer*' (New York: Charles Scribner's Sons, 1946), 60-1)

1923 he found reasons to 'deplore[s]' the 'unfortunate relation between Harvard and Tech [MIT]' with respect to the School of Public Health.[18] Only one Harvard student had taken any course at MIT, something that Gunn learned from his discussions with Edsall.

In September 1923 Edsall sought funds from the Foundation for a plan to improve 'the teaching of the preventive aspects of medicine during the course of the regular teaching in several departments of the medical school'.[19] Frederick Russell[ii], who had taken over from Rose the directorship of the International Health Board (IHB)[iii] earlier that year, and Vincent replied that they saw this project as 'one of great fundamental importance and distinctly one in which our Board might interest itself'.[20] Furthermore, they understood it to be **'the connecting link'** between the activities of the Foundation in the development of medical education and of the IHB in the development of public health.[21](Emphasis added) When Gunn visited the Boston area in 1927 he found that, while MIT personnel still believed that 'non-medical men had and can play a useful role in practical public health', the Harvard people felt 'that public health is essentially for doctors, and have a rather disdainful attitude towards the Institute'.[22] Furthermore, the Harvard school depended on RF fellowships for its students, without which, it 'would be a farce as a school and simply be a research institute'. On his next visit (1928) he judged that the Harvard staff did 'not really understand public health work in the field'.[23] Edsall seems to have been more preoccupied with raising the Harvard School of Public Health to a level equivalent to that of the Hopkins school, as Welch had proposed in 1920, rather than in preparing health officers and technicians, as the joint Harvard-MIT school had done. Hence, the stress on the word 'research' in all Harvard's proposals to the IHB during this period.[24]

Meanwhile, it had become clear that the idea that advanced training in public health would interest medical doctors, as Welch had imagined in 1914, had been in error.[25] Furthermore, these visits demonstrated to Gunn that America had not solved the problem of developing practical training programmes geared to serving public health officers in the field (with or without MD degrees). In short, America had little to offer Europe in this regard. European countries would have to develop their own approaches to the problem. When Gunn consciously realized this is not clear. What is clear, however, is his interest in both issues from the moment he moved from France to Prague in 1920 to take on the position as IHB advisor to the Czech government in all matters pertaining to public health.

---

ii Russell was a military physician whose main interest was in the laboratory side of public health. When he left the US Army Medical Corps his rank was that of Colonel; in the reserve it was that of Brigadier General.

iii The new name for what had been the IHC.

The Gunn-Rose Dialogue

Gunn and Rose knew each other in 1915 when Rose was a member of a committee that guided Gunn's survey of organizations interested in public health in America.[26] It was during Gunn's stay in Prague, however, from October 1920 to June 1922, that the two had an extensive correspondence which reveals the similarity of many of their views.[27] Not surprisingly, given the central role that he placed on an educated public, Rose fully supported Gunn's initiatives in health education. The experience of the Foundation had convinced him that it was possible to educate the people 'however illiterate they may be, and to secure their interested cooperation in public health measures.... An illiterate peasantry may, after all, be pretty intelligent.... Getting officialdom in line, I should regard vastly more difficult than creating health interest on the part of an illiterate peasantry'.[28] Furthermore, Rose hoped to see the 'methods that you developed in France', which he regarded 'as the most successful public health educational work that has been done anywhere', developed in some other country.[29] In fact, he wished to see it 'tried in our own country'.[30] Rose was referring to the health education work that Gunn had undertaken in the Foundation's anti-TB programme in France.[31] Gunn's campaign in France focused on school children, with the aim of getting them to adopt hygienic measures that their parents would also be encouraged to adopt. Its essential feature was a travelling exhibit mounted on motor trucks from which movies and slides were shown. Punch and Judy shows were incorporated as well. There was also full agreement concerning the value of demonstrations. Alluding to the early days of the Foundation's involvement in health, Rose informed Gunn that 'as a means of educating and stimulating people to action there seems to be no substitute for the convincing demonstration'.[32] The purpose of such work was less to control a disease than 'to make a demonstration which will lead ultimately to the enlistment of local agencies in the work'.[33] Gunn too was 'convinced that a good demonstration in health work in a carefully selected district will be the most useful thing to do'.[34] While Gunn encouraged demonstrations, the few that did begin while he was in Czechoslovakia tended to focus more on general health education endeavors, rather than on the control a specific disease, although studies of tuberculosis and typhoid fever were initiated.

It was first envisaged that Gunn's assignment to Czechoslovakia would be to study the work being done concerning TB and the 'public health situation in that country'.[35] But following a trip taken with Rose, a number of 'urgent needs' were identified, including emergency aid in the control of infectious diseases; competent counsel in public health administration; aid in establishing an efficient public health laboratory service, which was seen as 'the beginning of a school of public health'; the keeping of accurate vital statistics; young men and women trained for higher positions in the Ministry of Health; short practical courses in public health; and, a training centre for public health nurses.[36]

The programme approved by the Trustees in May 1920 only partially met these needs, being confined to the loan of an American advisor (Gunn), nine fellowships[iv], cooperation in the development of an efficient public health laboratory service (State Institute of Health), and provision for a commission of up to five representatives from the Ministry of Health to examine public health administration in England and the US. Russell, whom Rose had engaged in 1919, was sent to Prague in August 1920 for several months to initiate work on the institute; Gunn arrived in October that year. Unlike the mandate of the Foundation's hookworm commission, Gunn's responsibilities were rather open-ended, as best illustrated by his intense interaction with numerous organizations operating in public health, some of them with significant international funding, such as the American Red Cross. This led him to suggest to Alice Masaryk, head of the Czech Red-Cross and personal advisor to the country's president, her father, that she bring together representatives of these organizations for the purpose of discussing coordination and the establishment of a National Public Health Association.[37] In time this became a National Council of Social Hygiene.

Gunn's assignment was fraught with difficulties including the tenuous health of his wife and daughter.[38] Among the many serious obstacles that he encountered were the poor pay, limited authority and lack of education of the health personnel. Furthermore, 'the medical profession here as a general thing is out for the money. They have absolutely no social sense and the teaching they get at the present time is such that questions of this kind never enter their heads ... the future of health work in this country is in the hands of the medical profession'.[39] Rose noted that the 'attitude of indifference and quiet hostility on the part of the physicians is not novel ... this attitude must in the end yield to the public good'.[40] Russell, too, was optimistic concerning the future attitude of the medical profession towards public health. Writing to Gunn in 1921, he expressed his personal view that he was 'not at all sure that curative medicine should be separated from preventive medicine and as the socialization of the medical profession increases, I think we are more apt to bring the two things together than we are to separate them'.[41] Although full-time health officers constituted one of the basic tenets of the Foundation's programme, Gunn judged this to be 'entirely impossible until conditions are radically changed'.[42] What was needed was educational work in health matters '(primarily) among the medical profession, the governing officials, and (secondarily) among the people. A strong demand for adequate health service will have to be created; it is only through this that we can hope for full time trained health officials'.[43] The words 'primarily' and 'secondarily' were crossed out before posting this letter. Rose agreed that the full time public health officer was 'for the future'.[44]

iv The Foundation's fellowship programme was one of its most important activities. More than 10,000 fellowships were offered between 1913 and 1948.

Gunn expressed his inclination 'to push energetically the question of creating a School of Public Health' and wondered how this might be viewed by the Board.[45] This proposal was clearly linked with his desire to find some way to develop educational work among the medical profession. Rose suggested that the Institute of Hygiene 'might perhaps be considered as the nucleus of what might in time grow into an Institute of Hygiene and Public Health'.[46] Not only do the two 'mights' stand out, but Rose's next two sentences both stressed the modesty of whatever was begun: 'I am sure that Colonel Russell has guarded against committing the Board in any respect whatever.'[47] Nevertheless, Gunn brought this subject up several times, before conceding that it would 'have to wait the development of the Institute of Health'.[48] For the time being, at least, priority was given to the Institute, which was essentially a laboratory-related affair, rather than one geared to public health training. The priority status of the institute, which did not open until 1925, when it was still not fully operational, led Rose to suggest to Gunn that 'no additional proposals be brought to the attention of the Foundation until this matter of the Institute [had] been definitely settled'.[49] Another initiative that grew out of Gunn's presence in Prague was the establishment of a Bureau for Study and Reform of Public Health Activities, an idea that Rose did not encourage. After discussing this matter with the Czech commission visiting the States, he reminded Gunn of several 'fundamentals': 'the importance of a demonstration in the field as against a Bureau in the Ministry', 'the importance of securing the right man to direct the field demonstration', and 'the importance of beginning modestly'.[50] Gunn managed to use the Bureau to provide a place for returning fellows who could not be secured a place immediately. Rose later judged Gunn's action one of the 'most important services' that he was rendering.[51] The expectation that older staff in the Ministry would resign to cede their positions to returning fellows proved naïve; the Bureau served as a kind of waiting room from which much useful work could be done.

After 11 months in Czechoslovakia Gunn raised the question whether it was a 'good policy for the IHB' to send an advisor to serve in a capacity such as his.[52] He thought it was 'somewhat of a debatable question' as demonstrations were far easier than what he was doing.[53] In response, Rose pointed to the long-term potential of his work, arguing that Gunn had no occasion to be discouraged. Work of the kind that he was doing 'moves with the deliberation of an iceberg; one is not so much interested in the rate of progress as in its direction. We are working on the roots of a plant and must look for the fruitage through a long period of years'.[54] Interestingly enough, Russell too used a root-related analogy to describe the work of the IHB, but his message was different: 'Plant an acorn and eventually you have to take care of an oak tree'![55]

Advice From Afar

Gunn received several job offers that his wife would have been pleased to have had him accept, as they were all positions in America: Directorship of the American Red Cross health services, an 'important position with the new Child Health Association', Director of the National Health Council, and a position with the committee on Municipal Health Department Practices.[56] Rose supported his applications while indicating at the same time that 'so far as we can see we should like to continue you in Europe for some time to come'.[57] Gunn opted to stay with the Foundation. As expressed to his friend Charles Winslow, 'the programme of the work which I have the privilege of conducting in Europe at the present time is so important that I cannot relinquish it'.[58] At this point Gunn had settled down in Paris and was deeply involved in seeing what kind of service he could provide to other countries. While stationed in Prague, Gunn had visited nearby countries including Poland, Romania and Hungary. Now he found himself making extensive visits to a good number of new countries, sometimes more than once, including

1922: Ireland
1923: Bulgaria, Ireland, Sweden, Yugoslavia
1924: Romania, Yugoslavia, Hungary, Denmark, Ireland, Algeria
1925: Yugoslavia

Gunn's report on the situation regarding IHB work in Europe at the end of 1924, for obvious reasons, began with France, where the earlier anti-tuberculosis work had been transferred to the *Comité National*. As cooperation with the central health authorities of France had been 'very slow' to develop, a cooperative programme had been initiated with one of a government departments which, it was judged, would in five years time have a 'modern health services'.[59] Gunn also expressed the hope that a project would be developed for the creation of a school in Paris for the training of health personnel closely related to the Faculty of Medicine of Paris, under a special board of directors for the 'post-graduate work, with special courses for non-medical personnel'.[60] Gunn also helped in the creation of a national office of social hygiene, which resembled that of Czechoslovakia in many ways.[61] The other countries reported on in 1924 were England, Ireland, Denmark, Norway, Sweden, Austria, Czechoslovakia, Hungary, Poland, Yugoslavia, Turkey, Greece, Albania, Bulgaria, Romania, and Algeria. Several others were also included where no concrete action had yet been taken, including Russia, Belgium, and Germany. With respect to Czechoslovakia, despite confessing that he was 'somewhat discouraged', Gunn voiced the opinion that it was 'bound to be one of the most progressive and important countries from the point of view of public health in Central Europe'. He was also upbeat concerning prospects in Hungary, Poland, and Bulgaria, but it was Yugoslavia that he found 'the most interesting in Europe today'.[62]

Gunn and Russell had jointly visited Yugoslavia in 1923, by which time Russell had taken over from Rose the directorship of the IHB. Both were much impressed by the programme led by Dr Andrija Štampar, Director of the

Division of Hygiene of the Ministry of Public Health. When Gunn returned in the spring of 1924 Štampar accompanied him during most of his visit. His observations led Gunn to conclude that: 'without any assistance from outside and with limited and inadequately trained personnel they have been able to accomplish much within a short period of time'.[63] In fact, he doubted if there was any country in the world in which such strides had been made in 'so short a period of time'. As Gunn understood it, this was exactly the kind of situation the Board was looking for, 'to help those countries which are both anxious and capable of helping themselves'. Without such help Yugoslavia would continue on its path but with help 'we can accelerate it very materially'. Of perhaps even greater importance was the fact that 'by showing our interest in a material way we can undoubtedly assist in stabilization of the whole public health program'.[64]

It was through Štampar that Gunn extended his understanding of the intimate links between the social and economic condition of the rural poor and their health. Perhaps of even greater significance, reinforcing the conclusion he had already reached while working in Czechoslovakia, was Štampar's views on the importance of undergraduate training in public health in medical schools. Štampar believed that the development of public health services 'required a great number of properly trained physicians'.[65] In his opinion the separation of undergraduate and postgraduate training in public health was 'not a good thing'. Furthermore, undergraduate training was 'more important' and postgraduate training should be a continuation of the former and confined 'mostly to the doctors who have shown a great deal of interest in public health matters during their undergraduate studies'.[66] Undergraduate studies, as Gunn was to later tell George Vincent, would develop in Europe under professorships of 'social medicine in important medical schools' and would have a 'stimulating effect upon public health work in general'.[67]

Gunn continued to explore new possibilities in 1925 but late that year Russell expressed doubts concerning the Foundation's ability 'to undertake any program involving a considerable expenditure at this time'.[68] A limited number of fellowships was the best he could offer. Accepting Russell's directives would have reduced Gunn to a bureaucrat whose major responsibility would have been limited to the administration of fellowships in Europe, something that was clearly unacceptable to him. Instead, he raised the stakes by pushing for a unified programme involving the other programmes of the Foundation. At the same time, he continued to work with Štampar to see whether the Foundation could be persuaded to support more broadly conceived programmes applying the social sciences to health as well as agriculture.[69]

A Unified programme in Public Health for Europe

One of the major problems that Gunn faced in developing what he thought of as a unified programme for countries in Europe was the division of labour between the IHB and the Division of Medical Education (DME).[v] What particularly disturbed him, as he described in a long letter to Russell written in April 1925, was how this affected 'the undergraduate teaching of hygiene in medical schools'.[70] And, as the teaching of preventive medicine in the medical schools in Europe 'has been very poor in the past ... and ... remains so in most of the medical schools', Gunn judged the 'whole matter' to be of 'very considerable importance'.[71] Gunn described the rising importance of the professor of hygiene and the efforts being made in various places to improve the laboratories for the practical teaching of the subject. He introduced the question of the relationship of the Chair of Hygiene to postgraduate courses and special courses in public health, concluding, despite the fact that there were exceptions, that it was 'more logical that the postgraduate and special courses should be also tied up in some way with the Institute of Hygiene of the Medical Faculty'. He observed that the programme of the DME had, until then, been essentially 'of an emergency character' but that this was drawing to an end. There was 'already a tendency – as for example in connection with the development of the teaching of hygiene in the medical schools – for the DME to develop a constructive program'.[72] As events would shortly demonstrate, Gunn was somewhat over-optimistic in reaching this conclusion.

Gunn informed Russell that this subject had been discussed with Pearce during the latter's visit to Paris. On that occasion they concluded that 'it would be wiser if the undergraduate teaching of hygiene in the medical schools was transferred' from the DME to the IHB.[73] This would lead to a more unified programme of public health in a given country. A similar case was made for public health nursing, which Gunn thought should also be moved into the IHB from the Division of Studies, established a year earlier, whose responsibilities included nursing education. Gunn ended his letter with Pearce's suggestion of 'the three divisions represented in Paris making a joint report on new countries which are to be surveyed' as well as a similar report for countries in which the Foundation was already operating.[74] Russell's reaction was clear, as indicated by his note in the margin: 'reports should be made **after** instructions from NY. Joint action **to be in NY**' (emphasis added).[75] Clearly, Russell was not about to delegate any of his authority to the Paris office or to share it with Pearce, with whom he neither collaborated nor had a friendly relation.[vi]

Nevertheless, Pearce's visit to Paris had immediate consequences. A conference of officers was held the following month in New York to discuss the teaching of

v The DME was created in 1919 as a new division in the Foundation with Richard Pearce, whose pre-Foundation career was that of professor of pathology and research medicine, as Director.

vi Simon Flexner, one of the Board of Directors of the IHB, wrote of the 'friction' between Russell and Pearce, [that] on occasion led Russell to lose his temper. (Flexner to Fosdick, 19 June 1926, RAC, Record Group 3, Series 900, Box 17, Folder 122).

hygiene, closer cooperation among the divisions in working out plans in a given country, nurse training (division of labour), and the administration of the Paris Office.[76] The present arrangement, where Gunn conducted 'complete surveys' of public health, was no longer satisfactory to Pearce. He did not believe Gunn would send in reports on undergraduate education unless he was 'held directly responsible for such reports'. One possible solution, noted by Pearce, was that all hygiene, graduate and undergraduate, be turned over to the IHB. But this would 'interfere enormously...with the development of the medical curriculum', for which he was responsible. In the end, it was agreed that the unity of the undergraduate medical education should be preserved and that the IHB had the responsibility 'on the educational side **only** for the special training of health officers' (emphasis added).[77] For Gunn, this was tantamount to no solution at all, since it avoided what he considered to be of basic importance: the introduction of public health in the undergraduate curriculum for medical doctors.

An important development was the arrival in Paris of Alan Gregg, Pearce's representative for Europe.[vii] Gregg's first European assignment was Italy where he conducted a detailed survey of medical education before settling down in Paris in late spring 1925. He was thus present when Vincent visited in July, when two points of 'special importance' that had emerged from the May meeting in New York were discussed.[78] The first related to administrative matters, during which Gunn's status as 'senior officer in Paris' was noted. The other concerned 'methods to obtain closer organization between the divisions on programs in varying countries'. By stressing that 'the Paris office represents the Rockefeller Foundation' Vincent was hoping to obtain from the Paris office what he had been unable to develop in New York, namely, unity of action.[79] Vincent was obviously impressed by the team spirit that was clearly in evidence in the Paris Office.[viii] He encouraged the office to present unified programmes. With this in mind he created the position of Vice-President at the Paris Office, for which he first approached Gunn, with Gregg next in line, should Gunn refuse. Gunn accepted in early 1927.[80]

Vincent supported unity of thinking in other staff new to the Paris Office. But more important was his support of Gunn's position on medical education, as shown by his urging upon Daniel O'Brien, Assistant Director to Gregg, the

---

vii Gregg, a Harvard Medical School graduate, had joined the Foundation in 1919. He worked 3 years in Brazil on a hookworm project before Pearce offered him the position of Associate Director of Medical Education.

viii Gregg, in a letter to Gunn written shortly after his move to the New York Office (early 1931), wrote: I'm particularly grateful to you for all the help you've given me and indeed a good many others in Paris as well for you...are the principal cause of the developments that became the Paris Office. (Alan Gregg Papers, MS C 190, National Library of Medicine, Bethesda, Maryland) 'importance of stressing the preventive idea in all our medical education work – we entered this field for the sake of promoting public health interests – more important to educate the average doctor than even the special public health Officer ... we should aim at as intimate team-play as possible between the 2 aspects of medicine'.[81] Pearce, however, had other ideas. Now that the 'frankly emergency' period was over, it was time to start on 'definite programs based on my own ideas'.[82] He wanted Gregg to be free by the end of 1927 to take up what he had in mind. He advised Gregg 'not to be obsessed with the idea of helping medical students only in the undergraduate school'.[83] This idea had been inherited from earlier days; there was no reason now to not get away from it. Pearce chose, instead, to concentrate 'stipends and supplies in certain medical school departments ... to contribute to the progress of science and to train men in research and teaching'.[84] The major project was in London, where several universities received aid. Another priority was the 'Latin'-speaking countries (French, Italian, Portuguese, and Spanish).[85] This excluded almost all the countries that Gunn had hitherto concentrated on, except France, where there was perhaps least interest on the part of the national government in the kind of unified programme he had in mind. One cannot help but wonder what Gunn and Gregg might have constructed if left to their own devices, especially given their close friendship. They did, however, utilize other means to bring their case to higher authorities, beginning with Raymond Fosdick[ix], who was in charge of the ongoing reorganization resulting from informal discussions several years earlier.[86]

Fosdick, in a confidential letter dated 19 April, 1926, asked Gunn for his views on a wide range of issues related to the working and administration of the various Boards which the Foundation ran. Gunn, in reply, stressed the fact that the investigations and studies carried out by the Paris office were based on the 'principle of developing a unified program'.[87] He thought the 'inflexible' policies of the IHB to be 'most unwise'. The IHB would be better served by an 'opportunistic attitude', one that would allow 'different types of work to be carried out in different countries (or even in different parts of the same country)'. Furthermore, he was not convinced that 'American methods in public health work [were] necessarily the best for European countries...', in view of the existence of men and women in the countries themselves with 'a better understanding of the local problems and the means to be used to meet them than we have'. These points made it 'quite plain that a serious difference of opinion' existed between himself and Russell.[88] Gregg, in his confidential memorandum on reorganization, indicated that 'divisional identity (had) been emphasized to the point of isolation. Rather than adjust our organization to cope with problems

ix Fosdick was a Trustee of the Foundation and a very close advisor to John D. Rockefeller Jr., Chairman of the Board of Trustees of the Rockefeller.

as they occur ... we cut and trim opportunities to fit the narrow and apparently inelastic limits of Divisional or Board policy'.[89] Advantage was taken of both Gunn's and Gregg's presence in New York to organize a four-day conference on European policies and programmes in late February 1927, just after Gunn had been made Vice-President for Europe. At this conference it was agreed that 'hygiene, public health, medical education and nursing shall always be thought of in relation' and that the 'procedure would differ according to situation'.[90] However, the directives emerging from this meeting made it clear that decision-making powers still remained in the hands of the Directors in New York. Vincent's efforts to create an independent, mini-Foundation in Paris that worked on a unified programme had not yet borne fruit.

Gunn continued to promote the idea of increased integration of public health and medical training in the hope that the upcoming reorganization could serve to bring this about. To this end, he provided Vincent with ammunition in support of a strategy.[x] In a special memorandum written to Vincent on his return to Paris Gunn focused on a point that he had already raised with Fosdick earlier, namely the Foundation being perceived as having 'set out on a definite program of "Americanization" of European public health'.[91] 'Are we not dogmatists and too much sold to our dogma? Are we developing the same weaknesses as are attributed to missionaries? Too much faith in our particular brands of public health, medical education, nursing, etc.' He reminded Vincent of the high quality of the nationals with whom the Foundation dealt, using several examples to illustrate his point, including: 'Does Štampar know more about the best way to develop public health nursing training in Yugoslavia than Miss Crowell'?[xi] 'Is it right for RMP [Pearce] to decide not to help medical education in Prague while there exist two medical faculties...?'[92]

Vincent continued to report positively to Gunn on developments in New York, while never directly indicating that the changes taking place would bring about reforms Gunn was pushing for. In some ways they hinted exactly the opposite. Thus, while informing Gunn that it was 'practically certain that the Foundation will be set up in the complete form that we have been planning', he went on to advise him to become 'more and more familiar with the personnel and centers of research which have to do with all the major forms of human knowledge'.[93] Vincent may have had conflicting hopes of the reorganization. On one hand, he preached the kind of integration that Gunn sought. On the other, he and Fosdick were actively seeking through the organization to reduce the powers of the so-called Medical Barons of the Foundation, Russell and Pearce.

---

x Vincent and Gunn were very close, as witness the numerous times that Vincent stayed with Gunn on weekends in Cannes where Gunn had set up his wife and daughter owing to their continuous state of ill health.

xi Elizabeth Crowell was a nurse and staff member of the IHB.

In the end, neither was achieved, for after the reorganization the 'medical barons were still firmly in the saddle'.[94]

Fosdick, it would seem, never responded to Gunn's criticism, although he incorporated some of it in his own critiques. He had preoccupations beyond the question of whether or not the Foundation was overly dogmatic in its approach to countries. His major concern was how to bring together diverse programmes run under the various philanthropic bodies, of which the IHB was only one, i.e. 'to rationalize the messy administrative structure of the boards'.[95] It was decided that the Foundation 'should be built around a central idea, i.e., the advancement of knowledge'.[96] The reorganization that followed took the shape of five divisions: international health, medical sciences, natural sciences, social sciences, and humanities. Despite the new orientation of the Foundation towards individuals carrying out research, Vincent still encouraged Gunn to bring his ideas to the attention of two study committees that had been formed to guide the transformation of the IHB (Simon Flexner, chairman) and the DME (David Edsall, chairman).[xii] Flexner, with whom Gunn was expected to meet, fell ill and decided, instead, to request someone to undertake a study of the IHB activities in Europe. In the course of events, this study did not take place, as neither Andrew Balfour nor Arthur Newsholme, who had been asked, were free to take it on.[xiii] Gunn heard from Edsall, but there is no evidence of him having replied.

On his visit to New York in October Gunn learned of the plans for the IHB and the DME. He found the general plan for the IHD to be 'excellent'.[97] His reaction to that of the DME was otherwise. Meeting first with Vincent, he expressed the hope that aid to medical education would not be 'suddenly or wholly abandoned in Europe', arguing that 'country physicians need much better training (since) their co-operation in public health work (is) essential'.[98] He next raised the issue with Pearce and was not pleased with what he learned:

> SMG [Gunn] wonders whether the new policy of the RF in connection with medical education would mean that the program to develop strong departments of hygiene and preventive medicine in strategic medical faculties would be abandoned. RMP [Pearce] says that it will not necessarily be abandoned but will be approached

xii Flexner, in addition to being on the Board of Directors of the IHB was Director of the Rockefeller Institute for Medical Research.

xiii Several months passed, involving extensive correspondence, before this visit fell through. Balfour was with the London School of Tropical Medicine, while Newsholme was a very eminent (retired) English Public Health Administrator who had been engaged by the Milbank Fund to study state medicine in 13 European countries. Gunn had made it clear to Vincent that he thought Newsholme to be far the better choice of the two, Balfour being too highly specialized on laboratory and tropical medicine.

> from a different point of view, namely in the form of possible aid in research, etc., in bacteriology and immunology, etc. SMG [Gunn] doubts if such aid would really materially affect and modernize teaching of hygiene in the medical schools.[99]

The new policy Gunn referred to had been developed by Edsall's special committee. While Gunn may have protested, this direction could not have come as a surprise to him as it was totally consistent with the policies that Edsall had carried out at Harvard. Edsall's report indicated that the particular functions of the DME (which was in the process of becoming a Division of Medical Sciences) 'should be to develop opportunities for aiding men in and training others for research in those fundamental sciences that bear upon the problems of Hygiene and Preventive Medicine'.[100] The role of the DME should be 'largely confined to aiding those sciences upon which Public Health is built, and furthering research and advanced training in these'. As for the training of health officers, this should not be a 'matter of special interest unless unexpected peculiar opportunities with especially fruitful promise appear'. It was acknowledged that some support was being provided by the IHD, but by and large the training of 'actual governmental employees in Public Health...would seem to be properly the function of government'. At the same time, Edsall admitted that the training of physicians had been 'very inadequate almost everywhere in the practical applications of Hygiene and Preventive Medicine'.[101] The DME had supported research in the past, but the new strategy called for a 'shift away from reforming medical schools toward the support of researchers themselves'.[102] This direction was consistent with the new orientation of the Foundation (advancement of knowledge), but it effectively meant that all hope of the Foundation addressing the complete range of public health training needs of a country was lost. As recognized by the Executive Committee in January 1929 'the changes implied lessened concern with medical problems of backward countries ...[with] the development of teaching centers in hygiene and public health to be discontinued...'.[103]

At this point in his career Gunn turned to the social sciences in search for more comprehensive strategies for health and human welfare, a development that became possible with the creation of the Division of Social Sciences in 1928 within the Rockefeller Foundation. He became Associate Director for the Social Sciences in Europe in 1930, and thereafter had virtually no further responsibilities in European countries concerning either health services or health manpower development.

Conclusion

Before joining the Foundation, Gunn had served as a health officer (New Jersey), a teacher (MIT, Harvard-MIT school), a public health administrator

(State of Massachusetts) and an editor (AJPH). He had professional contacts with all of the leading public health figures in America at the time. The courses that he taught included bacteriology, industrial hygiene, municipal sanitation, sanitary biometrics, and immunology.[104] His students at the Harvard-MIT school included medical doctors as well as those without a medical degree. Gunn's prime interest was in strengthening public health. He obviously took particular pleasure in working as a health educator, but that no more defined him than any of the other functions and duties that he carried out during his long career. His work in Czechoslovakia convinced him of the necessity of training medical doctors in public health; no alternative existed. Unlike America, Czechoslovakia did not have sanitary engineers and non-medical health officers. The notion that public health could be a profession independent of medicine did not exist.

When the Foundation first entered the field of public health education it pursued an ambivalent course. While Rose and Vincent gave priority to the training of public health officers, others, led by Welch, gave priority to developing public health leaders endowed with a research mentality. These two potentially complementary approaches never came together. How otherwise can one explain Gregg's lament that 'Pearce did not want undergraduates in public health', that both Rose and Russell disregarded that they had 'a graduate school for a subject in which there was no undergraduate course', and that 'Rose was throwing away his best source of new material', because no effort was made to influence capable medical students during their undergraduate course to consider a career in public health.[105]

Gunn's contact with Štampar was of critical importance for many reasons, not least in demonstrating to Gunn, if he needed such demonstration, that it was feasible in the European context to link medical education and public health; this was precisely what Štampar was able to do in Yugoslavia. Ironically, it was Pearce who funded Štampar's 'new method' of teaching hygiene to medical students by enabling them to get direct field experience of public health work in the villages under expert direction.[106] The IHD funded the School of Public Health at Zagreb. Here was a demonstration of what could be done, but it was not one that was driven by the Foundation's officers. It was all Štampar's doing. Welch, speaking at the Zagreb school's opening said that it represented a 'radical break with the past', one that England and the US might study.[107] The school mixed administration, research and teaching, a combination that did not exist elsewhere. Welch had intended to protest against such a school, but now was prepared to accept it as a worthy experiment.[108]

While Russell was generally sympathetic to Gunn's desire to link medical and public health education, he and Pearce had other priorities. It obviously did not help that Russell had a poor working relationship with Pearce. It is perhaps revealing that after Pearce's unexpected death in early 1930 Russell indicated that there were 'important things in public health' which he hoped would 'be aided more than they' had been by the Foundation in cooperation with the Medical Sciences Division, whose director was now Gregg.[109] However, this was too late to benefit Gunn. By then, he had moved, one could even say been forced to move, into a different field, that of the social sciences, a move that soon took him to China. Even if Gunn had retained responsibilities for public health in Europe, the reorganization had so biased the Foundation in favor or research that it probably would have been impossible for him to mount a successful programme, even with Russell and Gregg cooperating with him. It is not even obvious that Gunn could have succeeded if no reorganization had taken place and Russell and Pearce had been supportive of his efforts, for the simple reason that the Foundation lacked qualified staff for the kind of work that he had in mind. This was the crux of Gunn's difficulty; his vision of what should be was far greater than what the Foundation was capable of pursuing. While it would be tempting to say that Gunn was ahead of his times, what has since transpired, regarding the difficulty of blending public health and medical education, suggests that Russell's sense of what could be done was far more realistic than his. However, this does not reduce the importance of Gunn's ideas. There can be little doubt that the Foundation could have done better had it adopted more flexible policies, better adapted to the needs of each country.

Acknowledgments

This paper is part of an on-going study of the life of Selskar Gunn supported by two grants from The Rockefeller Archive Center. I thank their support and invaluable assistance given me by Robert Battaly, Senior Archivist. Comments received on early versions of this paper from Ted Brown, John Farley, Pierre-Yves Saunier and William Schneider, led me to totally overhaul its contents. Then Iris Borowy provided invaluable suggestions for improving the structure of this paper and eliminating unnecessary text. Finally, exchanges with Benjamin Page helped me better understand what conclusions could be drawn from this history.

---

1 R.B. Fosdick, *The Story of the Rockefeller Foundation* (New York: Harper & Brother, 1952), 38.

2 R.M. Acheson, *Wickliffe Rose of the Rockefeller Foundation: 1862-1914 The Formative Years* (Cambridge: Killycarn Press, 1992), 70.

3 Rose to Jerome Greene (RF Secretary at the time), 30 September 1915 (Cited in RF History, 1278). Quoted in B.B. Page, 'First Steps: The Rockefeller Foundation in Early Czechoslovakia', *East European Quarterly*, 35 (2001), 26.

4 Acheson, *Wickliffe Rose,* 81.

5 See E. Fee, *A History of the Johns Hopkins School of Hygiene and Public Health 1916-1939* (Baltimore: The Johns Hopkins University Press, 1987); E. Fee, Designing schools of public health for the United States, in E. Fee and R.M. Acheson (eds) *A*

History of Education in Public Health: Health That Mocks the Doctor's Rules (Oxford: Oxford University Press, 1991); R.M. Acheson, 'The medicalization of public health; the United Kingdom and the United States contrasted', *Journal of Public Health Medicine*, Vol 12, No. 1, 31-8; G. Williams, Schools of Public Health – Their Doing and Undoing, *Milbank Memorial Fund Quarterly*, Fall (1976), 489-527.

6 Fee, *A History*, 66.

7 Quoted in J. Farley, *To Cast Out Disease: A history of the International Health Division of the Rockefeller Foundation (1913-1951)* (Oxford: OUP, 2004), 203.

8 See B.G. Rosenkrantz, *Public Health and the State: Changing Views in Massachusetts, 1842-1936* (Cambridge: Harvard University Press, 1972), 147-9.

9 Quoted in Fee, *A History*, 66.

10 For an account of the Foundation's TB programme in France, see L. Murard and P. Zylberman, 'L'autre guerre (1914-1918) La santé publique en France sous l'oeil de l'Amérique', *Revue Historique*, 560 (Octobre-Décembre 1986), 367-98; L. Murard, P. Zylberman, 'La mission Rockefeller et la crèation du Comité national de dèfense contre la tuberculose (1917-1923)', *Revue d'histoire moderne et contemporaine*, 34 (1987), 257-81; *Hommage à la Mission Rockefeller (1917-1937)*, RAC, RF, RG 1.1, Series 500, Box 28, Folder 267; Farley, *To Cast Out*, 44-58.

11 Rose, entry for 19 April 1919 (London), Notes on a journey to France, 19 March – 10 May 1919, RAC RFWR 1916-1922, 9. Quoted in Page, *First Steps*, 2.

12 Conference of Officers and Advisers, Gedney Farms Hotel, 17 and 18 January, 1920, RAC, RF, RG 3, Series 900, Box 22, Folder 165.

13 Ibid.

14 E.O. Jordan, G.C. Whipple and C.-E.A. Winslow, *A Pioneer of Public Health William Thompson Sedgwick* (New Haven: Yale University Press, 1924).

15 Hackett papers, RAC, RF, RG 3, Series 908, Box 3, 442.

16 J.A. Curran, *Founders of the Harvard School of Public Health, 1909-1946* (New York: Josiah Macy, Jr. Foundation, 1970); 25.

17 USPHS Conference on the future of public health, 14 May, 1922, RAC, RF, RG 3, Series 908, Box 7F, Folder 86, 73.

18 Vincent diary entry, 5 July 1923, RAC, RF, 12.1 diaries.

19 Edsall to Russell, 11 September 1923, RAC, RF, RG 1.1, Series 200, Box 20, Folder 233.

20 Russell to Edsall, 25 September 1923, RAC, RF, RG 1.1, Series 200, Box 20, Folder 233.

21 Ibid.

22 Gunn diary entry, 7 November 1927, RAC, RF, 12.1 diaries.

23 Vincent diary entry, 23 November 1928, RAC, RF, 12.1 diaries.

24 See Curran, *Founders*, 22-54.

25 See Fee, *A History*, 36.

26 S. M. Gunn, *The present condition of public health organization in the United States; being a report of the Central Committee on Public Health Organization based on a voluntary survey of organizations interested in public health* (Chicago: American Medical Association, 1915)

27 For technical details of the programme in Czechoslovakia, see B.B. Page, 'First Steps: The Rockefeller Foundation in Early Czechoslovakia', *East European Quarterly*, 35 (2001); B.B. Page, 'The Rockefeller Foundation and Central Europe: A Reconsideration, *Minerva*, 40:3 (2002), 265-287; P. Weindling, 'Public Health and Political Stability: The Rockefeller Foundation in Central and Eastern Europe between

the Two World Wars', *Minerva* 31:3 (Autumn 1993), 253.
28 Rose to Gunn, 17 January 1921, RAC, RF, RG 1.1, Series 712, Box 1, Folder 3.
29 Rose to Gunn, 29 October 1921, RAC, RF, RG 1.1, Series 712, Box 2, Folder 12.
30 Ibid..
31 See endnote 10.
32 Rose to Gunn, 9 December 1920, RAC, RF, RG 1.1, Series 712, Box 2, Folder 10.
33 Rose to Hackett, 25 April 1917, RAC, RF, RG 5.3, Series 305, Box 107, Quoted in Farley, *To Cast Out*, 37.
34 Gunn to Rose, 9 December 1920, RAC, RF, RG 1.1, Series 712, Box 2, Folder 10.
35 Gunn to Rose, 19 August 1919 (RAC, RF, RG 1.1, Series 712, Box 3, Folder 6)
36 W. Rose and S.M. Gunn, 'The Public Health Situation in Czecho-Slovakia', a report of their visit of February 17-26, 1920, RAC, RF, RG 1.1, Series 712, Box 3, Folder 6.
37 Gunn to Rose, 6 May 1921, RAC, RF, RG 1.1, Series 712, Box 2, Folder 11.
38 These difficulties are well described in Page, *First steps*.
39 Gunn to Rose, 9 Dec 1920, RAC, RF, RG 1.1, Series 712, Box 2, Folder 10.
40 Rose to Gunn, 10 Feb 1921, RAC, RF, RG 1.1, Series 712, Box 2, Folder 10.
41 Russell to Gunn, 31 March 1921, RAC, RF, RG 1.1, Series 712, Box 1, Folder 3.
42 Gunn to Rose, 31 Dec 1920, RAC, RF, RG 1.1, Series 712, Box 2, Folder 10.
43 Ibid.
44 Rose to Gunn, 17 January 1921, RAC, RF, RG 1.1, Series 712, Box 1, Folder 3.
45 Gunn to Rose, 31 Dec 1920 (RAC, RF, RG 1.1, Series 712, Box 2, Folder 10)
46 Rose to Gunn, 6 Jan 1921, RAC, RF, RG 1.1, Series 712, Box 1, Folder 3.
47 Ibid.
48 Gunn to Rose, 29 March 1921, RAC, RF, RG 1.1, Series 712, Box 2, Folder 11.
49 Rose to Gunn, 15 April 1921, RAC, RF, RG 1.1, Series 712, Box 2, Folder 11.
50 Rose to Gunn, 4 Jan 1921, RAC, RF, RG 1.1, Series 712, Box 2, Folder 10.
51 Rose to Gunn, 2 Nov 1921, RAC, RF, RG 1.1, Series 712, Box 2, Folder 12.
52 Gunn to Rose, 26 Sept 1921, RAC, RF, RG 1.1, Series 712, Box 2, Folder 12.
53 Ibid.
54 Rose to Gunn, 11 Oct 1921, RAC, RF, RG 1.1, Series 712, Box 2, Folder 12.
55 Hackett papers, RAC, RF, RG 3, Series 908, Box 4, 1089.
56 Gunn to Winslow, 24 Nov 1922, Yale University Archives, Winslow Collection, box 12, folder 310.
57 Rose to Gunn, 28 Oct 1921, RAC, RF, RG 1.1, Series 712, Box 2, Folder 12.
58 Gunn to Winslow, 5 June 1923, Yale University Archives, Winslow Collection, box 12, folder 310.
59 Statement with regard to the Present Situation in the Different Countries of Europe which the IHB is Cooperating Selskar Michael Gunn, 1924, RAC, RF, RG 5, Series 2, Box 58, Folder 368.
60 Ibid.
61 See W.H. Schneider, *Quality and Quantity: The Quest for Biological Regeneration in Twentieth-Century France* (Cambridge: Cambridge University Press, 1990), 134-41.
62 Statement with regard to the Present Situation in the Different Countries of Europe which the IHB is Cooperating Selskar Michael Gunn, 1924, RAC, RF, RG 5, Series 2, Box 58, Folder 368.
63 Gunn to Russell, 5 Sept 1924, RAC, RF, RG 1.1, Series 710, Box 1, Folder 4.
64 Ibid.
65 Štampar to O'Brien, 7 July 1939, RAC, RF, RG 1.1, Series 710, Box 3, Folder 18.
66 Ibid.

67 Vincent diary entry, 11 July 1927, RAC, RF, 12.1 diaries.
68 Russell to Gunn, 17 November 1925, RAC, RF, RG 5, Series 1.1, Box 104, Folder 1437.
69 For more on this aspect of Gunn's career, see S. Litsios, 'Selskar Gunn and China: The Rockefeller Foundation's "Other" Approach to Public Health', *Bulletin of the History of Medicine,*79 (2005), 295-318.
70 Gunn to Russell, 6 April 1925, RAC, RF, RG 5, Series 1.1, Box 91, Folder 1290.
71 Ibid.
72 Ibid.
73 Ibid.
74 Ibid.
75 Ibid.
76 Vincent diary entry, Exhibit, 9 May 1925, RAC, RF, 12.1 diaries.
77 Ibid.
78 Vincent diary entry, Exhibit, 17 July 1925, RAC, RF, 12.1 diaries.
79 Ibid.
80 Vincent diary entry, 16 and 21 February 1927, RAC, RF, 12.1 diaries.
81 Vincent diary entry, 11 November 1926, RAC, RF, 12.1 diaries.
82 Pearce to Gregg 28 December 1925, Concentrated investigation of single subjects, RAC, RF, RG 3, Series 906, Box 1, Folder 3.
83 Ibid..
84 G. Vincent, *The Rockefeller Foundation A review for 1925* (New York: The Rockefeller Foundation, 1926), 29.
85 See W.H. Schneider, 'The Men Who Followed Flexner: Richard Pearce, Alan Gregg and the Rockefeller Foundation Medical Divisions, 1919-1951,' in W.H. Schneider (ed.), *Rockefeller Philanthropy & Modern Biomedicine: International Initiatives from World War I to the Cold War* (Indiana: Indiana University Press, 2002), 7-60.
86 See R.E. Kohler, *Partners in Science: Foundations and Natural Scientists 1900-1945* (Chicago: University of Chicago Press, 1991).
87 Gunn to Fosdick, 6 Oct 1926, RAC, RF, RG 3, Series 900, Box 17, Folder 122.
88 Ibid.
89 A. Gregg, Memorandum on Reorganization, 24 July 1926, RAC, RF, RG 3, Series 900, Box 17, Folder 122.
90 Conference on European Policies and Programs, 28 February–3 March 1927 (RF, RG 3, Series 900, Box 22, Folder 166)
91 Attached to letter from Gunn to Vincent, 16 May 1927, RAC, RF, RG 3, Series 900, Box 21, Folder 159
92 Ibid.
93 Vincent to Gunn, 28 March 1928, RAC, RF, RG 2, Series 700, Box 12, Folder 97.
94 Farley, *To Cast Out,* 165.
95 Kohler, *Partners,* 234
96 Fosdick to Rockefeller Jr., 16 January 1928, RAC, RF, RG 3, Series 900, Box 17, Folder 124.
97 Vincent diary entry, 29 October 1928, RAC, RF, 12.1 diaries.
98 Ibid.
99 Gunn diary entry, 31 October 1928, RAC, RF, 12.1 diaries.
100 Report of the Special Committee on the Division of Medical Education of the Rockefeller Foundation, 9 Nov, 1928, RAC, RF, RG 3, Series 906, Box 1, Folder 7.
101 Ibid.

102 Schneider, *The Men,* 33.
103 Hackett papers, Reorganization of the RF, RAC, RF, RG 3, Series 908, Box 7b, folder 86.22. 721
104 See Curran, *Founders,* 68.
105 Hackett papers, RAC, RF, RG 3, Series 908, Box 7H, Folder 86.112, 1087
106 A. Gregg, The Work of the Rockefeller Foundation in Medical Education and the Medical Sciences, 1920 to 1929 Inclusive, under the Direction of Richard Mills Pearce, Jr., M.D. *Quarterly Bulletin of the Rockefeller Foundation,* 5:2 (1931), 358-75.
107 Strode diary entry, 3 October 1927, RAC, RF, 12.1 diaries.
108 Gunn diary entry, 3 October 1927, RAC, RF, 12.1 diaries.
109 Staff Conference, 8 October 1930, RAC, RF, RG 3, Series 908, Box 12, Folder 125.

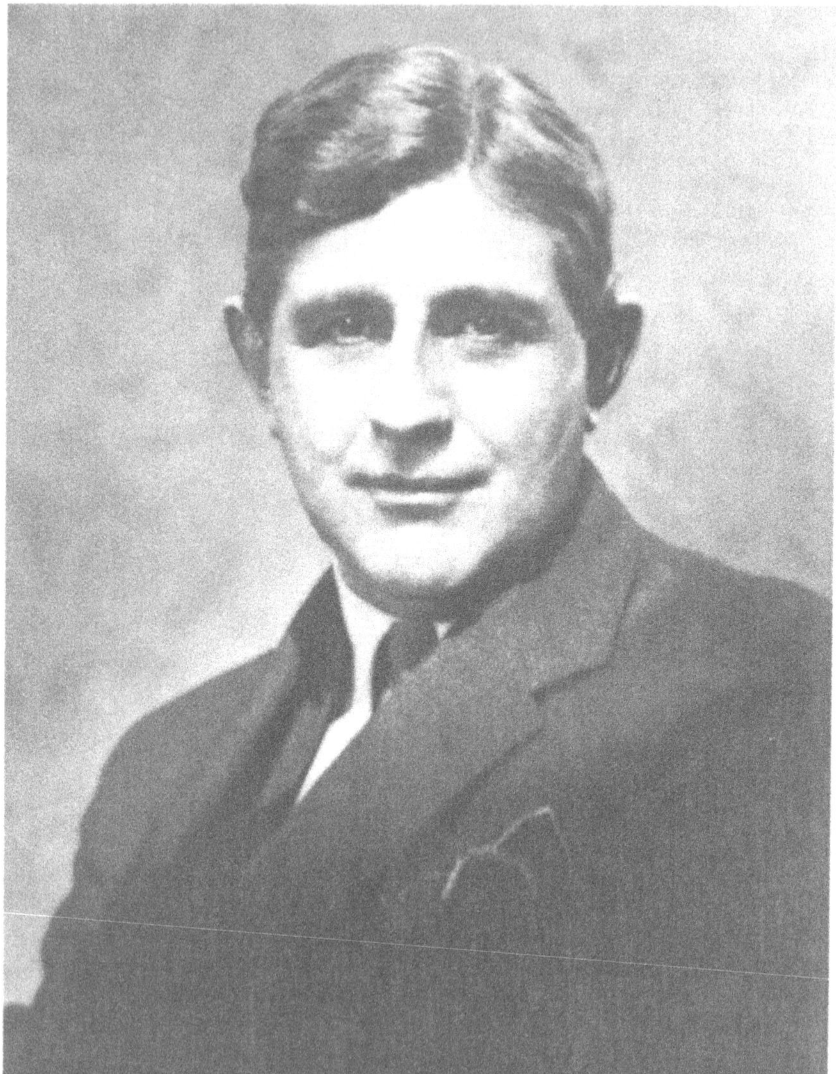

Selskar Gunn

Photograph Courtesy of the Rockefeller Archive Center

Béla Johan (1889-1983) and Public Health in Inter-war Hungary

Erik Ingebrigtsen

A noisy event taking place in an otherwise quiet Budapest street on 23 June 2006, put – at least temporarily – the end to a lasting controversy regarding inter-war Hungary's most influential public health administrator. With a pneumatic drill, workers effectively demolished the stone base that since 1989 had held the bust of Béla Johan (1889-1983) outside the institute he led in the inter-war years.[1] A number of decisions during the preceding months led up to this symbolic act: in February 2006 the Hungarian Parliament revoked a decision from April 2003 of naming a ten-year program for health-improvement after Johan. In the following month the Minister of Health announced that the National Epidemiological Centre also would cease to carry Johan's name. Opposition to the symbolic use of Johan as public health-icon was mainly based on his actions and inaction during the Second World War. Critics have argued that as state secretary in the Ministry of Interior until October 1944, Johan shared responsibility for the deportation and murder of several hundred thousand Hungarian Jews during May and June 1944. The Hungarian Holocaust was implemented under the direction of representatives from the Ministry in which Johan held a leading post. This crucial information was omitted from a biographical sketch presented to Parliament along with the proposal to dedicate the ten-year public health program to Johan's name in 2003. One sentence, in particular, which indicated that Johan was ousted after the German occupation of Hungary in March 1944, raised accusations of historic fraud: '...in 1944, after the German invasion, [Johan] was thrown out of his position; later he was interned.[2] As Johan, on the contrary, had kept his post under the German-imposed puppet regime for more than half a year after the invasion, and as he was never interned during the war or its aftermath, several Parliamentary representatives felt a deception was being practised. Furthermore, there were claims that Johan for years before the German invasion had implemented Anti-Semitic legislation within Hungarian health care, that he was a dear friend of leading Nazis[3], and that he actively contributed to the deportation of Hungarian Jewish medical doctors.[4] General opinion on Johan has now turned from laudatory praise to condemnation, making him unsuitable as symbolic figure for contemporary and future public health policies. The main topic of this paper is Johan's role in the inter-war years, but for context I will briefly sketch the controversy regarding his place in Hungarian collective memory.

Johan served simultaneously as state secretary of the Ministry of Interior and as director of the National Institute for Public Health until the seizure of power by the fascist Arrow Cross regime in October 1944. He was therefore regarded as a representative of the old order by the post war regime. As such, he was not considered suitable for similarly influential positions after 1945. He was, however, neither convicted nor charged for participation in war crimes, although he had to face two separate investigations.[5] Along with other inter-war medical leaders, Johan's name was expunged from public life and from Hungarian medical history after the communist takeover. For example, his name does not appear in a book published in 1959 on the history of the institute established under his direction. The author, quite characteristically, defined the whole inter-war period as 'the 25-year long night of Horthy fascism', when, from a Communist perspective, any progressive action was inconceivable.[6] This silence prevailed until the late 1970s, when medical historian Győző Birtalan set out to rehabilitate a number of medical leaders from the inter-war years. He regarded Johan's case as the most sensitive, given the close connection between public health reforms and the general political situation.[7] Birtalan's re-evaluation was presented in a public lecture, attended by both high-ranking officials and politicians, and the 90-year-old Béla Johan himself.[8] Although Birtalan stressed that the interwar public health reforms resulted from collective effort, Johan was for the first time since the war presented as a progressive force. Ten years later, at the centenary of Johan's birth, the National Institute of Health added Johan' name to its title, and the aforementioned bust was unveiled inside the institute's gates.[9] Although one newspaper-article from 1991 condemned Johan as 'nazi-collaborator',[10] resolute responses from medical historians and the Prime Minister's office silenced all criticism on the matter for more than a decade.[11] Criticism of Johan was dismissed as a continuation of communist injustice towards a great man. Most discussions of Johan during these years built on Birtalan's work.[12]

This truce proved temporary when, in 2003, the Hungarian Parliament approved the socialist/liberal government's proposal to name a ten-year health reform plan *'The Béla Johan National Program for the Decade of Health'*. Almost immediately, harsh criticism towards this decision appeared in an article ironically titled 'Professional with minor flaws'. The author claimed that Parliament had been deceived into naming this program after 'a dedicated Antisemite'.[13] The article appeared in a relatively marginal liberal weekly, but the leading right-wing daily newspaper seized the opportunity to embarrass the socialist Minister of Health, rhetorically asking if the health program had been 'named after a friend of the Nazis?'[14] Historian Krisztian Ungváry further undermined the 'official' presentation of Johan's war years.[15] Numerous futile efforts were made to defend the reputation and prestige both of Johan, and, not least, the embarrassed Minister. A succession of investigations into the matter were conducted by the Semmelweis Library for Medical History, by the Historical Institute at the Hungarian Academy of Sciences, and, finally, under the direction of the Presidency of the Academy. [16] While the medical historians at Semmelweis argued for the continued use of Johan's name, the Academy of Sciences concluded that the memory of Johan can not serve the purpose of present day health reforms.

Interpretations of Johan's role can roughly be grouped in three categories: First, there is the view that Johan was a brilliant scientist of wide international reputation and the initiator of tremendous progress in Hungarian public health. As an administrator he held no political responsibility for the regime's inhumanity, on the contrary, he is said to have used all his powers to help Jews and other victims of Nazi persecution.[17] By contrast, a second group portrays Johan as one of Holocaust's willing executioners, and as an enthusiastic collaborator to Hungarian and German Nazi-leaders.[18] The third view, which now appears to be the official stand, is that Johan was indeed an outstanding public health administrator, but that ambition made him blind to changing political realities. By failing to resign after the German invasion in March 1944, he became an accomplice in the horrors committed during the following summer. Keeping his post while aware of the atrocities committed by the Ministry in which he served makes him unsuitable as political symbol today.[19]

All these positions can be regarded as contributions to the construction of a Johan-myth in Hungarian collective memory. In a larger perspective, the changing fate of Johan's symbolic value comes under the general problem that post-communist Hungary faces in relation to its pre-communist authoritarian past. Although I may not be able to detach myself completely from this villain/hero myth-construction, this paper aims at a disinterested discussion of Johan's role in the development of an integrated state-run system of public health in inter-war Hungary. I will argue that a crucial factor behind Johan's significance was his ability to mobilise support for public health reforms from a divided medical community and from political leaders of divergent ideological positions. Similarly important, already from the early 1920s, Johan's work was conducted in intimate cooperation with representatives of the international public health community, primarily the International Health Division (IHD) of the Rockefeller Foundation (RF) and the League of Nations' Health Organisation (LNHO). Links to domestic medical traditions and to international influences were strategically used by Johan: At times he would stress the international origins of modernising ideas, at other times the essentially *Hungarian* character of the same proposals. It is impossible fully to analyse all Johan's multiple engagements within this paper.[20] To illustrate the complex development taking place under Johan's direction between the mid-twenties and the outbreak of war, I will focus in the following: institution-building within Hungarian public health in the 1920s, the establishment of a new rural health model around 1930, and the increasing importance of the institutions under Johan's direction in the late 1930s. First, however, I will discuss how the young pathologist Johan found his way into the field of public health.

Béla Johan in his 'second professional incarnation'

Johan grew up in Pécs in southern Hungary. His father was the city's Chief Medical Officer, and his mother came from an academic family. He was given a culturally ambitious upbringing, learning to play musical instruments, and – more relevant to the present discussion – studying English in addition to the obligatory German.[21] Johan is frequently noted as stating that he lived through three professional incarnations; first as a pathologist, then, between 1924 and 1944 as public health administrator, and finally in pharmaceutical production until he retired at the age of 90 in 1979. During medical studies and after graduation in 1912, he held assistant positions at the Institute of Pathology in Budapest. During the First World War he served in the laboratory of a garrison hospital, gaining his first experience in bacteriological and serological diagnostics, as well as the development of vaccines.[22] After demobilisation he returned to the Institute of Pathology, simultaneously acting as chief pathologist at a city hospital. In 1919 he received his *habilitation*, gaining the right to lecture in pathology at the Medical Faculty.

In spring 1921 the Dean of the Medical Faculty pushed Johan's career in the direction of his 'second incarnation', by recommending him as a candidate for a fellowship from the *Rockefeller Foundation* (RF). In the Dean's letter to the Foundation, Johan was said to have had a 'long-time ... desire to visit and to study the medical and hygiene institutions of the United States'.[23] The letter was sent just as the International Health Division (IHD) of the RF was in the process of extending its activities to Central Europe and Hungary.[24] Established in 1913, the RF's activities in Europe were initiated through war-relief and a post-war campaign against tuberculosis in France. While already active in the new republic of Czechoslovakia in 1919, the first proposal to send representatives to the former enemy-state Hungary was made in February 1920.[25] As post-war Hungary had neither fixed borders nor offered any political or economic predictability, the first RF reports concluded that 'constructive work'[26] would have to be postponed. However, two actions of 'academic emergency relief' were initiated already in 1920. The Medical Faculty's library was given back copies of all the English-language medical journals it subscribed to before the war, and the institutes were provided with necessary laboratory equipment.[27] According to Johan's recollection the donations were greeted with enthusiasm:

> I am sure there are many who share my recollection of the time when ... the new, excellent microscopes and other equipment procured with the first $10.000-donations from the Rockefeller Foundation arrived. Our holdings of scientific instruments, which had completely deteriorated during the war, were renewed and refreshed by this donation.[28]

Selskar M. Gunn, the director of IHD's program in Europe, visited Hungary in September 1921.[29] Gunn informed the Medical Faculty that a formal request from the government might lead to donations of RF fellowships to Hungarians.[30]

The Minister of Religion and Education personally applied to the Foundation for fellowships for study in the US. Presumably this request provided the background for a delayed evaluation of the Dean's aforementioned recommendation of Johan. Gunn probably interviewed and approved Johan during a visit to Hungary in March 1922.[31] Six months later, Johan travelled to the USA.[32] His travel companion was the engineer Aladár Jendrassik, who later became architect of the Institute of Public Health, and one of Johan's long-term colleagues.[33] Writing to his 'Dear Mother' after arrival in New York, Johan vividly described his journey.[34] Staying a night in Paris, he had enjoyed both the opera and an evening stroll in a city illuminated by electric lights. He was impressed by the density of cars in the streets of Paris, but this was vastly surpassed by the incredible Manhattan traffic. Of the transatlantic journey in *SS America,* the only aspect Johan found worth mentioning was the freely available abundance on the 'unbelievable' menu, illustrating the scarcity of such luxury in post-war Hungary. On arrival in New York, Jendrassik left for the RF-funded Johns Hopkins School of Hygiene and Public Health in Baltimore, the first of thirty-five Hungarians to study at this institution and the similarly RF-funded Harvard School of Public Health before the Second World War. Almost all these former fellows returned to leading positions under Johan's direction.[35] Johan started out in New York City's diagnostic laboratories. Thereafter, following a short stay at Harvard, he worked with Augustus B. Wadsworth at the New York State Public Health Laboratories in Albany. During his last months in the US, Johan visited a whole series of public health laboratories, and on the way home he also viewed the public health services in London and Paris. From available sources it is not clear whether he was already designated as director of a future state public health laboratory in Hungary before this journey. However, it is evident from the structure of this training program that it represented a break from his early career in pathology. Returning to Hungary, he first entered the semi-private company *Phylaxia* as head of a new department producing antitoxins and sera. The bacterial culture used in the production of diphtheria-antitoxin was supplied by Wadsworth at Albany.[36]

A survey of Johan's early scientific publications suggests that the year in the US was of fundamental importance for his scientific orientation. Until 1927 Johan had produced an impressive forty-six scientific articles. Even if his command of English was excellent prior to the stay in the US, he never referred to any English-language scientific literature before the fellowship. German and Hungarian texts were his only source of information and inspiration, and these were also his only languages of publication.[37] While still in the US he published his first English-language article.[38] A year later he discussed American bacteriology and serology solely based on English-language texts.[39] Extensive scientific publications during the following years referred to literature from the US and from a number of European countries.[40] It seems evident that the abandon of a purely

Hungarian and German orientation resulted from Johan's travels in the US and in Europe. It can be assumed that these new impulses influenced his general perspectives on public health, and on his future preferences for Hungarian public health-policies.

In Hungarian medical history, the establishment of the National Institute of Health has generally been portrayed as the realisation of genuinely Hungarian plans, which had been awaiting implementation due to lack of resources. The RF's role is reduced to that of a passive funding agency, whereas Johan enters the story as director after plans had already been made.[41] However, it can be argued that both Johan and the officers of the IHD fundamentally influenced the plans for the institution's architecture, purpose and place within the Hungarian public health machinery. Perhaps surprisingly, Johan seems to be "to blame" for diminishing his own and the RF's role in later historiography: Through a series of publications during construction and immediately after the opening of the institute, Johan presented the institute as the realization of plans awaiting implementation since the 1870s.[42] The idea of creating a public health institute in Hungary was credited to the country's first professor of hygiene, József Fodor, who did indeed make such a proposal in 1873. Fodor's successor, Leó Liebermann, presented revised plans in 1912, and Baron Kálmán Müller, long-time-leader of the National Public Health Council, was honoured for presenting the idea to the Upper House in 1918.[43] Although these early proposals are not available for scrutiny, it is likely that they were quite different from what eventually were adopted. Fodor's proposal was made before the fundamental breakthrough of bacteriology and serology. Liebermann's proposal was evaluated by S. M. Gunn in March 1922 and found in need of substantial reorientation before it could be presented to the RF's decision-making Board of Trustees.[44] After this 1922-visit, Gunn wrote to the Minister of Welfare, reminding him of crucial points agreed to in their recent negotiations, and asking that these aspects be incorporated in the revised plans. In particular, he mentioned 'practical work, training of personnel and research', indicating that one or more of these items were not included in the Liebermann-plan.[45]

In late 1923, a few months after returning from the US, Johan and Jendrassik presented a revised outline to Gunn and his superior, F. F. Russell.[46] This second version was also rejected, but led to RF-funding for the two Hungarians to study IHD-supported public health institutes in Europe during spring 1924.[47] Gunn returned in July to conduct a study of the public health situation in the country. On his arrival, he was presented with a third plan, thoroughly revised after Johan's and Jendrassik's study-trips, but this version was also regarded incomplete. After prolonged negotiations, agreement was reached on a revised version, which was forwarded to New York. This plan passed unaltered through both the Board of Trustees and the Hungarian Parliament. The three rejected proposals from 1922-24 are, unfortunately, not to be found either in American or Hungarian archives.[48] It is therefore impossible to define which elements of the realised institute resulted from new impulses. The experiences Johan and Jendrassik gained in the US and in other European countries probably shaped their professional preferences. The officers of the IHD influenced the outcome through the rejection of early drafts and the subsequent negotiations. However, as early as autumn 1925 when Parliament passed the law on the establishment and regulation of the institute's activities, all traces of trans-national influences on the outcome were forgotten: Gratitude was expressed towards the RF for its donation, but both the Minister and other speakers presented this funding as facilitating the belated realisation of plans existing for decades.[49] The myth of direct succession from the great Fodor, Liebermann, and Müller had become the dominant narrative. As the main architect of this construction, Johan seems to have understood that a genuinely *Hungarian* institute would mobilise enthusiasm better than one built on *American* inspiration. This incorporation of the new institute into a national medical tradition may have helped to encourage enthusiasm and a quite unusual consensual support towards the institute in a medical community tormented by conflicts. The respect paid to former (and already deceased) leaders may have given Johan more leverage in composing his staff of young, dynamic and internationally experienced experts. Already two years before the institute's formal inauguration, the IHD's representative noted with satisfaction:

> Dr. Johan already has his staff pretty well assigned. They will all be fellows of the I.H.B. with one exception. This, of course, applies only to the leading positions.[50]

Later, Johan always worked to provide international training for his leading personnel. From the late 1920s it was Johan's privilege to propose candidates for fellowships to the IHD. From the mid-30s it even seems that Johan himself made the selection, by the simple expedient of proposing only as many candidates as there were fellowships.[51] The RF consequently demanded that all fellows should have a post waiting for them upon their return. In effect, Johan recruited his leading staff by proposing candidates for fellowship. In a letter praising Győző Birtalan's rehabilitating article from 1979 for the emphasis the latter put on the collective endeavour behind the health reforms, the 90-year-old Johan took pride in one particular skill: his ability as a leader to select and to inspire a dynamic and highly competent staff. In old age, he regarded this as his most important contribution to the extraordinary development in Hungary's inter-war public health.[52]

The completion of the new institute took place between 1926 and autumn 1927. The RF contributed $290.000 towards the building costs. The state covered $20.000, in addition to the building site, some laboratory equipment, and a promise to cover salaries and maintenance after the first five years of gradually diminishing RF-support.[53] Already in 1925 the IHD-officer Leland W. Mitchell became permanent representative in Budapest, to oversee the building process and act as adviser to a RF-sponsored 'Health Reform Office' within the Ministry of Welfare. A number of successful applications for further IHD-aid during the following years were prepared in close cooperation between Mitchell and Johan. On the occasion of Mitchell's premature death in 1930, Johan described him as the most important link between Hungarian public health reformers and the international professional community.[54] The formal opening of the institute was a grand celebration, attended by Regent Miklós Horthy and a number of international guests. Experts from Brazil, Czechoslovakia, Great Britain, Poland, Italy, Portugal and the LNHO in Geneva attended an official LNHO conference on public health training in Budapest. After this event, all participants travelled to Zagreb to open a similarly RF-sponsored institute there. A specially honoured guest was the 77-year-old director of the Johns Hopkins School of Hygiene and Public Health, William H. Welch. Greatly appreciating the central role played in the region by his former students, Welch also praised these institutions' divergence from established organisational models:

> Dr. Welch stated that he had come with the idea of protesting somewhat against the development of Schools of Public Health independent of the University, but after what he had seen in Budapest and Zagreb, he felt that a protest of this character would be out of place.[55]

This administrative arrangement, placing the institute under the Ministry of Welfare, rather than making it a part of the Medical Faculty under the Ministry of Education was a Government decision, and not of Johan's making. However, he contributed to a smooth working relationship. He invited university professors to lecture in the training programme for Medical Officers, and established branch laboratories at the three universities outside Budapest. The most important consequence of the institute's subordination to the Ministry of Welfare only became apparent five years later: when the Ministry of Welfare was incorporated into the Ministry of the Interior in 1932, the Institute of Public Health became, in practice, a department of the most powerful Ministry. This transfer brought Johan much closer to the national political elite than he would have been as leader of an institute within a Medical Faculty. Initially the institute consisted of four divisions: Bacteriology, serology, pathohistology/parasitology, and a chemical division. In autumn 1928 the Division of Field Work was established, administering the organisation of five rural health demonstration districts established in cooperation with the International Health Division.[56] By the early 1930s a whole series of laws and regulations had expanded the mandates of the institute, e.g. the compulsory reporting of infectious diseases and testing of all pharmaceutical products. Laboratory activities remained central, but it was in relation to the institute's role in the education of public health professionals and the implementation of rural health work that Johan and his associates met with the fiercest opposition.

Johan and the reform of Hungarian Public Health professions

Johan played a significant part in the establishment of professional training for medical officers and public health nurses in Hungary. The idea that the National Institute for Public Health was to engage in the training of medical officers was suggested already in 1922. Johan took great interest in the development of curricula, in the integration of student facilities in the institute plans, and in the everyday running of the school. The first class of twenty-four students entered the nine-month course in February 1928. This marked a break with the existing situation: Since 1883, all medical officers had been legally obliged to pass an exam, but no training was offered, and the mandatory exam was often ignored as nobody ever failed to pass the test. Local medical officers were typically described as elderly and tired, adding to their incomes with part-time officers' posts.[57] Johan thought it important to educate medical officers both on public health issues and on bureaucratic routines, to overcome existing doubts about physicians' administrative skills. The minister of Interior expressed this view in 1934, arguing that lawyers such as himself were more fitted to administrative tasks:

> Medical officers cannot be given bureaucratic responsibilities. Doctors just don't understand administration, and they constantly make a mess out of everything...If all doctors were trained in administration there would be no reason to worry. But they're not.[58]

In response, Johan arranged for the Minister to attend the forthcoming oral exams in public administration, convincing him of the high standard of the candidates'. The training of medical officers paved the way for legislative reform, fundamentally altering Hungary's public health system in 1936. Most significantly, the Chief Medical Officers serving at county level were transferred from local appointment to the status of state employees. When linking these medical officers to the bureaucratic apparatus of the Ministry of Interior, they also received extensive bureaucratic authority.[59] This reform had a number of consequences. Johan regarded it crucial that the medical officers were no longer controlled or impeded in their work by local interests. The Ministry could also, if necessary, implement reforms by decree, without having to win the support of every single administrative unit. The Chief Medical Officer was put in charge of *all* public health work within the district, including that implemented by civil associations. Medical officers in the villages were still to be employed by the municipality, but the right to fill vacancies was transferred to the Ministry. This was regarded as crucial to the provision of health care in remote villages: accepting a post as medical officer in a remote village was, after 1936, no longer a one-way ticket to a place 'behind God's back'[60]. On the contrary, it marked the first step in an attractive career, exponentially increasing the number of applications for post which earlier was impossible to fill.[61] Johan regarded this integration of local medical officers into the state's administrative hierarchy as a fundamental prerequisite for continued reform.[62]

The second new profession introduced was the generally trained public health nurse. In 1925 the RF approved aid towards the establishment of nursing schools in Debrecen and Budapest, the latter to be operated by the Ministry in cooperation with the Hungarian Red Cross.[63] Almost instantly, however, the Red Cross refused all co-operation with the state, resenting outside involvement in the organisation's affairs. [64] In an attempt to mend the damage this Hungarian infighting caused to relations with the RF, the Ministry in late 1926 presented totally revised plans for a School of General- and Public Health Nurses under Johan's direction, connected to the National Institute of Public Health. From then on, Johan was deeply involved in the planning process for the Budapest nursing school. He became convinced that properly trained public health nurses were crucial to the planned public health reforms. Together with various representatives of the Ministry and the architect Jendrassik, Johan visited a number of European nursing schools developed in cooperation with the IHD. The future Directrice and several instructors simultaneously made prolonged study-trips in Europe and to the US. The IHD's nursing expert, Frances Elizabeth Crowell, influenced Johan's approach to nursing education during these formative years, for which she also took credit in her personal notes:

> Dr. Johan's house for dinner...until 1 a.m.. Excellent opportunity to educate Dr. J. re the fundamentals of nurse training. He has already learned a lot – believes that two years is a minimum training period – that bedside nursing experience is an essential part of the training for p[ublic] h[ealth] work and that standards of recruitment should be high.[65]

Already before construction started, bitter conflict erupted over the education of public health nurses, in relation to its implications for the organisation of local preventive health care. Civilian associations already in the field fiercely opposed the suggested state-run reforms. These organisations were defined as 'specialised', that is, each was handling one particular challenge to public health, e.g. tuberculosis, venereal diseases or mother- and infant care. Johan became the chief spokesman for the 'general' model, in which the state-employed, generally trained medical officers and public health nurses would take care of all of these tasks in each community. The opening of a new, RF-funded health demonstration district in Gödöllő, some 30 kilometres from Budapest, further intensified the conflict. This community was to serve as practice field for students in the medical officer program and public health nurses. Five other health demonstration districts were soon established nationwide with IHD funding. Already at this experimental stage, Johan named the general model *the Green Cross*. He presented these model communities as a more rational and modern approach to the country's massive public health challenges.[66] The suggestion that the existing specialised organisations be replaced by the Green Cross aroused great fury, in particular among *The Stefánia Association for the Protection of Mothers and Infants*.[67] To a great extent, opposition took the shape of personal attacks on Johan, since he was seen to be the general model's main protagonist. On several occasions, existing opposition made him investigate the possibilities of employment abroad. For example, during summer 1931, Johan was publicly accused of embezzlement.[68] Disillusioned by what he regarded an absurd campaign, he noted in his personal diary that, during a visit to Geneva, he had discussed the possibility of employment with the LNHO. Johan perceived the response from the LNHO's Medical Director, Ludwik Rajchman, as positive.[69] However, Johan's superior, state secretary Kornél Scholtz, on this and other occasions convinced him to stand the storm.

As indicated above, Johan and most of his close collaborators had strong ties to the US. Forty-three Hungarian medical doctors and nurses travelled to the US on IHD fellowship during the inter-war years.[70] An even larger number studied or visited RF-funded institutions in Europe, and several RF-representatives worked closely with Johan and his colleagues on various projects. In his initial public statements regarding the general model, Johan explicitly referred to the modern, American system as the source of inspiration.[71] It was not easy, therefore, to counter Stefánia's attack on the Green Cross for being 'foreign', and so 'ill suited' to national needs, that it was a 'violation of the nation's organic development' to use this 'alien implant' to replace the 'genuinely Hungarian' specialised model:

> Experiments and years of experience have proved that the question [of mother- and infant protection] cannot be solved through the adoption of foreign models. What is good in America is not necessarily good in Germany or France, but it is most certainly useless on the Hungarian countryside: There, we do not have electricity or good roads, we do not have cars or satisfactory housing, and first and foremost, we do not find mothers with sufficient intelligence to be of assistance to doctors and public health nurses in achieving their goals.[72]

For years, Johan attempted to counter the accusations that the Green Cross was an alien and ill-adapted intrusion in Hungarian public health with a variety of strategies. He once claimed that the general model could be seen as a continuation of the traditional Hungarian house-doctor system,[73] and, alternatively, that not only the US, but also countries similar to Hungary had introduced the general model with success.[74] Neither of these arguments could counter the Stefánia's attacks. Yet over the years the Green Cross over the years gained a steadily increasing reputation, not as part of a national medical *tradition*, but as a new, modern, and genuinely Hungarian rural health model. This transformation was primarily achieved through the great interest in and recognition of the Green Cross by the international professional community. Johan always paid close attention to the scores of foreign visitors, and made sure to let both press and colleagues know about them. The IHD covered the expenses of hundreds of experts travelling to Hungary, thereby indirectly supporting Johan's work by adding prestige for each visit. During the year 1930 alone, the institute received 91 foreign guests. Between 1927 and 1931, visitors came from all European countries except the Soviet Union, and from 14 non-European countries, representing all parts of the world.[75] Johan's awareness of the significance of this international attention to the internal Hungarian debate is illustrated by suggestions he made in connection with the opening of the new school for public health nurses in Budapest. IHD's leading officer in Europe, G. K. Strode, noted:

> J[ohan] has suggested […] desirability of League [of Nations' Health Organization] calling a conference on the training of p.h. nursing [sic], to be convened perhaps in the fall, at the time of the formal opening of the Budapest nursing school and the Gödöllő Health Dept. Headquarters. He believes it would strengthen his hand in Hungary. At present he is having much opposition to his program of training of general p.h. nurses. […] Scholtz and Minister are with J. but he needs outside support. GKS [Strode] believes J's suggestion to be excellent and timely.[76]

The opening ceremony of the nursing school and the ensuing conferences became propaganda successes.[77] The international congregation of leading medical officers and public health nursed concluded that the general Green Cross model was vastly superior to the specialised model. Through such endeavours, Johan made public health work relevant to one of the most central political programs in Hungary during these years: As post-World War I Hungary was dismantled and disarmed through the Trianon-treaty, many saw the best way to achieve revision of the peace treaty as through the demonstration of *Hungarian cultural superiority* as compared to the neighbouring countries. Progress in medical science and health care were indeed as expressions of cultural strength. In one particularly relevant example, Johan was interviewed on a matter directly linking public health reforms to national self-esteem: The LNHO had recommended Chinese experts to study Hungarian rural public health, and to conduct massive public health reforms in China on the Hungarian example. In an article titled *China, learn from Hungary!* 'the smiling Béla Johan' explained Hungary's contribution to reforms on the enormous Chinese countryside.[78] Socrates Litsios has demonstrated how Johan's long-term contact in the RF, Selskar M. Gunn, studied conditions in China to prepare a new rural health-program in that country at this period. Litsios argues that Gunn's experiences in East-Central Europe were of great significance to his perspectives for China.[79] In particular, Litsios mentions Gunn's contacts to the Yugoslav Andrija Štampar and the Pole Ludwik Rajchmann in the LNHO. However, at this particular time, Štampar was politically discredited in his homeland.[80] Rajchmann, on the other hand, was stationed in Geneva, but, unlike Johan, was not in control of practical public health work. It would therefore seem likely that the LNHO's advice for Chinese experts to visit Hungary was a result of RF initiative, but to establish this would demand further research. Within the Hungarian setting, the image that Hungary served as a model for Chinese public health reforms contributed to the idea of the Green Cross as promoting Hungarian cultural superiority. All traces of "Americanness" in the Green Cross had by now been wiped away.

The crisis in Hungarian state finances in the early autumn of 1931 placed all institutions under Johan's direction in jeopardy of dissolution. A six-member parliamentary committee, of which two were supporters of the Stefánia, proposed devastating budget-reductions for the National Institute of Health, the new schools for public health nurses- and officers, and for the Green Cross. [81] Two RF-representatives came to the rescue when they quite coincidentally arrived to Budapest the day after the cuts were announced:

> When we arrived in Budapest and met Johan his back was against the wall and he had admitted defeat. [...] Johan appealed to us to help him, and I felt that in an emergency of this sort we were perfectly justified in going to the Minister of Social Welfare and the Prime Minister.[82]

During their subsequent meeting with the highest-ranking Hungarian politicians and officials, IHD-officers Crowell and Chas N. Leach stressed the contractual commitments made by the Hungarian government on receiving RF aid, and, simultaneously, went far towards promising that the continuation of existing institutions would release extraordinary aid from the Foundation.[83] This carrot-and-stick-strategy seems to have done the trick, and the reductions Johan had to suffer were no worse than what other public institutions had to face.[84] Johan felt his work more secure after the incorporation of all institutions under his direction into the Ministry of the Interior in summer 1932. This placed Johan under the political control of an old acquaintance from youth in Pécs, Minister of Interior Ferenc Keresztes-Fischer. He supported Johan until spring 1944, including the years 1935-38 when he was out of office.[85] The British historian C. A. Macartney, has praised Keresztes-Fischer:

> As Minister, he paid great attention to [social policy], and several of Hungary's best social institutions, such as the Green Cross rural health service [...], were largely inspired by him.[86]

Although, as we have seen, the Green Cross was initiated from 1926 in the form of five health demonstration districts, Macartney's observation holds some truth. It was Keresztes-Fischer who lifted the Green Cross from a marginal experiment to core Government health policy. In 1933, he launched a 10-year program for rural health, in which the Green Cross had a central role. The Minister's statement to Parliament must have been music to Johan's ears, outlining the basic principles of the general model:

> In my opinion, our small villages are in need of a public health system, a prophylaxis, which includes all types of problems. In a small village there should be a village doctor and a public health nurse, and these two should be able to complete all tasks needing to be done in a village within preventive health care and social services.[87]

Urban public health was still to be implemented by specialised organisations, such as the Stefánia. Johan regarded it a final victory when the Green Cross gained responsibility for all communities with fewer than 6000 inhabitants in summer 1934.[88] As Hungary had a predominantly rural settlement pattern, this brought more than half the population and ninety per cent of all local communities under the general model.[89] The Stefánia was confined to urban communities where it was already well established, while the general model would be vastly expanded. IHD officers noted the development in Hungary with satisfaction: 'Recognitions of the things the IHD has aided has come about at last, but it took from 1926 to 1933 to reach that stage'.[90]

Béla Johan in charge of Hungarian public health

Johan served as state secretary in the Ministry of the Interior from summer 1935 until the introduction of the fascist Arrow Cross regime in October 1944. From 1935-37 he could rely on firm support from Minister Miklós Kozma, and from 1938 until March 1944 Johan again served under Keresztes-Fischer. Both ministers took a personal interest in strengthening the basis for state involvement in public health reforms, granting Johan extensive authority. As state secretary Johan appeared more as a minister without portfolio than as a functional bureaucrat under orders. Johan was first mentioned as a possible successor to Kornél Scholtz in a document from autumn 1927.[91] The matter was not seriously debated until summer 1932. Under pressure of constant opposition, Johan expressed a wish to devote himself to laboratory research. Scholtz explicitly removed all hopes of a quiet life outside the political turmoil: Johan's alternatives were, according to Scholtz, to assume ever greater responsibilities, or, alternatively, within few years to confront an antagonistic administration, dedicated to the destruction of everything he had achieved so far.[92] Following the announcement of the 10-year plan for rural health in 1933, the 62-year-old Scholtz agreed to postpone retirement for a few years on condition that he could prepare his own successor. Scholtz informed the Minister that only two men carried the necessary weight in the professional community: András Csilléry and Béla Johan. As Csilléry had on several occasions vehemently attacked Keresztes-Fischer in Parliament, Johan seemed an obvious choice.[93] Six months later, Johan was still expressing doubts about accepting this post to his IHD contacts:

> Dr. J[ohan] talked very frankly about his own personal problems in relation to problems which will arise with Dr. Scholtz' retirement. There is a question of how much he may be willing to undertake with the uncertainty of RF support. In 1925 he felt sure that the RF was back of him – without that backing, he says, he could never have succeeded to develop the Institute, its work and its influence to the point were it is to-day. Now he is uncertain how far the RF would support him supposing for instance he were to throw his chances for the future into an effort to re-organise the whole national health machinery.[94]

In contrast to the hostility which he had incurred in parts of the medical community since the late 1920s, Johan entered service as state secretary in 1935 with a unanimous backing of his profession. This change of attitude had complex causes. First, there was great dissatisfaction with Kornél Scholtz among organisations representing the *Christian* – i.e., *non-Jewish* – Hungarian medical men, making Johan seem like a lesser evil. In the autumn of 1934 a number of Scholtz' opponents approached Johan to let him know their wish that he should replace Scholtz.[95] Their attitude resulted from the Government's decision to reduce reimbursements for medical doctors serving the members of collective health insurance organisations, and, in addition, to deny them the right to practice privately on the side. This regulation predominantly affected non-Jewish doctors, because right-wing leaders in the late 1920s had blocked the approbation of Jewish physicians by the insurance associations.[96] The anti-Semitic 'National Union for Hungarian Physicians' (MONE) was deeply involved in the conflict, and Johan was repeatedly reminded that it would strengthen his position if he was to re-evaluate his 1932 decision to resign his membership in the organisation.[97] As a result, Johan expressed the wish to re-enter the MONE, stating that his resignation was caused by personal antagonisms, particularly towards its leader, Csilléry, and not by disagreement with the union's principles.[98]

Johan's relation to the MONE has been used in the Johan-debate during recent years. Critics have blamed him for joining the anti-Semitic organisation during the 1920s, while his supporters have claimed that he took a brave humanist stand with his 1932 resignation. Both sides seem to have misinterpreted the matter: Johan was probably collectively enrolled in the MONE along with all other Christian physicians in the early 1920s, neither actively seeking membership nor expressing the wish to be left out. And Johan never formally rejoined the MONE. In January 1935, however, a weakened Csilléry asked if the next state secretary might help him secure a teaching post in the University of Debrecen. Johan promised to do his best, probably satisfied to see one of his fiercest critics leave the political scene of the capital.[99]

In March 1935, Johan's appointment was again uncertain when the right-wing Prime Minister Gyula Gömbös reshuffled his government, replacing Keresztes-Fischer with Miklós Kozma. Word spread rapidly that the new minister was planning to appoint *a lawyer* as state secretary for health instead of a medical doctor causing uproar among physicians. Johan being regarded the strongest candidate within the medical community, all forces gathered in his support. Past antagonisms aside, anything would be better than a lawyer! High-standing physicians, professors, and leaders of professional organisations utilized all channels to express their support for Johan to Kozma, Gömbös, Regent Miklós Horthy and even to the Regent's wife. The latter was the source of alarming news revealed in early April 1935, seemingly reducing Johan's chances for appointment to an absolute zero: To his own great astonishment, a rumour spread that Johan was a freemason.[100] As part of the perceived international conspiracy towards the Hungarian nation, the freemasons were not only despised with an intensity that matched anti-Semitism and anti-Bolshevism, but their activities were formally outlawed in Hungary.[101] In what appears to have been a cleverly conducted smear campaign, Johan' name could not be cleared by investigation within Hungary: it was said that he had joined the freemasons in the US. These allegations further increased the likelihood that the physicians would lose this important position to the lawyers. A whole series of prominent medical leaders, some of whom hardly knew Johan, swore on their honour that the rumours were false. Quite remarkably, even the leaders of Stefánia, who had attacked Johan's name and reputation for the last eight years, offered to testify on his behalf to Minister Kozma.[102] Johan's eventual appointment was celebrated as a great victory for the medical community. He therefore entered service on a wave of support, even from former antagonists.

Before his appointment, Johan was summoned to an interview with Prime Minister Gyula Gömbös. Johan's recapitulation of their conversation illustrates both the importance of the freemason-issue, and the fact that the general model's focus on state involvement in public health was a perfect fit with the Prime Minister's plans for coordinated action in this and other policy fields:

> 11 June 1935. Prime Minister Gömbös called me to see him. He raised two questions: 1) had I ever been a freemason? My answer: no, and it's also a lie that I became a freemason in the USA. 2) Do I support his political line or do I believe in middle-of-the road politics?[103] I answered that up to now I haven't been member of any political party. He answered that I, in spite of this, probably had opinions. Did I share his view that Hungary's supremacy needed to be secured? I answered that if I hadn't thought his policies right, I would have declined the appointment as state secretary. ... He stated that in his opinion, our public health system is in the need of a radical, centralistic concentration of power, because there is much work to be done. Kozma wants to put me in charge of all health issues, and Gömbös concurs. He wants everyone serving in public health to belong to an army under my command. He urges me to face the challenge with great courage. I was told to develop a four year program and get to work.[104]

Among all the fascinating insights this passage gives into the workings of the Hungarian political system, the most relevant to the present discussion is that the right-wing political leaders and Johan shared some basic expectations of future health policies. The most specific common point of reference was the continued increase in the state's involvement in health administration at the expense of civil society and local administration. The quote also illustrates Johan's adaptability to changing political circumstances and ideological movements: In the twenties, he interpreted public health work as a part of the national-conservative policy for *cultural superiority*, while in 1935 the same policies were placed at the core of Gömbös more aggressively revisionist, right-radical political project. This flexibility to changing political programs was crucial to the exponential growth experienced in the public health system under Johan's direction between 1935 and the early war years. Public health-reforms gained mass support as well as a wide political mandate, as an important answer to major challenges facing the Hungarian nation. The late 1930s in Hungary were a period of increasing nationalism, militarism and anti-Semitism, providing a grim background to otherwise progressive public health reforms.[105] The appeal of these reforms to the radical right is particularly evident in the question of rural health, as the ideal 'village' assumed ever greater importance as the cradle of Hungarian national (i. e. – non-Jewish) blood and tradition. According to the 10-year plan of 1933, the Green Cross was designated to serve rural settlements, while the specialised organisations served the cities. With the growing concern for the well-being of rural Hungary, support for the Green Cross gained momentum. Johan actively participated in mobilising right-wing support for rural health work. For example, he lent his support to the anti-Semitic student union 'Turul', which undertook a large rural health survey during the autumn of 1935.[106] It should be mentioned in connection to the ongoing Hungarian debate, however, that in my study of all available texts from Johan's hand during the inter-war years, I have not come across one single anti-Semitic remark. Neither did he suggest that Jews should be discriminated against within the health profession or through being denied medical or social benefits distributed through the Green Cross apparatus. In light of the 'political correctness' of anti-Semitism in contemporary Hungarian political and medical discourse, this is remarkable indeed.

In 1933, the Green Cross was confined to the five demonstration districts financed by the IHD. Up to the mid-thirties the general model was extended to a few more communities, but from 1936 this growth escalated. Between 1936 and 1941, 270 health centres of various sizes were included in the Green Cross, at an average of 45 per year. To supply the necessary personnel, three new schools for public health nurses were opened. As an administrative hub and central laboratory, the activities of the National Institute of Public Health grew exponentially, necessitating the construction of a number of spacious new buildings. The aforementioned 1936 legal reform elevated all Chief Medical Officers from municipal employment to the status of state employees. In 1942 this status was extended also to the village doctors, creating one coordinated public health hierarchy stretching from the Ministry, via the National Institute of Public Health and the Green Cross out to local communities all over the country.

Ever-increasing investment- and maintenance costs were financed through various channels: Three private campaigns with an explicitly nationalist agenda provided substantial funding for rural health work, both in Trianon-Hungary and in the areas Hungary re-annexed from Czechoslovakia and Romania as a result of the country's co-operation with Nazi-Germany on the brink of Second World War.[107] Important though these campaigns were, the bulk of public health funding came from the state. In April 1938, the Prime Minister initiated a gigantic public investment program with an explicit militarist agenda. Around 200 million pengő out of a total 1 billion pengő were put into civil infrastructure, not least into rural health. The remaining 80 per cent was spent on armaments and strategically relevant infrastructure.[108] As this so-called *Győr Programme* was announced on the same day as the launching of Hungary's first explicitly anti-Semitic legislation, it serves as a prime example of the interconnection between militarisation, anti-Semitic sentiments and public health in Hungary during the late 1930s. All Ministers of Interior during Johan's brief decade as state secretary delegated substantial powers to him. Plans for legislative reforms and administrative reorganisation, and priorities within budget limits, were to a great extent made by Johan and his subordinates in the Ministry and at the National Institute of Public Health.[109] The media campaign against Johan from the years around 1930 was replaced by wide popular support. With the extension of the Green Cross apparatus to ever more local communities, Johan became an object of public celebration, often appointed honorary citizen of the village.[110] In her last visit to Hungary, the IHD's nursing expert noted Johan's optimism, tying recent developments both to the commitment of the present regime and to earlier Rockefeller Foundation support:

> Dr. Johan, at present, is like the happy country that has no history; everything is going well with him, he is getting everything he wants, and his Minister is backing him to the limit: he is justly proud of what has been accomplished in developing a public health scheme for the whole country and feels that the RF help has been justified by the results.[111]

A report made by the LNHO in the same period testifies to the interconnectedness of institutions under Johan's direction:

> The Budapest Institute of Hygiene is perhaps the most characteristic example in Europe of a great public health institute which is, at the same time, a school of hygiene and directly dependent on the central Government as a technical organ of health administration. ... As regards infectious diseases, epidemiology, medical statistics and measures for the prevention of endemic diseases and the organisation of rural health services, the Budapest Institute of Hygiene acts as a section of a Department of the Ministry.[112]

The final unification of local health care under the direction of the Ministry was implemented in January 1942, when all specialised public health organisations such as the Stefánia were dissolved, and all employees and assets were transferred to the Green Cross.[113] With Chief Medical Officers in state employment under the Ministry of Interior, all local preventive health care under the general model and a wide array of regulations implemented through the National Institute of Public Health, it is safe to say that Hungary entered the Second World War with a 'fundamentally reorganised' public health system under Johan's direction.

Conclusion

This discussion of Béla Johan's 'second incarnation' has focused on reforms in the Hungarian public health system during the years 1927-1942. Through the National Institute of Public Health, the Green Cross, and various educational programs for public health professionals, a new basis was created for the implementation of health reforms, both on a central level and in the local communities. Johan's entry into the field of public health, and his later work, was intimately connected to various international agencies, in particular the International Health Division of the Rockefeller Foundation and the LNHO. Johan and a number of his associates received training in Western Europe and the US through IHD fellowships. The most central institutions, such as the National Institute of Public Health, the nursing schools and the Green Cross were prepared and implemented in continuous interaction with foundation officers. For example, Selskar M. Gunn played a crucial part in the preparation of plans for the new public health institute between 1922 and 1924. W. L. Mitchell resided in Budapest from 1925-30 co-operating with Johan on a daily basis during the construction and early years of the institute, and in the establishment of the first health demonstrations. F. E. Crowell was Johan's main advisor on the question of nursing education. In the case of the local preventive health care, Johan's opponents used these foreign connections to discredit the general model. Eventually, however, international acknowledgement of towards the rural health reforms undertaken in Hungary added prestige to Johan's work. Johan strategically contributed to this construction of the image of a new, internationally recognised and genuinely Hungarian public health model. Both during the establishment of the central institute and at his appointment as state secretary, he was able to foster the enthusiastic support of a united medical community. He also contributed to a continuous reinterpretation of the meaning and significance of public health, adapting his arguments to the political currents of the day. This included connecting public health and the policy for *cultural superiority* in the 1920s, and the mobilisation of groups and individuals representing more aggressive, expansionist and even racist sentiments in the late 1930s. To different audiences, Johan would alternatively stress the international inspiration behind public health reforms and their connection to national medical traditions. Likewise, the political significance of these undertakings could be presented as both serving humanity in general, and as appealing to the more particularly oriented radical sections of the Hungarian political scene.

As public health reforms by default involve political commitment, and the mobilisation of a great number of professionals, as well as public endorsement, Johan's skills in creating such support may constitute the key to present-day controversies regarding his policies. While debate has centred on Johan's moral choices in the summer of 1944, the fact that his entire inter-war career involved a continuous fight for political support and the forming of ever-changing alliances around public health reforms has largely been ignored. In this perspective, Johan's decision to stay in his post until he was ousted in October 1944 seems a logical continuation of his past actions during troubled times, rather than a moral slip, to be excused by a temporary lack of clear vision.

---

1 I am grateful to the librarians at the National Epidemiological Centre in Budapest for informing me about this event per e-mail on the same day as it occurred. Johan's bust has been given sanctuary by the same librarians.

2 Document titled *Johan Béla életmű*, part of case file on Johan from 2003. The author of this one-page article has not been revealed. This and all other translations from the Hungarian are by the author. A few typological errors in Hungarian English-language documents have been corrected, to avoid the use of '*sic!*' within quotes.

3 K. Ungváry, 'Ki volt Johan Béla? Egy orvos pályaképéhez', *Magyar Narancs* 4 September (2003).

4 P. Felix, 'Johan Béla érinthetlensége', *Magyar Narancs* 23 Feburary (2006).

5 Semmelweis Orvostörténeti Múzeum, Múzeumi Adattár, Leltári szám: 1279-91 'Johan Béla igazoltatási ügyei (dokumentáció) újságcikkek 1991'. The file contains 128 pages, but of particular interest is the 'Kivonatos jegyzőkönyv', an 11-page resume of the questioning of Johan on 25 June 1945.

6 T. Bakács, *Az Országos Közegészségügyi Intézet működése. 1927-1957*. (Budapest: Medicina Kiadó, 1959), 11.

7 G. Birtalan, *Memoár orvosokról és történészekről (1943-1997)*. (Budapest: MedInfo, 1998).

8 G. Birtalan, 'Adatok a két világháború között magyarországon végzett szervezett egészségvédelmi munkáról, különös tekintettel az OKI tevékenységére.' *Orvostörténeti Közlemények-Communicationes de Historia Artis Medicinae*. xxv, 1-2 (1979): 181-218.

9 Z. Alföldy, 'Dr. Johan Béla, az országos közegészségügyi szervezet megteremtője'; M. Börzsönyi, 'Johan Béla, a patalógus'; L. Pillich, 'Dr. Johan Béla, az ipari mikrobiológus'. All in *Egészségtudomány* xxxiv, 2 (1990).

10 É. Vermes, 'Kollaborálás egy kollaboránssal? A kétszáz orvosból tizenöt maradt életben.' *Kurir*, 8 June (1991).

11 The Prime Minister was more involved in this matter than could generally be expected – József Antall came from a position as director of the Semmelweis Museum, Library and Archives in Budapest, and was familiar with Birtalan's work from the late 1970s. On the 1991-article, see letter fom J. Juhász to Prime Minister József Antall, 18. juni 1991. Semmelweis Museum of Medical History: Múzeumi Adattár, Leltári szám: 1279-91 'Johan Béla igazoltatási ügyei (dokumentáció) újságcikkek 1991'.

12 See, for example: G. Palló, 'Rescue and Cordon Sanitaire: The Rockefeller Foundation in Hungarian Public Health' *Stud. Hist. Biol. & Biomed. Sci.*, xxxi (2000), 433–45.

13 P. Felix, 'Szakember apró hibákkal' *Magyar Narancs* , 15 May (2003), 16-17.

14 M. Torkos, 'Egy nácibarátról elnevezett program' *Magyar Nemzet*, 16 May (2003). The article is based on Felix' article from the previous day. He has been the most persistent critic of Johan's inter-war role. See, for example, 'Dr. Feldmájer Péter a MAZSIHISZ elnökének levele Félix Péternek a Füstirtók egyesület elnökének' 10 April 2006. Publicised on Internet: http://www.mazsihisz.com/hirek.phtml?id=924

15 K. Ungváry, 'Johan Béla és a nemzet egészsége' *Magyar Narancs*, 26 June (2003); and 'Ki volt Johan Béla? Egy orvos pályaképéhez' *Magyar Narancs*, 4 September (2003).

16 'Törölték Johan Béla nevét az egészségügyi programból' 13 February (2006). Available on the Internet: http://www.origo.hu/print/itthon/20060213toroltek.html

17 This view is at present only voiced by Johan's former colleagues through the periodical *Magyar Epidemiológia [Hungarian Epidemiology]*. Between 1989 and 2003, however, this was the prevalent view.

18 Apart from Péter Felix, a number of journalists, historians and politicians have contributed to the condemnation of Johan. Péter Gustos, MP from the government coalition partner SZDSZ, has led the political process against the use of Johan's name, e.g. *Az SZDSZ kezdeményezi a népegészségügyi program nevének megváltoztatását.* http://www.szdsz.hu/hir.phtml?id=2049. Accessed April 2006.

19 This summarises the conclusion after the investigations under the auspices of the Academy of Sciences: 'Nem megfelelő személyt javasoltak (Pók Attila és Pótó János történészek Johan Béláról)' *Magyar Narancs,* 14 Oktober (2004). On the evening news show of the Hungarian Television (Magyar Televizió) Pótó gave similar statements regarding Johan's lack of political clear sight. Accessed April 2006: http://www.mtv.hu/cikk.php?id=5685

20 I have elaborated on this in my recent PhD thesis: E. Ingebrigtsen, *Revisjonismens fortsettelse med andre midler: Rockefeller Foundation og folkehelsen i Ungarn, 1920–1941.* (Trondheim: NTNU, PhD Thesis, 2007:42)

21 I am grateful to Johan's grand-daughter for giving me this information during our meeting in Budapest, 13 June 2004.

22 B. Johan, ifj, 'A védőoltóanyagokról' *Budapest Orvosi Ujság*, 3 (1917).

23 Letter from Dr. Kenyeres, Dean of the Medical Faculty at the University of Budapest, to the Rockefeller Foundation, 16 May 1921. Rockefeller Archive Center, Pocantico Hills, North Tarrytown, New York, USA, Collection Rockefeller Foundation, Record Group 5, Series 1.2, Box 125, Folder 1672, hereafter RAC.

24 B. Page, 'The Rockefeller Foundation and Central Europe: A Reconsideration' *Minerva* 40, 3 (2002), 265-287. Before a major reorganisation of the RF in 1927, this part of the Foundation was called the International Health Board, IHB. In its relation to Hungary, the change from IHB to IHD had no impact, as the Hungarians in general related to the RF as a whole, not to its subdivisions. Therefore, to avoid unnecessary confusion, I use the abbreviation IHD throughout.

25 Telegram from the President of the Rockefeller Foundation, G. Vincent, to the director of IHD, Wicliffe Rose, 2 Feburary 1920, and Rose's reply, 3 February 1920. Both in RAC, RF, RG 5, Series 2, Sub-series 700, Box 58, Folder 368.

26 Letter from Rose to Vincent, 3 February 1920. RAC, RF, RG 5, Series 2, Sub-series 700, Box 58, Folder 368.

27 Letter from Lajos Nékám to the Minister of Religion and Education, József Vass. The letter has no date, but an attachment is marked 20 November 1920; Letter from L. Nékám to J. Vass 24 December 1920. Hungarian National Archives, Bécsi Kapu tér, Budapest, hereafter MOL, K636-1924-4-33790

28 B. Johan, 'Adatok a M. kir. Országos Közegészségügyi Intézet felállításának történetéhez' *Népegészségügy* vi (1925), 861-867: 862.

29 From context it is clear that this was not Gunn's first visit to Hungary, but earlier visits were not documented. Letter from the Dean of the Medical Faculty to Minister József Vass, 9 September 1921.

30 Letter from the Dean of the Medical Faculty to Minister József Vass, 9 September 1921.

31 S. M. Gunn, 'Public Health Conditions in Hungary. Report of Visit to Budapest' (1924) RAC, RF, RG 1.1, Series 750, Box 1, Folder 1.

32 Béla Johan's fellowship card, from the Fellows registry at Rockefeller Archive Center. Unfortunately, Johan's original cards have been lost. The available card is a replica constructed from correspondence.

33 Both Johan and Jendrassik were finally approved on 31 July 1922. In a number of biographic articles Johan is praised as the very first Hungarian Rockefeller fellow, but this honour he has to share with Jendrassik. Johan's and Aladár Jendrassik's fellowship cards, RAC.

34 Letter from Béla Johan to 'Dear Mother', New York, 6 October 1922. In possession of Johan's descendants.

35 Ingebrigtsen, *Revisjonismens fortsettelse med andre midler*, 116-131.

36 Gunn 'Public Health in Hungary' (1924).

37 I will not provide full references to all of these texts, but they are easily available as special prints of Johan's scientific articles are collected in three volumes, kept in the library of the National Epidemiological Institute, Gyáli út, Budapest.

38 B. Johan, 'A simple and rapid method for preparing (macerating) macroscopic bone specimens. Presented at the Sixteenth Annual Meeting of the American and Canadian Section of the International Ass. of Medical Museums, Boston, Mass. March 29, 1923' *Bulletin no. X of the International Association of Medical Museums* (1924), 22-4.

39 B. Johan, 'A Bakteriologia és serologia az Északamerikai Egyesült-Államokban közegészségügyének szolgálatában. Az "Országos Közegészségügyi Egyesület"-ben 1924 február 20-án tartott előadása nyomán' *Egészség* xxxviii, 1-3 (1924), 11-22.

40 B. Johan, 'Az orvos és a modern közegészségügy (Jugoszlávia egészségügyi szervezete)' *Az Orvosi Hetilap tudományos közleményei* LXIC, 11 (1925); *Néhány külföldi óvodáról éz az óvónő képzésről orvosi szempontból.* Népegészségügy, 15 (1927); *Megjegyezés a közegészségügyi reformtervezet bírálatára.* Orvosi Hetilap, 7, 13 January (1927); 'A modern közegészségügy czéljai, eszközei, eredményei. (Előadta a Tisza István Társaskörben 1928. évi márczius hó 2.-án' *Népegészségügy*, 10 (1928).

41 T. Bakács, *Az Országos Közegészségügyi Intézet működése. 1927-1957.* (Budapest: Medicina Kiadó, 1959); G. Birtalan, 'Adatok a két világháború között magyarországon végzett szervezett egészségvédelmi munkáról, különös tekintettel az OKI tevékenységére' *Orvostörteneti Közlemények*, XXV, 1-2 (1979), 181-218; K. Kapronczay, *Fejezetek 125 év magyar egészségügyének történetéből* (Budapest: Semmelweis Orvostörténeti Múzeum, Könyvtár és Levéltár, 2001); and L. Kiss, 'Egészség és politika - az egészségügyi prevenció Magyarországon a 20. század első felében' *Korall*, 17 (2004), 107-137.

42 B. Johan, 'Adatok a M. kir. Országos Közegészségügyi Intézet felállításának történetéhez' *Népegészségügy*, 15 (1925); 'A létesülő M. Kir. Országos Közegészségügyi Intézetről' *Orvosi Hetilap tudományos közleményei* lxx, 8-9 (1926), 'A M. Kir. Országos Közegészségügyi Intézetről', in Z. Magyary (ed.), *A Magyar Tudománypolitika Alapvetése.* (Budapest: A Tudományos Társulatok és Intézmények Országos Szövetsége, 1927), 421-424; *A M. Kir. Országos Közegészségügyi Intézet* (Budapest: Egyetemi Nyomda, 1927).

43 József Fodor died in 1901 and Liebermann was 70 years old at the time when S. M. Gunn first was introduced to existing plans. Kálmán Müller was three years older. Both men died in 1926, one year before the opening of the new institute.

44 S. M. Gunn, 'Public Health Conditions in Hungary. Report from visit to Budapest, March 20 – March 23, 1922'. RAC, RF, RG 1.1, Series 750, Box 1, Folder 1.

45 Letter from S. M. Gunn to Minister of Welfare Nándor Bernolak, 27 March 1922. RAC, RF, RG 6.1, Series 1.1, Box 27, Folder 306.

46 Gunn 'Public Health in Hungary' (1924).

47 The fellowship files show that Johan travelled to Yugoslavia in May 1924. Jendrassik also visited Warsaw, Prague, Copenhagen and several German cities.

48 The RF did not file rejected proposals or requests. Most public health-related files from the Hungarian Ministry of Welfare and Ministry of the Interior are missing from the Hungarian National Archives. This has multiple causes, both destructions during the war as well as deliberate and accidental elimination of documents after 1945.

49 The Parliamentary debate lasted from 20-22 October 1925. The law was passed as Article XXXI:1925 *Regarding the establishment of the Royal Hungarian National Institute of Public Health.*

50 Letter from S. M. Gunn to F. F. Russell, 14 November 1925. RAC, RF, RG 1.1, Series 750, Box 1, Folder 3.

51 G. K. Strode, Diary, 4 December 1934. This and all diaries subsequently referred to are found in: RAC, RF, RG 12.1, Officers' diaries.

52 Birtalan, *Memoár orvosokról és történészekről.*

53 Report dated 1 January 1926. RAC, RF, RG 1.1, Box 27, Folder 306; and S. M. Gunn, Diary, 2 December 1926. RAC, RF, RG 12.1, Officers' diaries.

54 B. Johan, 'Leland W. Mitchell' *Orvosi Hetilap* , 48 (1930), 1253; also 'W. Leland Mitchell' *The Rockefeller Foundation. Annual Report* (1930). The Vienna-based Chas N. Leach covered Hungary after Mitchell's death. From 1936 to 1939 Richard M. Tyler represented IHD in Hungary, as director of an influenza laboratory at the National Institute of Health.

55 S. M. Gunn, Diary, 3 October 1927, RAC, RF, Record Group 12.1, Officers' diaries. See also the entry in G. K. Strode's diary for the same date

56 B. Johan (ed.), *Jelentés a m. kir. Országos Közegészségügyi Intézet 1928 évben végzett munkájáról.* (Budapest: OKI, 1929).

57 I. Weis, 'Tervezet az 1876: XIV. t.-czikk és 1908: XXXVIII. t.-czikk némely rendelkezéseinek módosítására (az egészségügyi közigazgatás szervezetére) vonatkozólag', *Népegészségügy* , 21 (1926), 1207-42.

58 Statement from Minister Ferenc Keresztés-Fischer, quoted in Béla Johan, Personal notes, 8. June 1934. These documents, compiled in a file titled 'Bizalmas tárgyalások' are in possession of Johan's descendants.

59 Theese regulations were formulated in:'1936. évi IX. törvénycikk. A hatósági orvosi szolgálatról és a közegészségügyi törvények és egyéb rendelkezéseinek módosításáról' (1936).

60 'Isten háta mögött', the Hungarian standard phrase for 'the middle of nowhere'.

61 B. Johan, 'Az orvosok elhelyezkedésének kérdése, A Budapesti Orvosi Kamara elökségének felkérésére dec. 2-án tartott elöadás' (1938) Reprint in Johan's collected works, stored at library of Országos Epidemiológiai Központ.

62 B. Johan, 'The Training of Physicians for Public Health Service in Hungary', *Orvosképzés* (1935), 340-347; 'Public Health Services in Hungary' *Hungarian Quarterly*, IV (1938).

63 F. E. Crowell, 'Memorandum re Study of Sick Nursing and Health Visiting in Hungary' (1923), RAC, RF, RG 1.1, Series 750, Box 2, Folder 21. Letter from F. E. Crowell to R. M. Pearce, 10 May 1927. RAC, RF, RG 1.1, Series 750C, Box 2, Folder 20.

64 Letter from the Hungarian Red Cross to the Ministry of Religion and Education, February 1928. MOL, K636-1928-9-38529.

65 Crowell, Diary, 14 November 1927, RAC, RF, RG 12.1, Officers' diaries. B. Johan, *Az ápolónő- és védőnőkérdésről. Különös tekintettel az ápolónők és védőnők képzésére.* (Budapest: A M. Kir. Orsz. Közegészségügyi Intézet kiadása, 1929).

66 B. Johan,' Az egészségvédelmi munka egységesítése és rationalizalása', *Népegészségügy*, 5 (1929)

67 Only the most important contributions number more than 70 articles. Johan published 22 articles directly related to this debate between 1928 and 1934.

68 These accusations were repeated, for example in spring 1933 when insinuations that Johan had skimmed Rockefeller donations were presented in a Parliamentary debate. The meticulous RF-comptroller did not share these suspicions, and from Johan's diary it is clear that he found the accusations most frustrating. See, for example "Az Eternitügy, a mátrai szanatórium és a Rockefeller-alap." *Pesti Hirlap*, 7 April 1933.

69 Johan, Personal notes, several entries during summer 1931. Johan, in fact, indicated in his note that he had a more or less standing invitation to come to work with Rajchmann. I am grateful to Iris Borowy for pointing out that, due to scarce funds at Rajchmann's disposal, this was probably a slight exaggeration on Johan's part.

70 This information is compiled from the fellows registry at RAC, where individual cards for all former fellows are held. Altogether seventy-two Hungarians received public-health related fellowships, in addition to eighty-two fellowships in other fields.

71 Statement made in interview: M. Pfeiffer, 'A gödöllői mintajáras' *MONE*, 6 (1927), 110-111.

72 L. Keller, 'A védőnőképzés problemája' *Anya- és csecsemővédelem,* I (1928), 515-516.

73 B. Johan, 'Meddig terjedjen az állami egészségvédelmi gondozás' *Országos Orvos-Szövetség*, 10 (1930): page 4 in special print.

74 B. Johan, 'Az egészségvédelmi munka egységesítése és rationalizalása' *Népegészségügy*, 5 (1929): page 3-4 in the special print.

75 The Hungarian National Institute of Health's Annual Reports for 1930 and 1931.

76 Strode, Diary, May 20, 1930, RAC, RF, RG 12.1, Officers' diaries.

77 Crowell, Diary, August 31, 1930, RAC, RF, RG 12.1, Officers' diaries

78 'Kína - tanulj Magyarországtól!' *Magyarország*, 3 December (1931).

79 S. Litsios, 'Selskar Gunn and China: The Rockefeller Foundation's "Other" Approach to Public Health', *Bulletin for the History of Medicine,* 79 (2005), 295-318. A similar observation is made in Q. Ma, 'The Peking Union Medical College and the Rockefeller Foundations's Medical Programs in China', in W. H. Schneider (ed.), *Rockefeller Philanthropy and Modern Biomedicine* (Bloomington, Indiana: Indiana University Press, 2002), 159-183.

80 See, for example, Gunn, Diary, 18 February 1929 and 20 May 1930, RAC, RF, RG 12.1, Officers' diaries.

81 I. Romsics, *Magyarország története a XX. században* (Budapest: Osiris Kiadó, 1999)

82 Letter from C. N. Leach to G. K. Strode, 5 September 1931. RAC, RF, RG 6.1, Series 1.1, Box 27, Folder 306.

83 The minutes from Leach' meeting with Prime Minister Károlyi are lost, but Johan recapitulated the most important points in his personal notes on 4 September 1931. See also letter from Minister of Welfare Sándor Ernszt to C. N. Leach, 13 November 1931. RAC, RF, RG 1.1, Series 750, Box 1, Folder 5.

84 Johan, Personal notes, 10 September 1931.

85 'Kivonatos jegyzőkönyv', an 11-page resume of the questioning of Johan on 25 June 1945. Semmelweis Orvostörténeti Múzeum, Múzeumi Adattár, Leltári szám: 1279-91 'Johan Béla igazoltatási ügyei'.

86 C. A. Macartney, *October Fifteenth. A History of Modern Hungary*. (Edinburgh: The Edinburgh University Press, 1957), 104.

87 'Vitéz Keresztes-Fischer belügyminiszter képviselőházi beszédéből 1933 május 18-án', *Orvosi Hetilap,* 24 (1933), 523-524.

88 Strode, Diary, 16 June 1934, RAC, RF, RG 12.1, Officers' diaries.

89 B. Johan, *Gyógyul a magyar falu* (Budapest: Országos Közegészségügyi Intézet, 1939), 2-3.

90 Strode, Diary, 20 January 1934; and Crowell, Diary, 13 January 1934, both in RAC, RF, RG 12.1, Officers' diaries.

91 Gunn, Diary, 2 October 1927 and Strode, Diary, 4 October 1927, both in RAC, RF, RG 12.1, Officers' diaries.

92 Johan, Personal notes, 18 June 1932.

93 Johan, Personal notes, several entries from May-June 1933.
94 Crowell, Diary, 18 January 1934, RAC, RF, RG 12.1, Officers' diaries.
95 Johan, Personal notes, several entries during 1934, in particular 27 August and 18 November.
96 This conflict is discussed at length in: M. M. Kovács, *Liberal Professions and Illiberal Politics: Hungary from the Habsburgs to the Holocaust* (Oxford: Oxford University Press, 1994).
97 Johan, Personal notes, 13 December 1933. See also: 'Johan Béla egyetemi tanár kilépett a MONE-ból', *Ujság*, 12 March (1932).
98 Johan, Personal notes, 27 August 1934.
99 Johan, Personal notes, January 1935.
100 Johan, Personal notes, 4 April 1935, several entries during the following weeks, and 25 May.
101 Ministry of the Interior, regulation BM1550/1920, also Zs. L. Nagy, *Szabadkőművesség a XX. században* (Budapest: Kossuth, 1977).
102 Johan, Personal notes, early June 1935. It was Stefánia's President, the former Minister of Interior Gábor Ugron and the director Lajos Keller who came to Johan with this offer.
103 The Prime Minister's words, 'középpárti politikának vagyok-e a hive', are not directly translatable. He referred to "the middle party", but the main division in 1935 went straight through the Government Party.
104 Johan, Personal notes, 11 June 1935.
105 These public health reforms were praised also outside Hungary. The most important example, due to the great publicity it received in Hungary, was a report written by a Danish statistician: K. Stouman, *Egészségügyi jelzőszámok egy magyarországi falusi körzet egégszségügyi felvételében. (Based on "Bulletin of the Health Organization of the League of Nations, no. 5, Vol. 6 1937.)* (Budapest: Athenaeum, 1937).
106 Special issue of the magazine *Bajtárs – A Turul mozgalom lapja*, 10 July 1935, in which Johan both gave an interview and wrote an article. On the right-radicals' enthusiasm for rural health, see: E. Ingebrigtsen, 'Right Radicalism and Rural Health in Hungary', in A. Andresen et al. (eds.), *Science Culture and Politics: European Perspectives on Medicine, Sickness and Health.*(Bergen: Stein Rokkan Centre for Social Studies, 2006), 187-201
107 P. Hámori, 'Kísérlet a visszacsatolt felvidéki területek társadalmi és szociális integrálására: A Magyar a Magyarért Mozgalom története (1938-1940)', *Századok* 135, 3 (2001), 569-624.
108 Macartney, *October Fifteenth,* 218.
109 Johan, Personal notes, 7 Februrary 1938.
110 To mention just one of dozens of similar examples: 'A mi díszpolgárunk' *Túrkevei Hirlap* 18 June 1939.
111 Crowell, Diary, 16 December 1939, RAC, RF, RG 12.1, Officers' diaries.
112 'Second General Report on Certain European Schools and Institutes of Hygiene', *League of Nations - Bulletin of the Health Organisation* VII, 2 (1938),191-407: 226
113 The reorganisation was legally regulated through BM730/1940 and BM1000/1940. See also L. Kiss, 'Egészség és politika...' (2004).

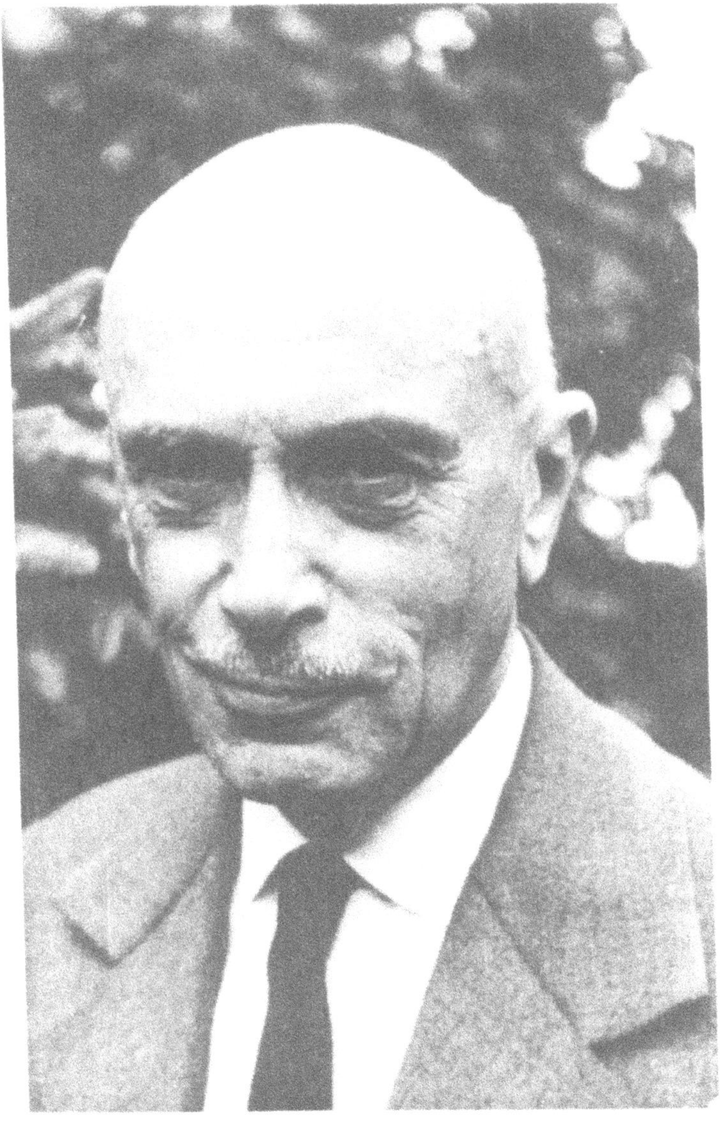

Bela Johan

Photograph Courtesy of the National Center for Epidemiology, Budapest

Andrija Štampar (1888-1958): Resolute Fighter for Health and Social Justice

Željko Dugac

In the introduction of the book Serving the Cause of Public Health: Selected Papers of Andrija Štampar (*U borbi za narodno zdravlje: izabrani članci Andrije Štampara*), the renowned historian of medicine and Štampar disciple, Mirko Dražen Grmek, wrote that Andrija Štampar's success was a triumph of ideology that put great trust in the value of health for the society, in the principal social role of health, and in the possibility to improve health using the methods of social medicine.[1] For Štampar, the interaction between human health and society was an obsession which persisted through his entire life. This obsession incited many conflicts with his medical colleagues and politicians, but also gave rise to great successes.

How did Štampar resolve organisational problems, fight dangerous enemies—including an entire political regime—and win the trust of his co-workers? How did he manage to achieve professional success whilst experiencing personal dramas: the death of his first wife, the raising of five children, spending years away from his home travelling or as a prisoner of war. To succeed, he must have possessed in ample measure the qualities that his colleagues and contemporaries saw in him: discipline, persistence, uncompromising attitude, exactness, steadfastness, courage, stubbornness, assertiveness, and, above all, honesty. He could not tolerate his own or other people's mistakes, and he never hesitated to say what he meant even if it displeased others. These two sides of Štampar were succinctly described by his long-term friend and colleague, Rockefeller Foundation fellow Selskar M. Gunn: 'Štampar in many respects is a big boy and he is somewhat petulant and very critical of people and problems that he does not approve of. He is, however, completely honest, even if occasionally not as tactful as he might be.'[2]

Štampar's tall, imposing figure often overshadowed other people physically and for that reason (and possibly because of the assertive and sometimes stern first impression he left) he was also called 'the bear of the Balkans'.[3] Henry van Zile Hyde recalled their intense collaboration in the post-World War II creation of the WHO in the following words: 'During the work in Paris, those of us who worked with him soon overcame our trepidation and found that the 'bear of the Balkans' was a very friendly bruin indeed—a friend of all mankind.'[4] The 'bear' could quickly turn into a 'friendly bruin', whose entire life was devoted to the health of human communities. His honesty, dedication and good intents, even if couched in open criticism, were immediately recognised by ordinary people, but also the authorities.

The life of Andrija Štampar may be divided into several chapters. The first chapter encompasses his childhood in rural Croatia and medical studies in Vienna. There and then he accumulated experiences that would inform his later career, established directions that would guide him through life, and formed principles he would never abandon. Following early hospital practice, Štampar embarked on the second chapter, from 1919–31, which was marked by his work at the Ministry of Public Health of the Kingdom of Serbs, Croats and Slovenes (from 1929, Yugoslavia). During that period he founded the public health system of the newly formed Kingdom. The third chapter began in 1931, when he was forced to retire from his post and from the public life in the Kingdom of Yugoslavia. In this period he pursued an active international career as an expert of the League of Nations Health Organisation and Rockefeller Foundation. Just before the Second World War, he again briefly resumed his public health work in Croatia, but was soon interrupted again, this time by Nazi imprisonment. The end of the war saw the beginning of the last and possibly the most active chapter of his life. In this period he completed numerous projects in the field of international health and occupied important posts in his homeland. In this article I will outline Štampar's biography and analyze in more detail certain key moments of his career, especially during those that took place in the interwar era. I will pay close attention to the political situation in Yugoslavia around 1930, when Štampar was forced to leave his position in the Yugoslav administration. Finally, I will discuss his collaboration with the Rockefeller Foundation and his international activity under the auspices of the League of Nations Health Organisation. The last chapter of Štampar's life, the post-war era, will not be examined in this article in detail.

Štampar's work has been well known to public health specialists, historians of medicine and wider medical audiences alike. In addition to an extensive literature in the languages of ex-Yugoslavia, there are numerous articles in English that discuss his life and career. Es early as 1939, Henry Sigerist dedicated to Štampar part of the text on his (Sigerist's) experiences at the International Congress of the History of Medicine in Yugoslavia.[5] Immediately after Štampar's death, Henry Van Zile Hyde published an intimate recollection of the most important events in Štampar's life. Although an obituary, this text manages to convey Štampar's optimism and the idiosyncratic sense of humour that people around him found so inspiring. Štampar's co-worker Branko Cvjetanović published a concise article that contains a good insight into his fundamental principles as well as key biographical data.[6] A short note on Štampar was published in JAMA in 1980.[7] Norman Howard Jones also wrote about him, as well as Theodore M. Brown, Elizabeth Fee and Patric Zylberman.[8] Because many of these authors did not read or have access to the literature and sources in Croatian, this essay hopes to contribute to the scholarship on Štampar by drawing the attention to Grmek's 1966 book, still a highly regarded analysis of Štampar's work, and by using hitherto little studied primary sources, especially those accessible in Croatian language only.

Successes and problems: the national politics and the public health
Andrija Štampar was born on 1 September 1888 in Drenovac, a village in the eastern region of Croatia, Slavonia. His mother's name was Katarina and his father Ambroz worked as the village teacher. In later years, Štampar frequently spoke of the traditional village life and in particular the poor sanitary conditions of Drenovac. There he first encountered poverty, backwardness, superstition, and vice. These early experiences helped him understand rural life, the improvement of which would later occupy a central position in his career. From 1898 until 1906, he attended high school in the nearby town of Vinkovci. Like many young Croatian men, he then left for the imperial capital of Vienna to pursue medical studies. His teachers at the University of Vienna School of Medicine included world-famous scientists and physicians such as Julius Wagner-Jauregg, Carl Toldt, Hans Chiari and others.[9] Štampar was particularly impressed by Ludwig Teleky, whose lectures and seminars in social medicine he heard in the ninth semester, 1910–11.[10] In addition to his university studies, Štampar attended lectures in social medicine at Vienna's 'people's universities' (Volkshochschulen).[11] Later he would refer to the anatomist and Social Democrat politician Julius Tandler, who in that period taught at these public institutions, as his favourite professor. In the 1930s, Štampar and Tandler travelled together as colleagues, studying health in East Asia and the Soviet Union.[12] Grmek writes that, as a medical student, the young Štampar was especially influenced by the work of the German evolutionist Ernst Haeckel, as well as the physician and founder of social medicine Alfred Grotjahn.[13] During this period, Štampar published several articles in which he clearly expressed his firm devotion to social medicine. As early as 1911 he wrote: 'Nowadays the benefits and successes of medicine are enjoyed solely by the rich. This means that medicine is individualized rather than socialized, and in that lies its biggest mistake. Its success will remain limited if it continues to monitor and assist ten out of hundred patients.'[14]

Immediately following his graduation on 23 December 1911, Štampar was appointed to the post of physician in the Municipal Hospital in Karlovac, Croatia. In 1913, he became the district physician in Nova Gradiška, from where he was recruited, in 1916, to the military sanitary corps. Following the end of the war in 1918, he returned to his old position in Nova Gradiška, Croatia, from where he was soon transferred to Zagreb, to work as a health consultant to the Department of Social Welfare.[15] In this period Štampar started a lively collaboration with Dr. Josip Lochert, head of the Health Service in Croatia. In Zagreb, Štampar was active in the Croatian Medical Association and was elected its vice-president in 1919. He used the Association as a platform to voice his views on the separation of health from political administration and the reorganisation of various forms of healthcare, in particular in relation to prevention.[16] In the process, he developed a 'manifesto', known among his co-workers as 'our ideology', in which he summarized his social medicine programme in ten points:

1. It is more important to inform the people than to conform to the laws.
2. The most important task in each community is to prepare the grounds for the correct understanding of health problems.
3. Improving people's health is not the monopoly of the physician but the task of the entire community. The people's health can only be improved by working together.
4. The physician should, for the most part, work as a social worker. Individual therapy achieves little. Social therapy offers means to attain success.
5. The physician must not depend financially on the patient.
6. In the matters of people's health, there should be no difference between the rich and the poor.
7. Health provision should be organized in such a way that the physician seeks the patient, rather than the patient seeking the physician.
8. The physician should be the people's teacher.
9. The people's health is of economic more than of humanitarian importance.
10. The main location of the physician's activity are people's homes, not his office or the laboratory.[17]

Štampar, therefore, placed the greatest value on correct information about health problems and the communication of medical and scientific knowledge to the widest social strata. Health education and promotion were, for Štampar, the key working methods—yet education alone did not suffice and concrete actions were required. A man of action, Štampar actively participated in the realisation of his goal, the improvement of health. Sigerist saw him as 'a fighter who is not content with teaching what should be done but wants to do it himself with his own big hands.'[18] In the process, Štampar did not shy away from conflict. For instance, by undermining the physicians' monopoly over health and by ending their financial dependence on their patients, and so eliminating differences between rich and poor patients, he effectively turned doctors into social workers and directly attacked the medical community and its commercialized attitude towards patients.[19] Convinced that efforts to improve health could achieve no results in communities where the living standard was below minimum, he insisted that increasing people's incomes and standards of living was the best health improvement program. This position made him critical of the political and social system, capitalism and exploitation.[20] At the same time, he tried—and failed—to stay away from politics. Politics punished but also helped him. Štampar knew how to use politics and politicians so as to serve the health interests of society. Van Zile Hyde noted: 'He had worked effectively under the monarchy and under the Tito regime. No one seemed quite to know his politics because perhaps his only politics were people and their needs.'[21]

In 1919, as the new state—the Kingdom of Serbs, Croats and Slovenes—was taking shape, Štampar left Zagreb for the new capital, Belgrade. Thanks to the efforts of the Serbian hygiene professor Milan Jovanović Batut, he was appointed chairman of the Department of Racial, Public and Social Hygiene in the newly founded Ministry of Public Health. This position, in which he would remain until 1931, provided him with the institutional basis for one of the most active and creative periods of his life. During this time, Štampar laid the foundation for national health legislation, launched a large-scale initiative to set up a number of public health institutions, and, more generally, produced diverse programmes to improve the 'people's health'. Between 1920 and 1925, he was instrumental in the establishment of 250 new social medical institutions. On 1 January 1931, the year of Štampar's retirement, the Kingdom of Yugoslavia had the following recently founded public health institutions: one School of Public Health, ten hygiene institutes, 44 polyclinics, 44 bacteriological stations, 52 anti-rabies stations, 81 school polyclinics, 28 infant outpatient clinics, 35 outpatient clinics for the control of tuberculosis, 66 outpatient clinics for the control of skin and venereal diseases, 17 outpatient clinics for the control of trachoma, 10 social-medical departments, 12 sanitary engineering departments, 19 chemistry departments, two biological-immunological departments, five parasitological departments, 16 anti-malarial departments, one department of veterinary medicine, one general departments, two hospital departments, 111 health stations, 10 public baths, 19 accessory stations and 20 sanatoria and resorts. There were 606 institutions in total.[22]

From 1922, he developed contacts and then collaboration with the Rockefeller Foundation, which resulted in numerous programmes. These included scholarships for physicians and other medical personnel, assistance for education in hygiene at medical schools, research projects into the biology and epidemiology of certain diseases, programmes in vital statistics, and help in the foundation and operation of new health institutions. A major result of this collaboration was the School of Public Health, opened in 1926 in Zagreb. The task of such institutions, established across Europe in the 1920s, was to put the theoretical concepts of modern public health into practice. At this time Štampar understood 'modern public health' as a system in which public health institutions actively participated in the social community by creating and implementing programmes that improved the everyday life of the community (health promotion, demonstrations, health education, various public health initiatives) and by encouraging the community to recognize and try to solve health problems. It entailed broad-based collaboration between different professions: physicians, nurses, sanitary engineers, urban planners, architects, teachers, artists and others. Such an approach aimed at replacing the hitherto prevailing bureaucratic perspective that viewed health and disease through the narrow framework of infectious diseases and their prevention. The new system was supposed to secure equal conditions for urban and rural, rich and poor populations.[23]

Political life in the Kingdom in the late 1920s was marked by dramatic events that profoundly influenced the society and, consequently, public health. In this period, members of the Croatian parliament, headed by Stjepan Radić from the Croatian Peasant Party, argued strongly for basic democratic norms and for social and economic equality between all regions and ethnic groups in the country, and against the Serb nationalist domination of the entire Kingdom. In a tense atmosphere in early 1928, Radić proposed to transform the country into a confederation. But at the parliamentary assembly on 20 June 1928, a member of the Serb National Radical Party, Puniša Račić, fired a revolver from the speaker's platform at the opposition benches, killing Pavao Radić and Gjuro Basariček, two members of the Croatian Peasant Party, and mortally wounding Stjepan Radić. Two other Croatian parliament members were also wounded. These dramatic and tragic events did nothing to promote democracy and equal rights for all the nationalities and regions. In contrast, Serb domination intensified: on 6 January 1929, King Alexander published a manifesto that abolished the parliamentary system and introduced a dictatorship. The king proclaimed himself the sole legislator and made the government responsible exclusively to himself.[24] As the president of that 'government' he chose General Petar Živković, Štampar's fierce enemy. In the early 1920s, Štampar's activity had been was criticized mainly by physicians who, by attacking Štampar, hoped to preserve the old system of values and privileges they enjoyed. By the end of the decade, the political situation presented a far more serious threat.

The tumultuous national politics of the Kingdom of Serbs, Croats and Slovenes/Yugoslavia around 1930 had a profound effect on socio-political life and consequently on national public health programmes and on their chief manager, Štampar. In 1931, he was forced to retire from his position in the Ministry of Public Health.[25] Štampar had been elected an associate professor at the University of Zagreb School of Medicine in 1922, so when his political position worsened in 1931, the School council decided to appoint him professor of social medicine. To support his appointment, the school solicited and obtained positive reviews of his work from leading authorities in the relevant fields, including the doyen of social medicine in Europe, Alfred Grotjahn; the director of the Danish State Serum Institute, Thorvald Madsen; the founder and head of the Institute for Tropical Diseases in Hamburg, Bernhard Nocht; and the Polish bacteriologist, Zygmunt Szymanowski.[26] Yet the central administration opposed his election. His enemies grew increasingly influential and he had to withdraw from public life in the Kingdom of Yugoslavia. Fortunately, he found a way out in the form of a new career beyond the borders of the Kingdom. His reputation opened him many doors, including that of the League of Nations Health Organisation.

Letters and memoirs of the employees of the Rockefeller Foundation, commenting on political problems in Yugoslavia, offer crucial insight into the socio-political situation there, its effects on Štampar's career and on the position of the Rockefeller Foundation in this increasingly volatile period. The tumultuous national politics of the Kingdom surprised the Rockefeller foundation. Did employees of the Foundation understand the country in which they invested, could they predict the course of political developments in a country with such fragile foundations? These questions are difficult to answer, yet one thing is certain: their early estimates were overly optimistic and, in time, the South Slavic labyrinth proved exceedingly complex. The Rockefeller Foundation's decision to fund programmes in the Kingdom of Yugoslavia was highly important not just because it made the implementation of Štampar's programme financially possible, but also because the Foundation represented a moral authority. In a country torn by internal tensions, it contributed coherence to Štampar's public health activities.

The Foundation was truly brave to start a new project in a country which had shown signs of political instability since its earliest days. Selskar Gunn's 1924 report on the Kingdom of Serbs, Croats and Slovenes—a key that opened the lock of the Rockefeller treasury—called the political situation in the country 'complex'. But he immediately weakened that statement by saying that the same applied to other Balkan states. Still, in the remainder of the text he listed a number of political problems. Explaining that the Radical Party, presided over by Nikola Pašić, was in power, he commented 'This is the party which has attempted to develop "Greater Serbia".[27] Yet the Foundation obviously failed to appreciate the ramifications of this statement. Gunn furthermore wrote that the political scene also encompassed the Democratic Party (lead by Svetozar Pribičević) that supported the idea of Yugoslavia in contrast to Pašić's 'Greater Serbia', and the Radić party, which he described as rather large and in favour of Croatian autonomy. That idea did not stand a chance, Gunn added. There was also the issue of Macedonians who argued for independence based on their difference from both Serbs and Bulgarians. Albanians were very numerous, continued Gunn, and the border with Albania difficult to oversee. Summing up, Gunn appreciated the problematic political situation in the Kingdom but did not expect an internal revolution. He ended on a cautious note: '(...) prognostications in Balkan countries are dangerous to make.'[28] Gunn also reported remarks and predictions he heard from his Yugoslav acquaintances.

They painted a picture of a weak king under the influence of generals and not particularly popular, suggesting the change of the country to a republic soon. Regarding ethnic conflict Gunn cautioned: '(...) [it] must be remembered that the different provinces which make up the Yugoslavia of today are very unlike. They have had all kinds of governments in the past and it cannot be expected that they will all settle down at once and live together happily.'[29] For him, the main reason that could prevent the country from falling apart was the fact that a united country of twelve million inhabitants offered a much better guarantee for peaceful future than a collection of tiny states. This view clearly reflected the well-established belief of the international community that one large state provided a stronger guarantee for peace in an unstable geopolitical area than many smaller ones.[30] According to Gunn, many believed that the solution to the Balkans problem required the formation of a confederation of South Slavs that would include Bulgaria and Macedonia. Bulgarians as well as supporters of Macedonian autonomy within Yugoslavia increasingly welcomed such a plan. Such a scheme would have solved the issue of Croatian autonomy. The states would enjoy a certain level of sovereignty with their own local assemblies, and the confederation could use the USA as a model. Gunn's reflections reveal the perspective from which the Foundation would develop its further collaboration with the Kingdom: the hope that this country would adopt the US organisational model and grow into a large and stable country, situated in a key geopolitical locale.[31] But the Foundation failed to fully appreciate the position of the Belgrade regime. It believed, naively and optimistically, that the king would withdraw and that the Serb politicians would happily relinquish the power at their fingertips.

Employees of the Foundation were, in a way, 'blinded' by what they heard from Štampar and Ivo Kuhn (who worked in the Ministry of Public Health with Štampar and reported to the Foundation). Hoping to implement the programmes they had started, these two painted the political situation in the country in much rosier tones than it deserved.[32] Only after the events of June 1928, the Foundation came to appreciate the instability of the Kingdom of Serbs, Croats and Slovenes. They paid more and more attention to analyzing the political situation. Gunn's record of his conversation with Štampar in Paris at the time reveals that Štampar found the situation bad and getting worse. He faulted the King for having 'missed a really big opportunity by not coming out definitely for a united Yugoslavia." for being 'too much of a Serb and too much under the influence of the military clique.'[33] When Gunn asked if he feared a civil war, Štampar admitted that such a development was indeed possible. Gunn commented upon Štampar's status as a Croat in the Yugoslav administration, seeing his position as 'apparently somewhat jeopardized'. Yet Štampar, Gunn continued, did everything in his power to make sure the activities that he started would proceed regardless of changes that might take place in the country. If the

Kingdom survives this crisis, Štampar thought, the Ministries of Public Health and of Social Affairs should be united under his authority.[34] The kingdom did not fall apart, but the dictatorship did happen. The Ministries of Public Health and of Social Affairs were indeed merged, just as Štampar hoped, but his position in the new ministry was diminished when he was transferred to the post of the general inspector, a position without any real power.

Soon after the introduction of the dictatorship, in February 1929, Gunn arrived in Belgrade and learned that Štampar's view of the dictatorship was far from optimistic. Gunn himself found the situation in Yugoslavia not very different from that in Italy, where all conversations were taking place in hushed tones behind closed doors. In Yugoslavia, criticizing the government was punishable by five years in prison and open disagreement by twenty years of incarceration. Štampar now doubted that Croats would agree to any form of Yugoslav state, even under the best of governments, because they now strongly aspired towards a higher level of autonomy.[35] He felt the king had made a poor choice of new cabinet members, particularly regarding the new minister of public health, Dr Uroš Krulj, who was one of Štampar's opponents.[36] The budget of the Ministry of Public Health was reorganized so that a larger share was now allocated to hospitals, while the preventive measures and institutions suffered cuts.[37]

The Foundation continued to monitor closely the development of the political situation in the Kingdom under the dictatorship. In February 1930, Gunn noted that Štampar was still 'very pessimistic with regard to the dictatorship which he feels is not working to the benefit of the country—in fact antagonism is very widespread, but suppressed, as prison sentences are imposed very freely on persons who make any criticism of the government.'[38] He and the employees of the Foundation were still hoping for the confederation to resolve the problem; however, the situation deteriorated. The king started to distance himself from Štampar, which caused additional worries.[39] By April 1931, Štampar's position was extremely controversial: the military, which, Gunn felt, was responsible for the dictatorship, was highly suspicious of him. Štampar's phone conversations were tapped and his mail monitored. His professional authority was reduced, so he could no longer sign documents as general inspector. However, in practice, these restrictions appear to have had little effect because the person who replaced Štampar, Vladimir Katičić, did nothing without his approval. Furthermore, Gunn continued, Štampar was in close contact with the Minister of Finance Stanko Švrljuga who secured an increase in public health funding, regardless of the budget restrictions that affected everything but the military. In 1931, Gunn believed that public health in Yugoslavia, in which the Foundation had invested so much effort, had reached the point at which it would resist destructive attempts. The peasants were very interested in the new processes, which appeared to secure good foundations for future work. Yugoslavia, he wrote, was an interesting country with intelligent people and good natural resources. He hoped that one day it would become a republic, which, of course, would not guarantee significant progress in itself, but with the current militarism and under Serb leadership, prosperity and advancement of all the Yugoslav peoples were unlikely to take place.[40]

In this period, Štampar was also again attacked by powerful medical circles for neglecting hospitals and all non-preventative health measures and, consequently, for spending almost the entire budget on prevention. The introduction of free treatment against tuberculosis and syphilis significantly reduced the profits of private practitioners. This tension tied into the conflict with physicians active in the Health Cooperatives (Zdravstvene Zadruge) in which Štampar became embroiled. Štampar believed that, while cooperatives might have offered some health services, they were not sufficient and that other health institutions, such as those in other parts of the country and within the remit of the relevant ministry, should co-exist with them. The Cooperatives, in contrast, argued that they were neglected by the Ministry and that Štampar intentionally ignored their needs. In reality local strongmen supported cooperatives because they saw new institutions organized by Štampar as competition. They furthermore feared Štampar's authority over their domains and possibly also worried over financial losses, as the cooperatives were financed by overseas foundations such as the Milbank Memorial Found and Serbian Child Welfare Association of America. Conflicts with the Cooperatives and powerful Serbian physicians such as Stevan Ivanić, who after Štampar's departure became the most powerful man in the national public health system and who was close to the Cooperatives, were one of the main reasons of Štampar's dismissal from the Ministry of Health.[41]

In a country plagued by national tensions and constant comparisons between the relative favours extended to different parts of the country, the Croat Štampar found himself under great pressure from the Belgrade regime. Building the School of Public Health in Zagreb rather than in the capital Belgrade—an exception to the general rule, since in all other countries these schools were built in the capitals—irritated the Belgrade regime, who persistently tried to impose its control over all segments of social and political life. These tensions spread into the international scene when, in 1931, the Rockefeller Foundation invited Štampar to a study trip around the U.S. Belgrade circles became worried. The Yugoslav representative in New York, Radoje Janković, visited the head of the International Health Board of the Rockefeller Foundation, Frederic Russell to express his concern. He was nervous that Štampar might use the American media to publicize his criticism of the Yugoslav government. Russell explained to Janković that Štampar had no political ambitions and suggested a meeting with him upon his arrival to the US, to discuss these concerns in person.[42]

Furthermore, George Radin, a pro-Serb U.S. lawyer, sent a letter to the Foundation accusing Štampar of working against Serb interests.[43] Štampar replied to these accusations citing official data obtained by the Ministry of Public Health and Social Policy, countering Radin's claims that Croats received a disproportionately more Rockefeller scholarships than Serbs: of 48 Rockefeller scholars 25 were of Serb, 15 of Croat, 5 of Slovene and 3 of some other nationality. Štampar stressed the political roots of these attacks by writing that 'The chauvinist blindness of these people is best confirmed by the rumour they recently spread overseas that I took one million Swiss francs from the Foundation for my personal use. This alone gives you an insight into the morals of these people.'[44] Next, as Štampar's opponents were intent on curbing his financial independence, which he enjoyed thanks to the Rockefeller funding, the Yugoslav representatives in New York and Paris asked the Rockefeller Foundation to submit a report on financial activities under Štampar's management. Gunn stated that the Foundation had always been fully satisfied with Štampar's financial management and trusted him completely. Štampar suspected that more initiatives of this kind were to be expected and thanked the Foundation for the trust they displayed.[45] But Štampar's enemies applied similar pressure on John Adams Kingsbury of the Milbank Memorial Fund, who was active in the American-Yugoslav Society and the Executive Committee of the Serbian Child Welfare Association of America.[46]

The case of the School of Public Health illustrates well problems that emerged in the Yugoslav public health sector upon Štampar's departure from the Ministry of Public Health. In 1932, Berislav Borčić, the School's director, applied to the Foundation for financial assistance because the school found itself in a difficult situation. The government had reduced funding by 60% in comparison with 1931. According to Borčić, all hygiene institutions in the country suffered from severe financial cuts, except the Central Hygiene Institute in Belgrade. In Belgrade, Stevan Ivanić, Štampar's enemy, was the director of the Central Hygiene Institute as well as Head of the Public Health Department in the Ministry. He thus held a position unimaginable under normal circumstances: as director of the Institute he proposed the budget to—himself, this time in the capacity of the chief administrator in the Ministry. At the same time, Ivanić delayed the process of agreeing on two candidates for the Foundation scholarship by insisting that for each scholarship granted to a Croat, a Serb must be granted a scholarship too.[47]

But regardless of the political persecution of the ruling political circles and individuals in Belgrade, Štampar had the support of his Serbian colleagues who appreciated his work. Thus, a young public health specialist Miodrag Popović assured him: 'Your current mission overseas worries all of your well-intentioned enemies who know that this is disgraceful for them. They thought that they could pension you overseas too.'[48]

The whole world as a new homeland: making interwar international health

'I suffer when I hear news about our institutions because I love them like my own children; but our thoughts are scattered all over the world and appreciated everywhere....rest assured, we have not laboured for nothing,'[49] wrote Andrija Štampar from Xi'an, China, in February 1934. His words reveal sadness that the efforts invested in his home country might have been wasted, but also satisfaction that his work was appreciated abroad. Štampar could no longer work in his own country and so he embarked on a world tour. His knowledge, experience and personal qualities earned him the trust of the League of Nations Health Organisation (LNHO), which, in 1931, employed him as its expert.[50] Andrija Štampar's collaboration with that institution went back to its earliest days. With Berislav Borčić, he represented the Kingdom of Serbs, Croats and Slovenes at the European Health Conference in Warsaw in March 1922. That conference was the most important meeting of the new LNHO after the London conference of 1920. Its task was to solve important problems of post-war Europe, which included the protection from epidemics and especially typhus arriving from Russia, Belarus and Ukraine to Europe. But one of its committees also stated the need for other health issues, including social hygiene and tuberculosis, venereal, occupational and other diseases, as well as the cooperation and exchange of experts, declarations, which seem to go back to Štampar's influence.[51]

In the following years, Štampar continued to work actively within the LNHO, both as a member of various specific commissions and, after 1930, as a member of the Health Committee, its central decision making body. [52] In 1930, Štampar took part in a study trip organized by the League, to study the public health system of the Netherlands and Scandinavian countries.[53] Together with his co-worker Berislav Borčić, he participated actively in the meetings of directors of European schools of public health, organized by the LNHO, for instance in Paris in May 1930.[54] At the European conference on rural hygiene in 1931, Štampar lectured on the most effective methods of organizing healthcare in rural areas.[55] He continued to work for the League in 1931, when he travelled to Dresden to help organize an exhibition on rural hygiene in the German Hygiene Museum.[56]

Štampar's visit to the USA and Canada in 1931 was his first major trip in his new role as a League expert. He visited many medical institutions, centres of health administration such as National Health Council, educational establishments such as the Vanderbilt University and the Rockefeller Research Institute. Štampar was especially interested in the living conditions of African Americans in the then largely rural American South. He travelled by car through the south-eastern rural regions of Louisiana, then populated by a predominantly African American population and troubled by a major agrarian crisis. He visited African American schools and wrote that they were not located in suitable premises.[57] His great interest in the health and social status of African Americans is not surprising: Štampar had always been primarily interested in the poorest and most disadvantaged social strata. Štampar stayed in the US and Canada until 2 January 1932, when he sailed across the Pacific Ocean via Hawaii to Japan. From there he continued his journey to China. During the following years, he repeatedly stayed in the country to assist the Chinese government in their fight against mass infectious diseases and, more generally, in their efforts to reform their public health system. From the fall of 1932 to the summer of 1933, Štampar was back in Europe to teach at numerous European universities and Schools of Public Health. At this time Štampar collaborated with almost all the important people in the field of public health in Europe including Bela Johan, Bohumil Vacek, Alica Masaryk, Josef Tomcik, Carl Prausnitz, Norman White, Witold Chodzko etc. Štampar lectured from his rich experiences and on wide-ranging topics, such as rural hygiene, town planning, industrialisation, and the comparison of morbidity and mortality in rural and urban districts.[58] Štampar was a highly charismatic lecturer. His students later recollected that his lectures, often accompanied by pictures and films, were very impressive. He knew how to attract and keep the attention of the audience, and how to earn their trust. Štampar's lectures in European countries followed the contemporary LNHO idea on encouraging collaboration across disciplines. Štampar was supposed to be one of the links between the League and the local experts. His task was to collect material and data on the activities of various public health institutions, to take part in the organisation of the League conferences (such as the one on European rural health) and to prepare reports on conditions in countries and institutions for the LNHO.

In 1933 and 1934, Štampar visited China again. Once more, he acted as an expert of the League of Nations, placed at the disposal of the Chinese government to continue his work in the organisation of the health service. While traveling extensively, seeing major Chinese cities, including Hong Kong, Shanghai and Nanjing, as well as remote areas in the Chinese west, he repeated what he once had done in the Kingdom of Serbs, Croats and Slovenes: establish new social-medical institutions and schools for training health personnel. During his stays, he formed an emotional attachment to the Chinese people and to the colleagues he met there. He commented in his diary: 'When I first arrived here my thoughts were constantly in the West, with my children and friends; every day lasted an eternity. But now when I left these parts I feel sad for them, for the river banks and the rivers, for the fields, peasants, hills, lakes, the eternal snow, new acquaintances: who could understand our souls?'[59]

In 1935, he briefly stayed in Zagreb before leaving, in the early spring, for his third trip to China. Before the ship departed from Venice for Shanghai, he observed the ongoing preparations for the Italian attack on Abyssinia (today's

Ethiopia). Repelled, he noted in his diary: 'Italy is getting ready to occupy an independent indigenous African country and one feels a kind of a warrior spirit everywhere. The newspaper and radio reports are full of militant speeches and great hopes in the superiority of the Italian military power and the civilizing mission of fascism; yet this warlike atmosphere on the boat somehow does not suit me.'[60] Once again travelling extensively, he saw some of the poorest parts of China. He was particularly impressed with his visit to mines in southwest Yunann where he found what he considered the worst forms of human exploitation, practically slavery. He had several conversations with Chiang Kai-shek's Western educated wife Soong May-Ling, which he used for frank and critical descriptions of social conditions in China as he saw them.[61] During his stay in China he worked with Chinese colleagues: the national health administration director Dr. J. Heng Liu, Dr. Marion Yang, the director of the Beijing School of Midwifery, as well as the pioneering activist for the improvement of rural health conditions and former of the National Association of Mass Education Movements (MEM) Dr. James Yen, and Dr. C. C. Chen from the Health Department of the Ting Hsien Mass Education Experiment.[62] After a thorough analysis of the Chinese situation, Štampar suggested to the provincial authorities that they focus their attention on the rural population. He proposed establishing the rural health centres as central units of the health system, served by all other institutions. The purpose of the provincial health centres in urban communities would thus be the provision of services not only to the urban population but to the entire province, by supervising and assisting rural health institutions.[63]

Indeed, in many ways, Yugoslavia appears to have 'served as a model for rural health care reform in the 1930s.'[64] The public health model that Štampar developed for Yugoslavia in the 1920s became a blueprint for China during the rule of the Nationalist Government (1927–1937). Štampar, as usual, began his trip with a tour of the provinces, where he made himself familiar with local problems. Then, in cooperation with the government administration, he started the process of establishing a network of institutions designed to implement a variety of programmes in the field. Simultaneously, and with the assistance of various philanthropic organisations, he established medical educational programmes for the training of specialized personnel. The trainees were sent, if necessary, to study overseas, for instance to Yugoslavia.[65] Yet Štampar was well aware that health could not be improved in a country of such large social differences without a profound social reform. This attitude was not always popular among Chinese administrators. In October 1935, he expressed his irritation about the Chinese national health director, Dr. Liu, in a letter to his friend and teacher Julius Tandler: 'It makes little sense to write about Dr Liu because you know him well: he is miles away from our ideology and we must cope with that (…) You must know how I think and where my sympathies lie in

China, not with the rulers but with the oppressed.'[66] But he was equally frustrated with his European colleagues, particularly the League of Nations' ignorance of the conditions in China: 'The organisation of the League of Nations activities in China is so poor that all of my results lose value tremendously; we are here to do something but we have no real tasks and no real contact with the League of Nations organisations, like lost children in the large world.'[67] The League of Nations, however, valued his work. After he reported on his activities in China in January 1937, the League of Nations Council noted that Štampar had visited China three times between 1932 and 1936, amounting to a period of nearly three years, and had 'made a very careful study of the local conditions. ... This had been found of great value to the rural construction work which the Chinese Government had undertaken in recent years.'[68]

Štampar left Manchuria in 1936 on the Trans-Siberian Railway at 'an average speed of 40 kms/hour' for Moscow, together with the Japanese who travelled to the Berlin Olympic Games. He was invited by the Commissariat for the Protection of People's Health of the Soviet Union to study the problems of rural hygiene. Besides Štampar, the Russians invited other experts such as the nutritionist Elmer Verner McCollum, the expert in public health education, Charles Edward Winslow and Marcin Kacprzak. Moscow also hosted a session of the Bureau of the League of Nations Health Committee chaired by Jacques Parisot. Štampar took part in the discussion by elaborating on two important problems: 1. Finding the best methods to secure the collaboration of rural populations in the course of public health programmes, and, more importantly, 2. Whether it was possible to solve health problems in the current socio-economic order. He supported his theses with examples from China and India. In his diary, he noted that the Russian delegates were much interested in his contribution to the discussion, and that they asked him to write a piece for a health journal.[69] The public health experts were supposed to tour the country in the group, which Štampar, who was not in favour of group visits, disliked. But his stay did prove an opportunity to meet several colleagues. For a while, Gunn joined their company but then decided to leave them for a tourist trip. In Moscow, Štampar met Tandler[70], who had arrived there at the invitation of the Soviet government and also Nikolai Semashko, then the commissioner for people's health in the Soviet Union. Štampar and Semashko communicated well because Semashko had worked for a while as a district physician in Paraćin, Serbia.[71] According to Henry E. Sigerist, whom Stampar met as well, Štampar and Nikolai Semashko shared the same concept of public health: they both emphasized the crucial impact of the economic system on healthcare.[72]

Štampar made many new and interesting observations in the Soviet Union, starting with the seemingly banal one that he could not get a room service outside the working hours of 9 am to 5 pm. He noted in his diary ironically: 'Of course, I was ashamed of my ignorance of the social system and of my brain that still thinks in a bourgeois and capitalist way.'[73] However, he was unaware of – or unwilling to notice – the irony inherent in the fact that he and other Western guests were wined and dined by their Soviet hosts as in any capitalist country just a few years after collectivisation. In his diary, he merely wrote that he ate the finest food from the china engraved with the initials of the executed Nicolas II and the imperial code of arms. But Štampar's remarks and comments stretched to more serious issues of health economics. His diary brims with data on the organisation of health and social care in the Soviet Union, obtained from the Commissioner for People's Health of the Federal Republic of Russia, Grigoriy Kaminskiy, or from Levko Medved who was the deputy Ukrainian Commissioner for People's Health. Štampar recorded statistical data, or indeed anything that came his way, including conversations with ordinary people he met in the streets or on public transport. He tried to note down people's living conditions in the Soviet Russia down to the smallest detail. After a visit to a kolkhoz, a colleague from the group, annoyed by the number of questions that Štampar asked as well as the stench that spread from a nearby cowshed, said: 'My friend, your questioning was thorough, but you forgot to ask the names of each of the cows.'[74] Štampar was a highly precise observer but at the same time he was rather naïve concerning the real advancement of the public health in Soviet Union.

After the trip to China and Russia, Štampar was once again invited to Geneva and Paris. As he had already suspected, the dark shadow of fascism was spreading over Europe and enthusiasm in the League of Nations was on the wane. He became painfully aware of this development during the meeting of the Health Committee, where the French Minister of Health, Henri Selier enthusiastically announced the establishment of a School of Public Health in Paris. Bitterly, he noted in his diary: 'It was painful to see that the speech by the French minister of public health was not received by the members of the hygiene bureau with the attention and enthusiasm it deserved. It seemed to me that the issues of international collaboration are not understood as they should be and that the attitude towards them has cooled down.'[75] Štampar also criticized that Committee members largely failed to grasp the problems under discussion and appeared to hold superficial and old-fashioned views. He felt lonely and sad, thinking that in most countries governments were full of people who thought similarly. 'Everything seemed to me like a wilderness with no way out.'[76]

Two months later, having spent time with his family, Štampar left for a research tour of European Schools of Public Health, which the Health Section of the League of Nations had organized for him, Wilson Jameson and Gustavo Pittaluga. Štampar looked forward to that trip and wrote: 'I planned to study the work of the schools of public health in other countries in order to compare it with the Zagreb school, into which I invested so much of my heart and soul.'[77] He met with Pittaluga and Jameson in Paris, and started the long trip. Štampar was greatly affected by the fate of his old acquaintance Pittaluga, whose family he had met during his stay in Republican Madrid. Now Pittaluga was in a difficult position: his family fell apart in the wartime Spain, and all the effort he had invested in his home country came to nothing. Štampar understood him well because he too was a refugee of a sort. Their other companion, Jameson, had no problems of that kind: he was content and, as Štampar noted, happily fortified himself with wine and whiskey.[78] The three colleagues travelled to Budapest, Prague, Warsaw, Bucharest, Sofia, Athens, Ankara, and finally Rome, before returning to France.[79]

In 1937, Štampar repeatedly visited his homeland to lecture and to represent the League of Nations at the international agriculture conference in The Hague. That year he married Dr. Desanka Ristović, head of the Outpatient clinic for school children in Zagreb, who had been his close colleague for many years.[80] Their friendship had developed into romance, and Desanka had taken care of his children while he had been away from Zagreb. In a letter from Nanjing, Štampar wrote: 'Your exceptional attention to my orphans brings tears to my eyes, my dear ... only God can repay what you are doing for me and for them.'[81] But he kept up his intense travel pace. After another lengthy tour across Scandinavia to Moscow and then across France to London in 1937, [82] he left for a new and highly significant trip through the US and Canada. Alan Gregg of the Rockefeller Foundation sent him an invitation on 23 August 1937 to visit several leading American and Canadian medical schools to talk about his experiences and observations.[83] Rather than an ordinary lecture tour, it was designed to consist of "leisurely visits to a few important and strategically located medical centers— important particularly from the standpoint of teaching public health to undergraduates" including "information meetings with students and teachers". The main objective was to stimulate interest in rural hygiene.[84] Between February and May 1938 Štampar followed an impressive itinerary, lecturing, at Columbia University and Cornell University Medical College in New York, at the Harvard University Medical School in Boston, at John Hopkins University in Baltimore, the Cincinnati Medical School, the School of Medicine of Vanderbild University in Nashville, Tulane University in New Orleans, the University of Texas Medical Branch, the Universities of Berkely and Stanford in California, the Medical School of Minnesota in Minneapolis and the schools of hygiene at the Universities of Toronto, Ottawa and Montreal. While his lectures focused on rural pathology, using examples from various countries, he also tried to learn about conditions in North America, particularly regarding rural health activities and the lives of African and Native Americans.[85] Following Štampar's visit to Tulane University School of Medicine in New Orleans, a member of the faculty W.H. Perkins summarized his impressions of Dr. Hercules (as Štampar was often called) and especially of his idiosyncratic behaviour, his almost painfully open and critical attitude, and the impression he left on his audience:

> Dr. Štampar has come and gone and I am sure we are all the gainers from his visit. He is a man with a wealth of information in the line of his main interests and possesses an interesting philosophy behind his attitudes on medical science... However, Rural Health was on his tongue so much and presumably also on his mind that I played it up at every opportunity. It came back on us like a boomerang for Louisiana Rural Health is not something to bring out on parade. And when the good doctor turned the responsibility for the deplorable state of affairs back to medical education and particularly to training in preventive medicine, I felt extremely uncomfortable. He spared no words and no one's feelings but did it in such a way as to make you like him more and thank him for it. It was altogether a delightful experience to know Dr. Hercules and I thank you on my own behalf for sending him here and giving me the opportunity to be associated with him so intimately even for so short a time.[86]

Indeed, Štampar gained rather an unfavorable view of American public health, which he found too timid in the face of the interests of private physicians and generally less vigorous than its European counterpart. He criticized the American model of expensive medical education, affordable only to the rich. He further condemned existing social, sex and race discrimination.[87]

At the end of the 1930s, Štampar returned home, enriched by experiences of China, the Soviet Union, the US and other countries where he had lived and worked in the previous decade. He found his native country undergoing profound change that resulted in a more extensive autonomy for the Croatian regions and the establishment of the Banovina of Croatia in 1939. After the eight years of waiting, Štampar was finally confirmed as full professor of hygiene and social medicine at the Zagreb School of Medicine.[88] The new political atmosphere allowed Štampar to resume his activities in public health. He drew on his experiences to write articles for Liječnički vjesnik, the organ of the Croatian Medical Association, as well as other publications, such as the well-received book on Health and society ('Zdravlje i društvo').[89] In 1940, he published a university textbook on Hygiene and social medicine ('Higijena i socijalna medicina'), which summarized his social-medical viewpoints.[90] In 1940–41, he was elected dean of the School of Medicine and immediately launched an educational reform.[91] Yet the halcyon days of the Banovina of Croatia were short. In 1941, the German army occupied Yugoslavia, the country fell apart, and a new quisling 'Independent State of Croatia' was formed on parts of the Croatian territory. Štampar was arrested on 17 April 1941 under the suspicion of possessing illegal material. He was released on 11 May but on 15 June he was arrested again, on the orders of the Gestapo.[92] He was then transferred to the internment camp in Graz where he remained until the arrival of the Red Army.[93] We know little about Štampar's years in the internment camp. Apparently, he enjoyed a somewhat better treatment and was actually imprisoned in a house in Graz 'thanks to a German professor'.[94] Nevertheless, upon his return to Zagreb, his closest friends failed to recognize him because he had lost so much weight. Yet no matter how physically weak, he still possessed the same desire to work.

In May 1945, Štampar returned to Zagreb and immediately continued the work interrupted by the war. He also resumed contact with his colleagues overseas which had been temporarily interrupted. Without any pause or rest Štampar participated in the Yugoslav delegation at the conference of the ministers of foreign affairs in October 1945 and, in early 1946, at the UN conference in London. He was then elected the first Vice President of the Economic and Social Council of the UN and a member of the Preparatory Committee, whose task was to lay the foundation of the World Health Organization (WHO). As early as March 1946, the committee met in Paris to write the constitution of the future WHO. Štampar influenced the content of this document substantially. At the international health conference in New York, in the summer of the same year, representatives of 51 states accepted, with some alterations, the proposed draft of the constitution. An Interim Commission composed of representatives of 18 countries was elected to act in place of the World Health Organisation until its formal establishment on 7 April 1948. The commission initially chose Feodor Grigorievich Krotkov from USSR as its chairman but two days later he was replaced by Štampar. The commission was the direct predecessor of the WHO, as it took over the business of international health in this critical post-war period, but it was not allowed to bear the name of the WHO until the UN ratified it. Štampar skillfully managed the Interim Commission and succeeded in bringing order into the disorganized post-war international health. He unified existing and established new organisations, stimulated the foundation of new programmes, and, more generally, created conditions in which the WHO could function. The first assembly, under Štampar's presidency, took place from 24 June to 24 July 1948 and it ratified the constitution of the WHO.[95] In addition, these active post-war years saw Štampar elected the chancellor of the University of Zagreb (1945–6), professor of the School of Medicine in Zagreb, and director of the School of Public Health. Extensive organisational reforms of medical education were launched and the School of Public Health became part of the Zagreb School of Medicine. It was precisely in this period (1947–58) that the school, under the influence of Štampar and his younger colleagues and future successors, saw its second renaissance. At the same time, Štampar continued to publish widely, for instance a book on *The physician, his past and his future* ('Liječnik, njegova prošlost i budućnost').[96]

During this last period of his life, Štampar was elected to a number of influential positions in his country. In 1947, Štampar became member and then, in the same year, the president of the Yugoslav (today Croatian) Academy of Science and Arts, to be re-elected three times. Under his leadership the Academy developed into a major research institution with a considerable publication output in a variety of academic disciplines. Numerous independent institutes and research units were established under the umbrella of the Academy, including the Institute of Work Hygiene and the Department of the History and Philosophy of Science in Zagreb. In 1947, Štampar was elected a corresponding member of the Slovenian and, in 1948, of the Serbian Academy of Sciences and Arts. From 1952 until 1957 he served as the dean of the School of Medicine in Zagreb. He received numerous recognitions for his work. At the meeting of the WHO assembly in Mexico in 1955, he received the Léon Bernard Foundation Prize for his work in the field of international public health. The last years of Štampar's life were also dedicated to travel to countries such as Afghanistan, Egypt, Sudan and Ethiopia, where he offered expert advice on the reorganisation of medical education and on the organisation of healthcare. He remained active in the thematic work of the WHO.
He died in Zagreb on 26 June 1958 from stroke.[97]

Human community and social medicine measures
After many years of travelling in various parts of the world, including the last big tour of the well known American university centres, Štampar summed up his impressions of the American public health and medical education for the Rockfeller Foundation employee Alan Gregg:

> Public health is nowhere understood correctly [...] Practical exercises in public health institutions lack imagination and vision. These centres are lifeless. Their purpose should be to bring the postgraduate students into touch with everyday life, to let them study it, to let them seek and find problems, to ask themselves what a physician should do. Too divided, too much epidemiology, and not enough community-related questions. They learn how to examine the body in detail, why don't they learn how to study a community?[98]

To study the human community, to recognize problems, to examine them, to keep one's eyes open and to separate the trivial from the important. Furthermore, not to limit oneself, not to think that a physician alone is capable of solving a problem, to open up the opportunities for collaboration, to create dialogue, to make the environment interested, to let other professions do their task. To recognise the inability of medicine alone to improve human health. To understand that the physician, along with the nurse and ancillary health personnel, also needs engineers, agronomists, architects, urban planners, social workers and economists to work together. Furthermore, to act within the community and to inspire the community to work with oneself, to turn the passive objects into subjects of joint action in which all parts complete part of the task. To be clear and simple, active and lively. These were all principles advocated by Štampar, principles he found neither in American students nor in their professors. He found that discovery painful because he always placed his hopes into young people, equipped with good education to tackle problems. Štampar expected much from his co-workers. He expected them to dedicate their entire lives to their work. Josip Škarić, his Dalmatian collaborator and the director of the Hygiene Institute in Split, wrote: 'Everyone worldwide, intellectual or a manual worker, must have several weeks of holidays in each year. To us, each holiday was interrupted, either by an epidemic, or by Štampar's sudden appearance. This is what being a physician—a conscientious, constructive, knowledgeable physician—is like.[99]

In the United States, Štampar encountered the problem he had come across earlier in other parts of the world including his homeland. Of this problem, he wrote: 'Public health is too weak and it withdraws when it notices a threat to the interests of private practitioners. [...] Professors are closer to students than in Europe, but they do not form future members of the community, but members of a commercialized profession.'[100] The commercialized profession had no interest in improving the health status of the population; indeed, a healthy individual was of little interest to it as it was not a source of profit; a healthy community even less so. Štampar was entirely opposed to the close link between the physician and the profit, against market in medicine. In his view, physician was under no circumstances to depend economically on the patient. The solution lay in etatization of medicine. For him, the most effective and the most just system was such in which all people had health insurance. The physician would not be paid by the patient but by the system. Štampar, utopistically, hoped that health insurance would in time grow to include all the people of the world: health for all. While visiting California, he noted with sadness that plants' health seem to be more protected than human.[101] For him health was inextricably linked to using the benefits of science, accessible through various medical institutions. These medical or social-medical institutions were supposed to be staffed by well trained professionals, but they were not to be the only site of their activities. Institutions, according to Štampar, were supposed to be accessible to people and distributed so that they cover the most remote areas, like a network spreading through the landscape: from hygiene institutes, to general polyclinics and finally health stations. He advocated the model developed in the Kingdom of Serbs,

Croats and Slovenes for the use in Chinese provinces, where he had the opportunity to start once again with the health system organization. Štampar built the system in a pyramid form, from a single central institution on the top to the whole range on the bottom. The professional competition followed the same scheme, but not the sources of financing. To protect the system from possible turbulences, Štampar developed methods of decentralization, and looked for ways of reducing the financial dependence on the centre as much as possible. He also considered the opportunities for self-financing and collaboration with the local community, which was supposed to recognize the benefits from such institutions.

The economic progress of the community was for Štampar a key condition for the improvement of health. The progress could, however, not be achieved on the expense of people's health, by exploiting the majority of population and by throwing them into direst poverty. In contrast, the progress was supposed to ensure decent living to all, bigger expenditure for social needs and larger support to social-medical institutions. His experience in China made him realize that no constructive work on the improvement of community health is possible if the economic power of population is falling beyond the lowest tolerable minimums. Štampar continually emphasized the link between social injustice and community health. That problem became his chief preoccupation, especially after encountering the most drastic form of exploitation in European colonies in Asia and pewter mines in China. It was there that he saw the most extreme forms of human misery and powerlessness. At the same time, as a foreigner, expert of an international organization, he moved among people who belonged to a different world, where money mattered little. The encounter with two extreme sides impacted his sensitive personality strongly. Štampar criticized the emptiness of the expatriate life, the easy life at the expense of a foreign country and its people. He also criticized European and American experts who used their positions for work often incompatible with the needs of host countries. He discussed the work of missionary communities in China, arguing that in many cases their chief goal was material gain. He criticized the work of medical and educational institutions in China, set up for the needs of the 'white man' rather than the local population. He was especially opposed to the Beijing Medical School pursuing education wholly unsuited to Chinese needs, and churning out physicians incapable of and without interest in working with Chinese peasants. They then mostly looked for work in cities, ideally those under foreign concessions.[102] Štampar here reinforced his belief that physicians needed, in his words, a clear ideology to take them out of the nineteenth century and prepare them for the new era, for future challenges. As early as after his first trip to the United States (1931), Štampar stated: 'Today's general medical education is in my opinion not capable of training physicians for reforms of medicine that will happen, willingly or unwillingly, no matter how physicians think of them. The times always win and physicians will do nothing but lose, if they do not get ready for the changes.'[103]

These thoughts were not entirely original. There were other intellectuals in this era that equally strongly emphasized the importance of examining the role of the physician and medicine through the prism of society. For instance, Sigerist studied Soviet medicine in this period and approved of their healthcare system organization.[104] Štampar's close colleagues John Grant and Julius Tandler followed the same ideology. But, Štampar was more aggressive and assertive than others, and he acknowledged no obstacles that could stop him. Cvjetanović wrote about Štampar's ideas: 'Some like to call Štampar's ideas revolutionary, but they were actually reformist, because he developed them from earlier knowledge, seeing himself and his ideas as a continuation of earlier thoughts and experiences, of hundreds of years of traditions, which he hoped to use as foundations rather than to dismantle. To build on, in accordance with the people's traditions and needs.'[105] True, as noticed by Grmek, Štampar added on and built. He cared more for effectiveness than originality; he preferred ideas that passed the test of real use.[106] Štampar's central idea was always strongly linked with the situation in question, and it entailed finding the best possible solution and being ready to work not for one's own, but for general good. For Štampar, society was an organism that suffered from disease, had a specific pathology and could be prescribed a specific therapy. His views built upon the heritage of the founders of social medicine in the late nineteenth and early twentieth century, especially his teachers Ludwig Teleky and Julius Tandler. His interest was always focused upon those social groups that suffered the greatest disadvantage, be it economical, racial, political or age-related. In summary, Štampar was a physician equipped with all the humanitarian characteristics associated with that profession—though not as physician of the individual but of society. To him, social welfare was a crucial element of health. To that end, he worked in the interwar era, participated in the formation of the WHO, and contributed to the international health order after World War II.

Acknowledgments
For comments on earlier drafts of this paper and for assistance with the English translation, I am grateful to Dr Tatjana Buklijas, Dr Iris Borowy and Dr Anne Hardy. Special thanks for allowing me to peruse their family archives go to the Štampar family, especially Andrija Štampar's daughters Professor Zora Lukovnjak and the late Dr Bosiljka Plasaj. For their assistance in collecting archival material and for useful conversations, I thank Professor Michael Hubensdorf of the Institute of the History of Medicine 'Josephinum' in Vienna, Mrs Bernardine Pejović from the League of Nations Archives in Geneva, and the staffs of the Croatian State Archives in Zagreb and the Rockefeller Archive Center in New York.

1 Throughout the text I will be using the original, Croatian edition of M.D. Grmek, *U borbi za narodno zdravlje: Izabrani članci Andrije Štampara* (Zagreb: Škola narodnog zdravlja, Medicinski fakultet, 1966). The English edition followed: *Serving the Cause of Public Health: Selected Papers of Andrija Štampar* (Zagreb: School of Public Health, Medical Faculty, 1966).

2 Gunn to Carter, 21 March 1941, RF, 710, 1.1, Rockefeller Archive Center, New York (henceforth: RAC).

3 The nickname was mentioned by Henry van Zile Hyde: 'And Štampar, who was known as the Bear of the Balkans(…)' (Oral History Interviews with Henry Van Zile Hyde, Truman Library, http://www.trumanlibrary.org/oralhist/hydehvz1.htm#72). Van Zile Hyde mentions the nickname in his excellent obituary to Štampar: H. Van Zile Hyde, 'A tribute to Andrija Štampar MD, 1888–1958', American Journal of Public Health, 48 (1958), 1578–82. Finally, the nickname is also mentioned by N. Howard-Jones, *International Public Health between the Two World Wars: The Organisational Problems*, (Geneva: WHO, 1978), 82.

4 Van Zile Hyde, *Oral History Interviews.*

5 H.E. Sigerist, 'Yugoslavia and the XIth International Congress of the History of Medicine', *Bulletin of the History of Medicine*, 7 (1939), 99–147.

6 B. Cvjetanovic, 'Homage to Andrija Štampar', *World Health Forum*, 11 (1990), 376-80. The author also used the *Chronicle of the World Health Organisation*, 9 (1955), 203–6.

7 R.A. Kyle, M.A. Shampo, 'Andrija Štampar', JAMA, 243 (1980), 2404. That text contains several factual errors: for instance, Štampar was born in Drenovac and not Brenovac, he gave a series of lectures on hygiene and social medicine in the United States in 1938 and not 1937.

8 Howard-Jones, *International Public Health,* 82; T.M. Brown, E. Fee, 'Andrija Štampar: Charismatic Leader of Social Medicine and International Health', *American Journal of Public Health*, 96 (2006), 1383; P. Zylberman, 'Few Parallels then Antitheses: Rene Sand and Andrija Štampar on Social Medicine, 1919–1955', *Social History of Medicine*, 17 (2004), 77–92.

9 On Vienna School of Medicine around 1900, see E. Lesky, *The Vienna Medical School of the 19th century* (Baltimore: Johns Hopkins University Press, 1976).

10 Nationale. Mediziner-Winter-Semester 1910–11(S).0. Universitätsarchiv Wien; Hubensdorf M. Ludwig Teleky. I am grateful to Professor Hubensdorf for allowing me to peruse the unpublished manuscript.

11 On Volkshochschulen, see K. Taschwer, Wissenschaft für viele. Zur Wissenschaftsvermittlung im Rahmen der Wiener Volksbildung um 1900, (PhD dissertation: University of Vienna, 2002).

12 The Archives of the Collections of the Medical University of Vienna hold correspondence between Tandler and Štampar, which testifies of their closeness and the shared standpoint concerning the socialization of medicine. Štampar also mentioned Tandler on several occasions in his Diary (Tandler-Štampar correspondence, Collections of the Medical University of Vienna; Štampar, Dnevnik (*Diary*), Osobni fond, 831, HDA). On Tandler's life and career see K. Sablik, *Julius Tandler Mediziner und Sozialreformer* (Vienna: A. Schendl, 1983).

13 Grmek, *U borbi*, 17.

14 A. Štampar, 'Socijalna medicina', *Zora*, 3 (1911), 126–31.

15 Grmek, *U borbi*, 21-22.

16 A. Štampar, 'Primjetbe k osnovi zakona o čuvanju narodnog zdravlja. Preventivni dio zakona', *Liječnički vjesnik*, 41 (1919), 424-9.; A. Štampar, *Nacrt zakona o čuvanju*

narodnog zdravlja (Beograd: Ministarstvo narodnog zdravlja, 1921), 4-16.; *Nacrti sanitetskih zakona* (Zagreb: Zbor liječnika Hrvatske, Slavonije i Međimurja,1921).

17 A. Štampar, *Pet godina socijalno-medicinskog rada u Kraljevini Srba, Hrvata i Slovenaca* (Zagreb: Institut za socijalnu medicinu, 1926).

18 Sigerist, *Yugoslavia and the XIth International Congress.*

19 More in: Ž. Dugac, 'Zbor liječnika, Andrija Štampar i javnozdravstvena politika u Kraljevini Srba Hrvata i Slovenaca-Kraljevini Jugoslaviji', *Liječnički vjesnik*, 127 (2005), 5–6; 151–7.

20 Štampar, *Dnevnik.*

21 Van Zile Hyde, *Oral History Interviews.*

22 Štampar, *Pet godina.*; A. Štampar, *Deset godina unapređenja narodnog zdravlja* (Zagreb: Narodne Novine. 1934).; Ž. Dugac, 'New Public Health for a New State: Interwar Public Health in the Kingdom of Serbs, Croats, and Slovenes and the Rockefeller Foundation', in: I. Borowy, W. Gruner (eds.), *Facing Illnesses in Troubled Times: Health in Europe in the Interwar Years* (Frankfurt am Main: Peter Lang, 2005), 277–304.

23 More in: Ž. Dugac, *Protiv bolesti i neznanja: Rockefellerova fondacija u meduratnoj Jugoslaviji* (Zagreb: Srednja Europa, 2005); Ž. Dugac. *'Like yeast in fermentation': public health in interwar Yugoslavia* (in press).

24 More in H. Matković, *Povijest Jugoslavije* (Zagreb: Naklada Pavičić, 2003), 165–76.

25 More in: Dugac, *Protiv bolesti i neznanja*, 129-47.

26 Dopis Ministarstva prosvjete Kraljevine SHS, 10 November 1922. Osobnik dr. Andrija Štampar, Arhiv Sveucilista u Zagrebu/ University of Zagreb Archives (henceforth: ASZ); Dopis medicinskog fakulteta Sveučilišta u Zagrebu Rektoratu univerziteta kraljevine Jugoslavije, 27 May 1931. Osobnik dr. Andrija Štampar, ASZ; Grmek, *U borbi*, 35.

27 Gunn, Report, *Public health in Yugoslavia*, 1924, 6.1,1.3, RAC.

28 Ibid.

29 Ibid.

30 A version of this belief played greatly informed the Western policy during the tragic war on the ex-Yugoslav territories in the 1990s.

31 Gunn, Report, Public health in Yugoslavia, 1924, 6.1,1.3, RAC.

32 See for instancde Gunn, Diary, 15 February 1928, RF, 12.1, RAC.

33 Ibid.

34 Gunn, Diary, 15 February 1928, RF, 12.1, RAC.

35 Gunn, Diary, 18 February 1929, RF, 12.1, RAC.

36 Uroš Krulj was the first Minister of Public Health of the Kingdom of Serbs, Croats and Slovenes. After the establishment of the dictatorship and the appointment of the General Petar Živković as the prime minister, Krulj was reappointed to his former position. He was a Serb physician from Mostar, famous for his eugenic interests.

37 Gunn, Diary, 10 February 1930, RF, 12.1, RAC.

38 Ibid.

39 Gunn, Diary, 11 March 1930, RF, 12.1, RAC.

40 Gunn to Manson, 22 April 1931, 710, 1.1, RAC.

41 More in: Dugac, *Protiv bolesti i neznanja*, 81-2; 134-5.

42 Frederic F. Russell, Diary, 2 September 1931, RF, 12.1, RAC; Minutes of the International Health Department meeting, 13 January 1932,710, 1.1, RAC.

43 Radin to Gunn, 30 July 1931, korespondencija, Osobni fond, 831, HDA. Zagreb.

44 Štampar to Gunn, 7 December 1931, korespondencija, Osobni fond, 831, HDA. Zagreb.

45 Gunn to Manson, 22 April 1931, 710, 1.1, RAC.; George Strode, Diary, 25 March 1931, RF, 12.1, RAC.; Štampar to the Rockefeller Foundation, 30 March 1931, 710, 1.1, RAC. Štampar was seen by the Foundation as a very good collaborator. They proved their trust in him on multiple occasions by supporting him and entrusting him to manage financial resources granted by the Foundation. Senior RF members also repeatedly expressed their appreciaton of him. Vincent, 25 November 1929,710, 1.1, RAC; Gunn to Russell, 1 May 1925, 710,1.1, RAC.

46 Radin to Kingsbury, 31. July 1931, korespondencija, Osobni fond, 831, HDA. Zagreb.

47 Strode, Diary, 15 December 1934, RF, 12.1, RAC.

48 Popović to Štampara, 7 June 1931, korespondencija, Osobni fond, 831, HDA. Zagreb.

49 Štampar to Ristović, 28 February 1934. Courtesy of Bosiljka Štampar.

50 Rajchman to Štampar, 14 July 1931, Osobni fond, 831, HDA. Zagreb.

51 Report, European Health Conference. Warsaw, 20-28 March 1922. (League of Nations Archive, Geneva) LONA.

52 He was a member of the Committee for Hygiene Education, Committee for Social Insurance, and Sub-committee for Preventive Medicine. Grmek, U borbi, 35. See also Annual Report of the Health Organisation for 1930, April 1931, LONA, A.7.1931.III, 60, 62.

53 Štampar to Boudreau, 24 Octobar 1930, LONA, R 8B/18878/1218.

54 Health General, LONA, R 8A/20164/3073 and 8A/20827/3073.

55 Minutes, European Conference on Rural Hygiene 1931, LONA.

56 Štampar to Rajchmann, 28 May 1931, LONA, R 8B/18878/1218.

57 Štampar, *Dnevnik.*

58 Grmek, *U borbi,* 36.; Štampar to Rajchmann, 1 November 1932, LONA, R 8B/ 18878/1218.; Communication concerning the lectures in Warsaw and Smokovec, 7 February 1933, Osobni fond, 831, HAD; Štampar, *Dnevnik.*

59 Štampar, *Dnevnik.*

60 Ibid.

61 Ibid.

Štampar usually went to Ting Hsien, a model county that boasted an innovative project model of hygiene and general education, developed after the ideas of the Chinese public health and educational legend, James Yen. It was there that Štampar met Ch'en Chih-ch'ien (C. C. Ch'en), head of the public health programmes in Ting Hsien, whom Štampar later recommended for further education overseas. So in 1935, Chen went to the Soviet Union, Kingdom of Yugoslavia and India, with the support of the League of Nations. In a later book, this highly active Chinese physician stated that he was deeply impressed with the achievements in the area of rural health in Croatia. (More in C.C. Chen, *Medicine in Rural China* (Berkeley: University of California Press, 1989).

Štampar to Liu, January 16, 1936, korespondencija, Osobni fond, 831, HAD, Zagreb.; Grmek, U borbi, 36–8.

63 Štampar, 'Zdravstvene i socijalne prilike u Kini', *Liječnički vjesnik,* 59 (1937), 372–379.

64 A.E. Lucas, *Chinese Medical Modernization Comparative Policy Continuities, 1930s-1980s* (New York: Praeger, 1982), 59; see also Chen, *Medicine in Rural China,* 102-5.

65 Chen to Watson, with Expenses Account, 15 February 1936, korespondencija, Osobni fond, 831, HAD, Zagreb.

66 Štampar to Tandler, 2 October 1935, The Archives of the Collections of the Medical University of Vienna.

67 Ibid.

68 Minutes, Ninety-sixth Session of the Council of the League of Nations, 25 January 1937, LONA.
69 Štampar, *Dnevnik.*
70 Tandler was a political refugee and persona non grata in Austria after 1934. See more in Sablik, Julius Tandler..
71 Štampar, *Dnevnik.*
72 Sigerist, *Yugoslavia and the XIth International Congress.*
73 Štampar, *Dnevnik.*
74 Ibid.
75 Ibid.
76 Ibid.
77 Ibid.
78 Ibid.; Not only was Štampar a sworn teetotaller but he frequently made jokes about his abstinence. He was greatly amused by the reactions of people when they realized he would not even taste an alcoholic drink.
79 Ibid.
80 Grmek, *U borbi*, 40.
81 Štampar to Ristović, 29 October 1933, Courtesy of Bosiljka Štampar.
82 Report, 1937, Osobni fond, 831, HDA. Zagreb.
83 Gregg to Štampar, 23 August 1937, RF, 710, RAC.
84 Lambert to Dickson, 17 December 1937, RF, 710, RAC.
85 The tour was reconstructed using the following documents: Štampar's Diary; Itinerary of the trip, 1938, RF, 710, RAC.; Willard C. Pappleye to Lambert, December 10, 1937 RF, 710, RAC.; Russell to Gregg, 4 February 1938, RF, 710, RAC.; Lambert to Lowell J. Reed, 20 November 1937, RF, 710, RAC.; Lambert to W.S. Leathers, 20 November 1937, RF, 710, RAC.; W.S. Leathers to Lambert, 23 November 1937, RF, 710, RAC.; Lambert to W.G. Smillie, 17 December 1937, RF, 710, RAC.; Lambert to Ernest C. Dickson, December 17, 1937, RF, 710, RAC.; Lambert to Harold S. Diehl, 22 November 1937, RF, 710, RAC.; Lambert to R.D. Defries, 27 May 1938, RF, 710, RAC.; Lambert to Grant A. Fleming, 27 May 1938, RF, 710, RAC.; R.E. Wodehouse to Lambert, 3 June 1938, RF, 710, RAC.; Lambert to Burke, 12 April 1938, RF, 710, RAC.; Lambert to Štampar, 12 April 1938, RF, 710, RAC.
86 W.H. Perkins to Lambert, 6 April 1938, RF, 710, RAC.
87 Memo, Gregg's interview with Štampar, 24 May 1938, RF, 710, RAC.
88 Dopis Ministra prosvjete, 5 March 1939. Osobnik dr. Andrija Štampar, ASZ.
89 A. Štampar, *Zdravlje i drustvo,* (Zagreb: Hrvatska naklada, 1939).
90 A. Štampar, *Higijena i socijalna medicina*, (Zagreb: Narodne novine, 1940).
91 Gremk, *U borbi,* 40-1.
92 Karton Andrija Štampara, Redarstvena oblast za grad Zagreb, HR HDA 259, K.36. HDA. Zagreb.
93 Gremk, *U borbi*, 41.
94 Oral communication, Bosiljka Štampar Plasaj
95 Gremk, *U borbi*, 46–7.
96 A. Štampar, *Liječnik, njegova prošlost i budućnost*, (Zagreb: Preporod, 1946).
97 M. Kraljević, 'In memoriam. Akademik prof. dr. Andrija Štampar', *Liječnički vjesnik,* 80 (1958), 505–7; Grmek, U borbi, 49.
98 Greggov intervju sa Štamparom, 24. svibnja 1938. RAC, Col.RF., RG 710, S.1.1, RAC.
99 More in J. Škarić, *Uspomene jednog liječnika* (Split: vlastita naklada, 1965).
100 Greggov intervju sa Štamparom, 24. svibnja 1938. RAC, Col.RF., RG 710, S.1.1, RAC.

101 Štampar, *Dnevnik*.

102 During his Chinese travels he was accompanied by John B. Grant, professor of hygiene at the Peking Union Medical College (PUMC), founded by the Rockefeller Foundation. Grant was also the representative of the International Health Board for Far East. Grant was extremely knowledgeable about China, hygiene and social medicine. He and Štampar immediately found a common language. They criticized the curriculum of that medical school and requested its adaptation to suit the Chinese needs. In his diary, Štampar wrote about their activities and often repeated that the curriculum of the Peking Union Medical College was entirely unsuitable for China, because it trained physicians according to the criteria of Western medicine, using an elitist educational model suited for working in institutions equipped to Western standards that were few in contemporary China and used mostly by the rich. So these physicians were incapable of working in the contemporary Chinese conditions and among the mostly poor rural population. See M. Brown Bullock, *An American transplant. The Rockefeller Foundation and Peking Union Medical College* (Berkeley: University of California Press, 1980) and Štampar, *Dnevnik*.

103 Izvješće, 1931, Osobni fond, 831, HDA, Zagreb.

104 Cf.: H.E. Sigerist, *Socialised medicine in the Soviet Union* (London: Victor Gollancz, 1937).; Sigerist H.E. *Medicine and health in the Soviet Union* (New York: The Citadel Press, 1947).

105 Cvjetanović, Rukopis Štampar i svijet.

106 Gremk, *U borbi,* 13.

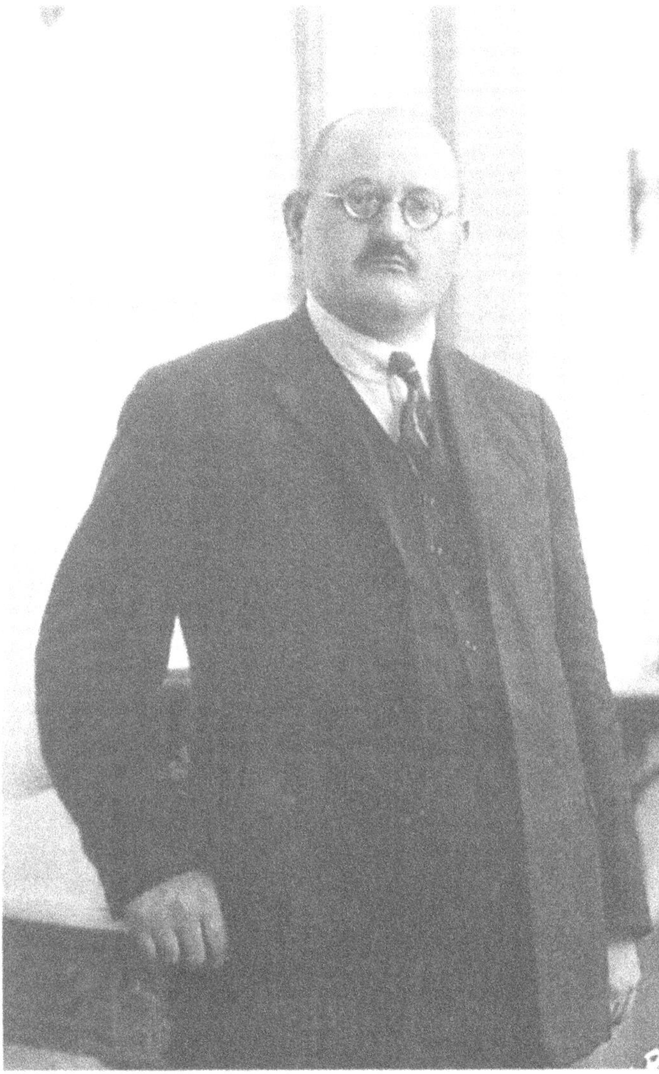

Andrija Štampar

Dr Melville Mackenzie (1889 – 1972) 'Feed the people and prevent disease, and be damned to their politics.'[1]

Zoe C. Sprigings

Introduction

The intertwined nature of politics and healthcare is now such an established concept that belief in their bifurcation is dismissed as a 'myth' belonging to a bygone age.[2] However, Melville Mackenzie steadfastly held onto this ideal as an achievable reality throughout his life and, as one of the founders of the WHO, his views merit some interrogation. The introductory quotation epitomises his functionalist argument that healthcare could and should be a politically neutral service guided only by concern for the patient's medical needs.[3] It was written in a rare outburst of passion in 1922, and another two decades passed before Mackenzie provided his one and only elaboration of this, his guiding principle:

> [medicine] has great power and influence, and for this reason is the easier to utilize for other ends than the purely medical welfare of the human race. Party political preoccupations may too readily become reasons for carrying out a particular piece of work which may achieve its non-medical object even if done in an entirely superficial manner, an effective face which can have no lasting benefit ... progress in the science of medicine, the good it can bring to all peoples of the world, and how each can benefit from the experience of others should be the only concerns of an international medical organisation. Administrative medicine necessarily has certain political aspects, but these need not be allowed, by undue development, to overshadow the goal in view – the cure of the sick and the prevention of disease.[4]

This statement was in itself political. The paradox is that, although Mackenzie prided himself on eschewing party politics, his life story serves to demonstrate the ineluctability of its influence. Throughout this chapter, his actions will be tested against the paradigm he proposed. He occupied numerous political roles as a doctor and held political beliefs which influenced his professional actions. Mackenzie's struggle for certainty despite surrounding contradictions is an illuminating case study of one man's attempt to make sense of international healthcare in its formative years. Moreover, he was not just any doctor but a founder of the WHO: he embodied the complicated dynamic between health and politics and this investigation of his inter-war development provides a new insight into a figure responsible for setting up the problematic 'conceptual division', which lives with us today through the WHO's statutes and is now under such scrutiny.[5] As well as being a key figure in post-war health, Mackenzie was equally important in the LNHO as a Special Commissioner on several occasions, as the Secretary-General's Special Representative, Acting Director of the Singapore Bureau and briefly of the LNHO Health Section.[6] Yet, he has received only a handful of one-sentence mentions in the history books, mainly from contemporaries or official historians of the organisations for which he worked. [7] This may partly be due to his retiring character, which was well suited to the anonymity granted by LNHO reports and research; unlike more public colleagues, Mackenzie maintained the lowest of profiles and rarely expressed his personal opinions. Perhaps, too, his later prominence in UNRRA and the WHO overshadowed his links with an organisation whose memory many were actively attempting to bury after the war.[8] However, as such a senior figure his influence was considerable and his story is an important part of the jigsaw of international inter-war health.

The total absence of secondary literature on Mackenzie means primary sources are of paramount importance and dominate this paper, and thus deserve some consideration. Contrary to what one might assume from the historical neglect of Mackenzie, there is a substantial amount of material on him scattered throughout various archives. It falls into two types, each with considerable limitations. The first is the official documentation: the extensive League of Nations Archive, his slim government file from the UK National Archive and his various publications. By their very nature, these sources are generally detached and formal in tone and make the individual behind them hard to identify, although it becomes clear that Mackenzie adhered to these conventions far more than most other colleagues. The second group is the personal documentation, and undoubtedly Major Jock Haswell's unpublished biographical manuscript 'The Doctor Who Stopped A War: The Adventures and Achievements of Dr Melville Mackenzie CMG' is the most precious of these. Written at the request of Mackenzie's widow and using material she furnished, this family friend provided a fascinating, albeit unreferenced and uncritical, account of Mackenzie's life. Sadly, all Mackenzie's papers were then destroyed. The only extant family documents are those copies which his widow provided to the archives of the School of Oriental and African Studies, SOAS, (on Liberia) and the Friends House Library, London (on Russia). The one exception to either group is a small collection of letters between Mackenzie and his friend Lord Lugard, held in the Rhodes House Library Lugard collection, Oxford. Like most historical figures, Mackenzie's image was carefully managed in both the official and personal documentation, and this must be borne in mind during attempts at reconstruction.

This chapter will focus on the four formative phases of Mackenzie's interwar career which had the most profound effect on his philosophy of international healthcare: his service in the Royal Army Medical Corps (RAMC) during and immediately after the war; his volunteering during the 1920s Russian famine; his diplomatic experience in Liberia in the early 1930s and his senior responsibility for China in the late 1930s. Although he spent most of his life working as part of the international, even transnational, medical community, Mackenzie always felt himself a member of the British Empire and Government.[9] This had a noticeable influence on his beliefs about functional co-operation between states on healthcare issues, and consideration will be given throughout the chapter to the interplay between the national and transnational elements of his identity.

Mesopotamia: Mackenzie's introduction to international medical work

Melville Mackenzie came from a comfortable middle-class background, born in 1889 to a Huddersfield general practitioner and a teacher, and he inherited great academic ability and a passion for education. He was extremely close to his family and was obviously much influenced by his father, whom he described thus in 1918: 'his whole life was his work for the sick and for his home and family ... his conscientiousness and love for his fellow beings made him an excellent doctor.' Mackenzie's later letters to his family suggest a man trying to prove himself cut from the same cloth.[10] He attended Epsom College, a boarding school, and then won a scholarship to St Bartholomew's medical school in London. He was forced to follow directly in his father's footsteps when the latter fell ill just after Melville graduated in 1911, so he returned home to his family to shoulder the entire practice aged 23.[11]

Service with the RAMC during the First World War, however, roused an interest in preventative medicine far beyond the parochial confines of curative general practice and revealed his talent for sanitary work and epidemiology. He was posted with the Basra Expeditionary Forces with responsibility for infectious diseases in the hospital, then the port and later across the region. Some RAMC officers struggled with the new disciplines of sanitation and hygiene, and the need to place state demands over the individual, but not Mackenzie.[12] The majestic scale of his task and the war operations appealed to him, and he wrote home that, 'it is great to feel that one's work is for the country and not for money. It gives life to the dullest job'.[13] He threw himself with success into epidemiological work, prompting his immediate superior Col. Fremantle (Chief Sanitary Officer) to call him 'a born sanitarian.'[14] Mackenzie recorded:

> My heart and soul are in preventative medicine and Public Health. Out here, medicine has been a new joy. During my five previous years of hard general practice, patching people up, nine-tenths of whom ought never to have needed it, I began to forget research and progress, and medicine did not have its full meaning, but here I have had opportunities to follow up diseases and to read and understand the vast possibilities of organized medicine.[15]

The potential for combating disease through practical and often simple measures was part of what attracted Mackenzie to preventative health, whether through building hospitals or digging wells, and he relished the physical freedom of outdoor work. He was appointed Captain whilst in Mesopotamia, and was 'mentioned in dispatches' for his famous Mobile Disinfecting Train Service, a practical steam-cleaning invention which he designed to combat the typhus and relapsing fever epidemics of 1918-19. He reported its use in several journals, marking the beginning of what was to be a prolific publishing career.

Although Mackenzie was anxious to reach the front line, he remained behind it throughout the war and was shielded from the real carnage of conflict. Probably for this reason he did not suffer the moral qualms of so many other doctors in the First World War, for he could fulfil his Hippocratic duty with a clear conscience without having to confront the paradox of preparing men immediately to die, like those on the Western Front.[16] It may also be why the 'gigantesque human tragedy' of the epidemics he encountered after the war in Mesopotamia and Russia then had such a profound impact on him and remained his definitive memory of the cost of war, as will be explored later.[17] The stimulating life of a doctor in the British Empire clearly appealed to Mackenzie, who wrote 'life here is full of interest and one is continually gaining new knowledge that alters one's outlook on Nature, mankind and religion'.[18] Although it appears paradoxical today in our post-colonial society, Mackenzie saw no conflict between his deep interest and respect for other cultures and his contribution to supporting Britain's control over them as her colonies. His aptitude for languages became evident whilst abroad: in a matter of months he was proficient in Hindustani and Arabic and moved on to Turkish. Mackenzie held that speaking the vernacular was essential for proper administration.[19] He was regularly invited to attend religious events and he threw himself into local life. The implicitly political nature of his healthcare, although he did not acknowledge it as such, is illustrated by his description of the pro bono service he provided to local children:

> My only hope is that it may help the child and also help to give the Arabs a good impression of their new conquerors. We want the Arabs to prefer us to the Turks, spontaneously. We want a second loyal India here, and every little helps. Unofficial doctoring also makes for variety in one's life and I love treating children, black, brown or white.[20]

Jennifer Beinart argues that from 1920 colonial paediatric care moved from dismissing the child as an irredeemably wild 'Child of Nature' towards a 'process of anglicisation' and although she focuses on Africa, Mackenzie's case suggest it could be equally relevant to other parts of the Empire and even earlier than 1920.[21] Like the majority of Britons of his day, Mackenzie felt latent support for the Empire, without ever reflecting on his justification of 'imperialism' as a philosophy. It does not emerge as his primary motivation, but he was undoubtedly pleased that his work contributed to the positive promotion of Britain and her Empire.

Throughout his time in Mesopotamia and afterwards, the influence of his parents' wish to have him in England with them is evident in Mackenzie's letters, as he struggled with his conflicting desires. Once he reassured them 'I am often afraid you may think the East will exert a claiming influence over me when you read my accounts of people and things... you can always be assured that home and England are first in my thoughts and desires'.[22] Despite his enjoyment of working abroad, strong family ties called him home with the death of his father in 1918 and kept him in England for several years while he settled his father's affairs. Between 1920 and 1921 he set about extending his medical education and succeeded in establishing himself firmly on the British medical scene. He amassed an impressive number of qualifications: a doctorate, bachelor's degree and many diplomas with a specialism in tropical medicine and hygiene.[23] Through achieving the highest marks (garnering another scholarship) and studying at the leading institutions Mackenzie was soon at the forefront of his field and had an considerable array of contacts at places as diverse as Cambridge, the medical schools of Liverpool and Newcastle and the London School of Tropical Medicine (LSTM).

He studied at the LSTM as it was turning its attention towards the broader topics of public health and preventative medicine around the world, and as these issues were rising up the political agenda. He graduated in 1921, the year that the Athlone Committee accepted Rockefeller Foundation (RF) plans and funding for the LSTM to merge with the University College Department of Hygiene to create the London School of Hygiene and Tropical Medicine (LSHTM).[24] He seemed accepted wherever he went and this description by his superior at the Newcastle Health Department was typical:

> Mackenzie is one of the finest men I have ever had to deal with, a brilliant student, a most capable and loyal officer, with high ideals, indomitable energy, wide prospective... coupled with good appearance, happy disposition and shrewd judgement and diplomacy.[25]

His RAMC service had also introduced him to influential men such as Sir Francis Fremantle and Sir George Buchanan (late Lieutenant-Colonel in the War Office Sanitary Committee in Mesopotamia) who were now in the new Ministry of Health and keen to help their old friend Mackenzie. Before he left Mesopotamia, Fremantle had assured him: 'we must not let you leave preventative medicine. Whatever you want when you come back to England I will see you get'.[26] It was an offer which he soon needed to take up in an unexpected way.

Russia: Mackenzie's reaction against 'politics'

It seemed that his various connections had set Mackenzie up for a promising domestic career. He settled down as Assistant Medical Officer to Liverpool Port Sanitary Authority, but it was not long before he ventured abroad once more, albeit in the very different capacity of international non-governmental volunteer. In the December 1921 issue of the Lancet he read about the disastrous famine which had struck Russia, and the Society of Friends' (Quakers) appeal for a doctor for their Russian Famine Relief Unit. He decided to offer his services. Mackenzie was neither Quaker nor Communist, but this opportunity offered the large-scale humanitarian purpose and adventure he had lacked since demobilisation. The need was particularly urgent as the Medical Officer appointed to the League of Nations Epidemic Commission, Dr. R. Farrar, another British epidemiologist, succumbed to typhus that month.[27] Although Mackenzie felt an obligation to help, his employers disagreed and rejected his application for six months' leave on the grounds that the UK's need of him was just as important. However, Mackenzie found full support from Fremantle and Buchanan, who arranged for him to receive leave as an RAMC reserve. He swiftly resigned, upset at the friction caused but reassured by local press praise for their doctor off to 'serve the cause of humanity'.[28] This dilemma of whether to serve nationally or abroad continued to worry Mackenzie, as he explained to his mother and brother once in Russia: 'It is difficult to know how far we ought with our suffering at home to be here – I am not convinced of which is our first responsibility but there is no doubt the suffering here is and will be great. And it is very hard to see deaths that we know how to avoid.[29] Russia was a crossroads for Mackenzie. His close family ties and feeling of obligation to his home country led in one direction, and his spirit of adventure and awareness of huge international health problems in the other. Ultimately the extent of the suffering in Russia, the professional satisfaction of countering epidemics, and the excitement of a grand humanitarian mission convinced him to pursue an international career.

Mackenzie relished the challenge which faced him, though he felt the responsibility acutely, and once again flourished in the outdoor environment which so appealed to his exploratory, practical side. His normal practice was Buzuluk, South-East Russia, an area the size of Wales with a population of 400,000 and only 26 Russian doctors and one microscope (Mackenzie's own). In collaboration with local medical workers, Mackenzie oversaw the successful defeat of cholera, typhus and malaria through inoculation programmes and other preventative measures. He then set about establishing an infrastructure which would continue independent of him, which was his chief ambition. He worked with ceaseless energy, as recorded in his diary: 'this week I have kept open 4 general hospitals, 4 cholera hospitals, and have taken steps for establishing a training centre for nurses.'[30] He also secured local doctors, built laboratories, initiated infant relief hospitals and care homes, and gave lectures in Russian to local practitioners. He maintained close links with Britain, collecting material for the LSHTM and relaying information to Oxford University and the Rockefeller Foundation, and also fundraising for the relief work. For a time he was acting head of the entire Nansen Relief Administration in Russia, to which the Quaker Mission was affiliated, and was Senior Medical Officer in charge of the British and American Quaker Relief Units in his last months.[31] Balinska makes no mention of Mackenzie, despite describing his countryman Dr Farrar and also the activities of the Quaker and Nansen Missions in Eastern Europe. Weindling refers to him once and briefly. He may have been overlooked because he never worked directly for the Epidemic Commission, only appearing at senior level on secondment, and was often in the field far from policy makers. However, Mackenzie's experience is a key example of the effect of the Russian relief work on medical staff who then went on to influential positions in the new LNHO, and beyond.

It was in Russia that Mackenzie encountered the nascent LNHO, in the form of the League of Nations Epidemic Commission, and he was inspired by this international co-operation to write 'There is something very fine in the united effort of nations to help the Russians... it is a wonderful spirit that co-ordinates all those other countries to help the stricken one'.[32] Two decades later, in 1942, Mackenzie ascribed the birth of international medicine to the relief and reconstruction work of the early 1920s, and he was clearly profoundly influenced by his participation.[33] The organisations also recognised his merits: the Quaker British Mission in Moscow approached him and the Epidemic Commission invited him to become the second of their two British doctors. Mackenzie rejected both on the grounds of family ties back home, but he had clear regrets about the latter post. In a letter to his mother he described the Commission's work as 'one of the most important functions of the League of Nations' and admitted that the job 'would be interesting from a public health point of view'.[34] Again he was forced to choose between practising at home or abroad: although he chose Britain this time, it was clear where his true interests lay.

Mackenzie's experience of Soviet Russia had a fundamental influence on his belief system, though he did not explicitly acknowledge it. The shock of what he witnessed produced a visceral reaction against the political situation which later hardened into personal dogma. Widespread cannibalism, hospitals clogged with dead children, desperate starvation, invasive government surveillance and the outlawing of religion convinced him that Communism was an inhuman and unworkable political system. However, he did not see his reaction as a political stance. For Mackenzie, the problem of 'politics' was caused by the Soviet authorities alone, and privately he was unusually outspoken on the matter. In his one uncensored letter from Russia he declared: 'I am much more afraid of political complications than of typhus because it is so difficult to get one's work done and not get involved in politics ... we went out to feed the people and prevent disease, and be damned to their politics'.[35] This reaction was not accompanied by articulated logic, and the context of its conception brought with it an implicit bias against left-wing 'radicalism' which emerged in his later life. It was Mackenzie's genuine belief that he was acting impartially, and his attempt to repress his views was part of a strenuous attempt at neutrality. He later wrote an article for The Times on his experiences but requested anonymity and refused to voice an opinion on the political situation, although he admitted in typically cryptic fashion 'I may say however that my own views on the matter are very definite'.[36] He also lobbied publicly in Britain for more funding, but he carefully focused on the symptoms of the problem, not the cause.[37] Nonetheless, it is clear that he did have very strong feelings and these had considerable influence on his later actions, however much he believed they did not. It is worth remembering that Mackenzie had not seen the political implications of his service in Mesopotamia, despite explicitly acknowledging that it could help promote the Empire. It is also striking that although his humanitarian impulse to aid Russia was real, the men who permitted him to go may have had strong political reasons for doing so. Weindling suggests that the Ministry of Health was concerned with 'propping up the post-Versailles European order' and that in fact 'epidemic prevention offered a pretext for political intervention'.[38] What emerges from both these cases is that until Mackenzie's latent principles and everyday work were challenged – and in the most dramatic way possible – he did not consider the political power of medicine. When these were challenged, he saw the politicisation of medicine as the problem, and violently rejected it.

As Mackenzie travelled home he developed paratyphoid, then relapsing fever and malaria, in what was very nearly a fatal combination. However, he survived and after a few months of recuperation he was back in Europe with the Friends' British Medical Commission, this time for a survey of children's health in Germany.[39] On his final return to England, thoroughly exhausted, he spent several years recovering and slowly returning to work in various British hospitals in a range of fields ranging from mental deficiency to venereal disease. Then, with Fremantle's enthusiastic support, he joined the Ministry in 1926 as a Medical Officer in the Department for Control of Infectious Diseases. Fremantle, a good friend of the first Chief Medical Officer Sir George Newman, had been especially impressed by Mackenzie's approach to preventative medicine, and provided a reference which described Mackenzie as combining 'professional ability and resource, practical common sense, tact and power in the command of all men of all rank, races and classes, with vision, zeal and personal charm...he has as wide a view of the potentialities and ideals of public health as any junior man that I know'.[40] He added in a personal note of recommendation to Newman that 'you couldn't have a better man for your department'.[41] There is no material in the UK archives on Mackenzie's activities during this period and Haswell's brief coverage suggests that Mackenzie's personal documents offered little in detail or interest. The job entailed some research and travel to epidemic loci, it does not appear to have greatly impacted on Mackenzie and it is no surprise that when the LNHO once more invited Mackenzie to join, he accepted.

In joining the League, Mackenzie was entering a new phase which would present him with conflicting ideas on what constituted 'international co-operation'. The Ministry of Health agreed to lend him on 'approved service', but it is revealing that they believed Mackenzie would be sent to India for malaria research and would therefore be 'of real value' to Britain's colonial interests. In fact, Mackenzie was initially posted as Special Commissioner to a malaria epidemic in Greece and never posted to India during all his time at the League. The Ministry official added that 'we do attach a good deal of importance to having a substantial proportion of Englishmen upon the League staff ... trained in our ways and conversant with our ideas'. [42] The British were wary of LNHO operations, and this was certainly the feeling of the previous UK representative and friend of Mackenzie, Sir George Buchanan, who was determined to limit LNHO 'transnational' powers and opposed even collaborative schemes. [43] Mackenzie was trusted by the British administration but although he remained loyal to Britain, he took his primary responsibility to the LNHO very seriously and did not share Buchanan's attitude in this regard. British administrator Lugard later described him as a 'servant of the League,' and commented from his example that those employed by the League 'must work "internationally"' viz. for the League and the country', meaning the country of deployment.[44] However, there is no sign that Mackenzie took a political stance on this point. In the next few years Mackenzie travelled a great deal, beginning with visits to Eastern European health centres and concluding eventfully when he was caught up in a wave of revolutions whilst touring South America and had to escape in a boat crate. His influence on policy back in Geneva appears to have been minimal, but it provided him with vast experience of many of the League's more distant countries.

Liberia: the challenge of diplomacy

Mackenzie's longest assignment for the League of Nations was with Liberia, and it marked his transition from medical officer into medical diplomat. He first became involved in 1931 as one of three Special Commissioners sent to make recommendations to the Liberian government after the Christy Commission in 1930 found widespread slavery and neglect of the native ethnic groups by the ruling elite. Moreover, the government's failure to repay a loan from the US Firestone rubber company was causing serious concern to the US government, which had traditionally supported the Liberians, but was now supporting League involvement. The 1931 Brunot Commission therefore visited at the official behest of Liberia, a League member, to provide a 'Plan of Assistance' and to advise on how the Liberians might implement it; Mackenzie's duty was to consider the medical issues. This meant maintaining League impartiality whilst keeping the government's trust despite his critical findings. Simultaneously, he needed to bear in mind the security concerns of neighbouring French and British colonial powers. Endemic yellow fever in the border areas, amongst other diseases, made Liberia's health problems an international health issue. His report was written with an eye to the League's dominant members, and their empires, so the humanitarian health crisis is also presented as one of 'economic' and 'international concern'.[45] During his work with Liberia, Mackenzie became very good friends with Lord Lugard, who became godfather to Mackenzie's first child. Lugard, after extensive experience as a colonial administrator, became involved in the LN through its Permanent Mandates Commission and Permanent Slavery Committee. Their correspondence reveals that Mackenzie's views on Liberia considerably influenced Lugard, especially on the issue of the sending a Chief Adviser.[46] Lugard frequently turned to Mackenzie for information about LNHO activities and through him Mackenzie had access to a large network of contacts and media outlets. In temperament, the two men could not have been more different, as Mackenzie's extreme discretion and obsessive struggle for impartiality found their opposite in Lugard's outspoken and pugnacious approach.[47] Twice, Lugard asked Mackenzie to take action: in 1934 he suggested a lecture tour in America to publicise the Liberia situation, and in 1936 he invited Mackenzie to join the British Ambulance in Ethiopia. And twice Mackenzie declined on the grounds of preserving his neutrality. This did not mean he was without interest or opinion, quite the reverse, but he refused to make them public. He told Lugard that America had a serious moral responsibility to Liberia, that his sympathies were wholly with the oppressed Kru ethnic group and that he was unimpressed by America's actions, but this is never evident from his official reports.[48] He was also deeply moved by the Ethiopian crisis, declaring 'it is only with the greatest possible difficulty that I resist the temptation to enlist'. Although he felt bound to the League, he began learning Amharic just in case.[49] This correspondence offers a rare glimpse of Mackenzie's strong feelings, and illustrates how he strove to separate his personal views from his official work. Unsurprisingly, this compartmentalization did not succeed in preventing his more subconscious thoughts from influencing his actions.

Mackenzie's reports and correspondence on Liberia display a strange mixture of conventional prejudice and progressive insights. He was undoubtedly a product of the Victorian Britain into which he was born, both supporting imperial Britain as a world power and having a keen sense of 'the white man's burden'. In his letters he referred to the Kru as 'childlike', and 'looking like arrivals direct from the inferno',[50] but he also commented in a private report that although one may be taught that different races are 'primitive', they may simply be different from – even superior to – Western societies.[51] Nonetheless he supported colonial rule and thoroughly enjoyed the role of colonial administrator whilst in the Liberian bush, and his administrative recommendations were very conservative. He was emphatic about the need to train native doctors in order to make Liberia self-sufficient, but he still believed that the solution to Liberia's problems was the introduction of a foreign (probably British) and explicitly white administration, at least in the short-term.[52] Mackenzie's attitude to colonialism did not constitute a very coherent philosophy, perhaps because he never really interrogated it.

Mackenzie's second visit to Liberia in 1932 was in full diplomatic capacity as the League Representative and with no connection to the LNHO, for this time he was charged with disarming the Kru and solving the internecine conflict – a deeply political challenge. The Liberian government accused the Kru of insurgency and threatened to seek harsh retribution unless they agreed to a ceasefire. The League was obliged to assist the Liberian government as the official authority, and also hoped to minimise the bloodshed by bringing about peace as soon as possible. Although Mackenzie succeeded in his task, it had a fatal legacy – one which he had suspected but which his optimistic nature perhaps glossed over. He was a peaceful man and even when travelling in war zones or among bandits he eschewed carrying a gun. His philosophy was that being armed 'destroys the confidence of a primitive people … after all, to be armed can be regarded as an insult and, rightfully, resented'.[53] He succeeded in persuading the Kru to disarm, using only negotiation, and in establishing 'the Mackenzie line' to define territorial boundaries. On his return home he was described in the national press as the doctor who 'stopped a civil war,' and Lord Cecil claimed he had saved hundreds if not thousands of lives.[54] At a time when Hitler and Mussolini were suspected of re-armament, and the memory of the First World War remained fresh, Mackenzie's success was regarded as a ray of hope. Cecil claimed Liberia was proof of the League's relevance, and one newspaper urged 'Politicians Please Copy'.[55]

However, events took a dramatic turn for the worse. In 1934 and again in 1936 the Liberian Frontier Force unleashed violent reprisals against the Kru and in their desperate petitions to the League, the ethnic leaders identified Mackenzie as the guilty party for making false promises about their security and leaving them helpless.[56] In his own defence, Mackenzie argued that he had repeatedly emphasised the need for further action to guarantee peace, but none was taken. He denied making false claims to the Kru, and the documentary evidence and his track record support this claim. In reality, the Liberian government was duplicitous, the world powers were lazy and the League was impotent – the situation was a true precursor to Abyssinia. Nonetheless, it does seem that despite his mistrust of the Liberian government Mackenzie was naïvely optimistic. Indeed, Lugard said as much in a letter to him.[57] His desire to see the best in everyone was key to his successes, such as the peaceful disarmament, but it could blind him to political reality.

UK: using domestic contacts to promote the LNHO

Mackenzie's British citizenship meant he had a natural affinity with many of the League's most senior figures: Eric Drummond, Lord Cecil and Frank Walters. He had personal and professional links to Ministry men who also served on the LNHO like George Buchanan and Neville Goodman, and earned the respect of seniors such as Fremantle and Arthur Macnalty (the second Chief Medical Officer). This situated him in a network of powerful men drawn from the most powerful country in the League. Despite Britain's financial support of the League, Raymond Gautier (senior LHNO colleague and good friend) commented that 'in the past it has been difficult to interest public health workers in England in the Health Section's work'.[58] Mackenzie spent much of his time tirelessly publicising the work of the LNHO and furthering connections between it and the UK. The biggest success in this respect was the British government's decision to allow him to conduct a two month investigation on behalf of the LNHO into the influence of the economic depression on health in 1934. The connection between health and economics was contentious, and at first the UK authorities vetoed the plan. After much negotiation they agreed, and it seems very likely that the designation of Mackenzie as investigator was a persuasive factor, as he was a trusted Ministry man. The Ministry agreed to the report because it would be of use to them, and when it was published it met with great acclaim. The British Medical Journal (BMJ) declared it 'a model of accuracy, selection and arrangement'.[59] Mackenzie's own views about the English health system are impossible to discern from the report, but this was the secret of its success. Like most of his other publications, it focused on practical details and only reported the observations (eg, the state of rooms, radiators, beds etc) without any attempt to speculate on causes or tackle controversies. The views of others and best practice were summarised, but no identifiable conclusion was drawn by the author. Hence the BMJ noted 'there is in the pamphlet no advocacy of any particular policy; it is an impartial statement of prevalent ideas, news and suggestions. As such, it forms a most valuable and almost indispensable basis for further discussion by committees or at conferences'.[60] The report was sent to 50 key figures in Britain and internationally, working for governments and NGOs; the LNHO received numerous extra requests for re-prints, and it was re-published in the Quarterly Bulletin of the LNHO.[61]

Mackenzie was passionate about sharing the LNHO's information with the world, for he believed its repository of comparative studies and expert reports to be among its greatest strengths. To this end, he proposed a 'Public Health Intelligence Service' in 1934 which would provide easy access to the LNHO's information bank. In a letter to C.L.Park of the Eastern Bureau, he enthusiastically championed the unique worth of the international data held by the LNHO.[62] Mackenzie was confident that the world would value the LNHO as much as he did, if only they knew about it. It is hard to tell from the record whether this eventuated or not, although it certainly received Rajchman's enthusiastic support and he wrote to medical publications and administrations all over the world announcing the service. However, the plan mainly consisted of formalising a service which already existed, and quantitative analysis is needed to establish whether the amount of correspondence increased as a result. Nonetheless, this episode offers an important insight into Mackenzie's personal ideal of international co-operation, and the importance he attached to information-sharing between countries and the LNHO as a facilitator of this function.

On the specific issue of Britain, Mackenzie used all his connections to publicise the LNHO, and never refused an invitation to speak about it. Given the reservations felt towards the League in various parts of the medical and political establishment, which Mackenzie was well aware of, his support represented a political statement although he presented it in functional terms. His old friend Fremantle invited him to address the Health and Housing Committee of the House of Commons on two occasions. In 1935 he outlined the history, aims and achievements of the LNHO and answered many questions. His report noted that several Members of Parliament strongly felt that the Health Organisation should be better publicised within the United Kingdom, 'in the interest of the future of the League of Nations, particularly in view of the attitude towards the League in a large number of influential quarters in England at the present time'.[63] Growing disillusionment with the League's Disarmament Committee was undoubtedly in mind, and this experience encouraged Mackenzie's campaign. When invited back in 1939 the outlook for the League was even bleaker but Mackenzie emphasised the 'fundamental necessity' of the LNHO's continued existence for political and economic reasons as well as scientific ones. He concluded by urging Members of Parliament to support closer co-operation between the UK and the LNHO.[64] Mackenzie reported that, once again, Members were interested and impressed by the LNHO's work. His other audiences included the British Hospitals Contributory Schemes Association and the British Medical Association, the latter being reported very positively in the BMJ.[65] Mackenzie even lectured the African Circle on the Liberian question, having been invited by his old friend and its chair, Lord Lugard.[66] The real impact of his work is hard to evaluate, but it illustrates his commitment to persuading the UK into international co-operation.

Although Mackenzie spent his life in transnational health organisations, this did not shake his belief in the sovereignty of the state, which placed him philosophically between his continental colleagues, like Gautier, and his British colleagues, like Buchanan. He firmly believed that because disease recognised no boundaries, every country was bound to each other 'as a member of a community of nations'; it was his regret that 'while the art of healing and prevention of disease is essentially world wide in its claims, the technical method of its application too often been limited by politico-geographic boundaries'.[67] And yet, this should not be read as a rejection of the sovereignty of the state or the value of nation-state borders. A deeper exploration of Mackenzie's idea of 'nationalism' in health reveals that for him it meant limiting information within national borders. This was what he opposed. As an epidemiologist, the idea of countries not sharing disease statistics, warnings of outbreaks or developments in vaccines was wrong on a moral and practical level because of the nature of infectious diseases.[68] It is essential to grasp his epidemiological perspective in order to understand how the idea of conventional national boundaries slotted into Mackenzie's vision of international co-operation.

China: the inevitability of politics

Mackenzie's final years with the League brought him his most prestigious postings, but it was a time of growing problems and uncertainty for the League. His focus shifted to the Far East, where LNHO Director Ludwik Rajchman was also active. Mackenzie's experiences provide an essential insight into the high-level tensions surrounding Rajchman and Avenol during this period. Mackenzie continued his work of promoting the LNHO's profile, a task which became increasingly important as military issues began to dominate international politics once more. In 1936 he was posted to Singapore to head up the Eastern Bureau Epidemiological Intelligence Service whilst the Director, C.L.Park, was on sabbatical. Although the job was primarily concerned with the collection and dissemination of epidemiological statistics, Mackenzie seized the opportunity to publicise the Bureau's achievements and explain the broader work of the LNHO. In a series of newspaper articles and radio broadcasts, he undertook to explain how 'essential' the Bureau was, and how much the Eastern countries relied on it because of its information sharing function.[69]

A far more exciting task awaited him. In November 1937 Secretary-General Avenol summoned Mackenzie to appoint him Chair of the China Committee. It was a reasonable choice given Mackenzie's experience and ability, but when placed in the context of internal League politics, Avenol's decision acquires new significance. It is well known that Avenol sought to drive Rajchman out of the LNHO, but rather less known is the part Mackenzie played in the process. Whilst Avenol was influenced by fascist sympathies, Mackenzie's motives are far harder to define. Rajchman appears to be the only colleague Mackenzie ever really disliked, as his discretion masked most of his other personal opinions. In many ways, Mackenzie's antipathy is explicable as typical of the British administration, but it was complicated by personal dogma and mitigated by sympathy by Rajchman's ambitious goals for the LNHO.

The British government was opposed to Rajchman's ambitions for LNHO expansion, which he expressed thus in a 1922 memo: 'the [Health] Section should regard as its duty the initiation of action which, at the present time, no single administration by itself can undertake, of investigations of international concern and importance'. [70] George Buchanan and others claimed that this approach threatened British sovereignty and encroached on the remit of the tamer *Office International d'Hygiène Publique* (OIHP). They were also uncomfortable with Rajchman's frequent trips to China: Buchanan suspected him of 'motives more political than hygienical' when Rajchman initiated co-operation with the Chinese, and generally disliked Rajchman's outspoken political views.[71] His anti-colonialism, support for the Spanish Republicans and opposition to appeasement flew in the face of most of British foreign policy and led him to be considered a dangerous 'activist' by the administration.[72] When his support for Russian rapprochement was added to the mix, there seemed sufficient evidence of Communist leanings. Balinska argues that 'his real attitude regarding the Soviet Union as a regime remains difficult to define' and suggests that the climate of suspicion and anti-Semitism in the 1930s was partly to blame for his being labelled a Communist.[73] She names M.T.Morgan of the OIHP as one of the British collaborators in his downfall, but omits Mackenzie's role. By the time Avenol approached Mackenzie in late 1937, two attempts had already been made to sideline Rajchman through reorganising the Health Section and forbidding his return to China. Mackenzie's account of his meeting with Avenol reveals a new tactic, whereby Avenol seized the opportunity of Rajchman's absence in London to create a post above and beyond his powers:

'He [Avenol] said he had specially selected me because he had complete confidence in my ability, tact and integrity. He said: "I have absolute trust in you and it is on my special instructions that you will undertake this work. You will be released from your Health Section duties, and, whilst on this work, you will be solely responsible to me and the Assembly". I said "Do I represent the Health Section?", and he said: "You have no connection with the Health Section now. You are not being made chairman of this committee as a doctor but as an individual whom I feel I can trust to act wisely, tactfully and efficiently to make this piece of League work successful, and it is not an easy job. You will be open to all kinds of criticism from League governments and financial controllers, but I know you can do it". He went on to say that he realised that during all my time at the League I had never allowed politics to affect my judgement. It means, of course, that as far as China work is concerned I am now far above Rajchman, because no expenditure can be made without my committee's sanction"'. Mackenzie went on to say 'Rajchman knows nothing of all this and he will be furious when he knows that everything connected with China must be approved by my committee and bear my signature'.[74]

Judging from this, Mackenzie shared Avenol's dislike for Rajchman and agreed with marginalising him. Haswell states, 'it is clear, from his correspondence, that Melville had very little time for his superior in the health section, a Dr Rajchman'.[75] Sadly, as the correspondence has since been destroyed, Haswell's impression is all that survives, and his is the only account of the incident. Although it is evident that Avenol respected and trusted Mackenzie (despite his general dislike of Britons) we have no indication of whether this was reciprocated. Mackenzie's moderate views, respect for Jewish colleagues and empathy with the Abyssinians make it implausible that he shared Avenol's fascist leanings. So, why the dislike of Rajchman? His one surviving description, via Haswell, of his Director is that he was 'always involved in intrigues and very Bolshevist in tendencies and sympathies'. In contrast, Mackenzie was wedded to the belief that healthcare and politics must be kept separate, though privately erring on the side of conservatism. Despite insisting that politics could be forced to serve healthcare, [76] he also warned against health developments which were too far ahead of political ones. [77] He never really articulated this as a coherent philosophy, and his high-ranking involvement in health policy and diplomacy illustrate that his definition of 'politics' was a narrow and inconsistent one. Nonetheless, he had been convinced of the dangers of explicitly combining a specific political dogma with health by his experience in Russia, and no doubt the Japanese rebuke of Rajchman's 'anti-Japanese' stance which lead to his grounding in Geneva had strengthened this belief. Furthermore, the harrowing sickness and poverty Mackenzie had witnessed in Russia had certainly persuaded him that the reality of Communism was no utopia. No surprise, then, that he disagreed both with Rajchman's suspected political beliefs and the way he allowed them to mix with health policy.

In many ways Mackenzie seemed to share the social and political conservatism of the British medical administration, and thus disliked Rajchman by default, but with an important exception. Mackenzie was a strong supporter of strengthening the LNHO and international collaboration, unlike Buchanan, and was subsequently a key figure in creating the far more powerful and autonomous WHO. He cannot have found Rajchman's activism in this field so unpalatable, and, indeed, in a rare academic mention Mackenzie is described as one of the able men around Rajchman who shared his ambitious goals for the LNHO.[78] Mackenzie must have respected Rajchman's talents and their professional relationship appears to have been successful one. Rajchman described Mackenzie in 1929 as 'a pleasant man of excellent character... you can trust him completely'[79] and he often addressed him as 'Dear Mackenzie'. However, unusually, Mackenzie's reply was always a more formal 'Dear Dr. Rajchman' and his letters lacked the family enquiries and suggested visits which sprinkle so much of his correspondence with other old colleagues.

The sizeable amount of money assigned for China by the League and Mackenzie's role in distributing it was widely reported in the press, although the exact figure is unclear.[80] The LN archive corroborates most of the practical details in Haswell's account, confirming that Mackenzie acted as the Secretary-General's representative whilst in China for about six weeks, and that he had freedom to act at his own discretion. His mission was to devise an anti-epidemic plan which suited both the League Commission and the Chinese government.[81] Correspondence with his friend Lugard also mentions that whilst in Geneva Mackenzie was heavily involved with equipping Chinese units and was preparing for a visit himself.[82] As in Liberia, although now dealing with a medical question, he was acting in a diplomatic capacity and had to handle issues such as Chinese accusations of LNHO espionage. He was in China for March and April 1939, a fraught time overshadowed by the imminent Japanese invasion, waves of refugees and epidemics, and the disappearance of valued colleague Boudrez. It seems that most of Mackenzie's time was spent worrying about dwindling finances and trying to make savings wherever possible. It appears that he was only appointed on a temporary basis, awaiting the appointment of his successor, but he had considerable influence on the choice and managed to persuade the Secretary-General to change his original decision in favour of his own preferred candidate.[83] It is unclear why he was only temporary, though it may be because he was needed back in Geneva, and his letters to Lord Lugard imply he was not happy to be based in China at that time. The LN archive does not provide positive evidence for Haswell's assertion that Mackenzie was Secretary of the China Committee, as there is only a letter which he signed as 'Acting Secretary' in 1938.[84] It looks as if Rajchman yet again deflected Avenol's attempt to sideline him and continued to be significantly involved. Mackenzie consulted him when the Chinese made allegations of espionage against the LNHO employee Dr Jettmar, and Rajchman's personal contacts with the Chinese Prime Minister appeared to play a vital role in resolving the affair satisfactorily to preserve LNHO presence in China. The international situation was worsening, and the League's survival seemed ever more precarious, but Mackenzie's continued activity into 1939 indisputably refutes assumptions such as Jürgen Osterhammel's, that every League organisation had ceased co-operation with China after Rajchman's departure in 1934.[85]

Mackenzie's return from China in 1939 brings us to the end of Mackenzie's interwar activities and his service with the League of Nations, although it was in fact the beginning of the most powerful and prestigious part of his international career. Secretary-General Sean Lester appointed him acting Director of the LNHO, but concerns for family safety and his desire to serve his own Government meant he only remained briefly.[86] It is revealing that in times of crisis, Mackenzie's allegiance to his homeland asserted itself. The family's car journey across France in mid-May 1940 was a hair-raising one, surrounded by refugees fleeing the approaching Nazi troops, and it was only when they reached England that they learnt about the Dunkirk disaster they had so narrowly escaped. It was not long before Mackenzie was recalled to international affairs, and once again his British nationality put him at the centre of action as a pivotal member of the United Nations Relief and Rehabilitation Administration (UNRRA). This inevitably led to him playing a major role in the Technical Preparatory Committee which crafted the WHO, and he then attended World Health Assemblies as the British Chief Delegate and was later on the WHO Executive Board, which he chaired 1953 – 54. However, despite ostensibly belonging to the 'new' organisations which sought so hard to distance themselves from their League predecessor, Mackenzie remained very aware of his inter-war past.[87] The LNHO 'epistemic community', or knowledge-based community, continued despite the decimation of its Geneva staff-base and Mackenzie remained an active member through his contacts with old colleagues and friends. This community succeeded in transmitting its experiences and beliefs from the LNHO to the WHO and thus created a direct descendant, with the help of actors like Mackenzie.[88]

Mackenzie was a firm believer in the lessons of experience,[89] and his determination to create an organisation buffered from political pressures was the most obvious example of what he had learnt from watching the crumbling League Disarmament Commission bring down the reputation of the LNHO. In 1945 he made this quite explicit: 'we must not overlook the problems attendant on harnessing medical work too closely to a world-wide political international body whose fate it must necessarily share'.[90] The result was a classic commitment to the functionalist separability-priority hypothesis, ie, that the technical concerns of health can be removed from politics and pursued separately.[91] In this respect, he was side by side with Buchanan. And yet, he also endorsed the concomitant idea of 'spillover', whereby successes in the health arena can bring about political successes. In words more reminiscent of Rajchman, he declared medicine to be 'the greatest of the sciences lending its help in the cause of peace'.[92] Yet again, Mackenzie characterised that which frustrated him in international medicine as 'political', but positive achievements were seen as 'peaceful'. During the inter-war years, Mackenzie had seen the great achievements in health which inter-governmental co-operation could produce, but he had also seen how governments could destroy a health system and bring down a health organisation. His contradictory beliefs about health and politics are an unsurprising reflection of his circumstances, and were shared by many contemporaries. It was their post-war hope (now seen as a dream) that the advantages of international co-operation could be extracted from experience without the disadvantages, and this hope shaped the foundation of the WHO.

Although it is increasingly anachronistic, the cliché of the British 'stiff upper lip' is apt for Mackenzie. His reserved reports, with their attention to practical detail and procedure rather than social ideology, admittedly make for less interesting reading than the manifestos of Rajchman. Mackenzie's preference for the anonymity of the League and his suppression of his views make him seem a less colourful character than those who used the League as a public podium. Nonetheless, beneath his studiously neutral exterior was a passionate and adventurous humanitarian motivated by high ideals just like his more outspoken colleagues. We must not take Mackenzie's carefully crafted image of a detached bureaucrat at face value. He did have strong personal views, and they did influence his professional decisions. In his quiet way he shaped the course of inter-war and post-war international health.

Acknowledgements
My particular thanks go to Mary May, nee Mackenzie, for all her help and in particular for providing the Haswell manuscript. I am also indebted to Bernhardine Pejovic and her colleagues at the League of Nations Archive in Geneva for their assistance with locating material. For editorial comments on this paper I thank Iris Borowy for her patient insight, and Peter Turner for his questions, and I am very grateful to Somerville College, Oxford for financial assistance via the Margaret Pollock Fund.

---

1 C.J.D. Haswell, *The Doctor Who Stopped A War*, (unpublished family manuscript), 63.

2 V-Y. Ghebali, 'The Politicisation of UN Specialised Agencies: A Preliminary Analysis', *Millennium: Journal of International Studies* (Winter, 1985), 322.

3 D. Mitrany, 'The Functional Approach in Historical Perspective', *International Affairs*, 537.

4 M.D. Mackenzie, *Medical Relief In Europe* (London: Royal Institute of International Affairs, 1942), 61 – 2.

5 J. Siddiqui, *World Health and World Politics*, (London: Hurst, 1995), 50-51; see ch. 6 for a discussion of the literature on functionalism and politicisation.

6 M.D. Mackenzie, Acting Director, LNHO to MacNalty, Chief Medical Officer, MoH, 26 September 1939 and MacNalty to Mackenzie 31 January 1940, The National Archive (TNA) file MH 107/56; see also M.D. Mackenzie, Acting Director of the Health Section, to the Secretary-General, 16 February 1939, LONA R 6118/8A/37224/15197.

7 See scattered references throughout the work of his personal friend N.M. Goodman, *International Health Organisations and their Work* (London: J.& A.Churchill, 1952); his photograph in *WHO, The First Ten Years of the World Health Organisation* (Geneva: WHO, 1958), 161; one mention in G. Woodbridge, *UNRRA* (New York: UN, 1950); one (inaccurate) sentence in M. Dubin, 'The League of Nations Health Organisation' in P.J. Weindling (ed.), *International Health Organisations and Movements 1918 – 1939* (Cambridge: CUP, 1995), 70; one brief reference in P.J. Weindling, *Epidemics and Genocide in Eastern Europe, 1890 – 1945* (Oxford: OUP, 2000), 172; extensive analysis in Z.C. Sprigings, *LNHO to WHO: From the Last of the League to the First of the United Nations* (Oxford University 3rd year thesis, 2007), chapter 2.

8 F.P. Walters, *A History of the League of Nations* (London: OUP, 1952), 814.

9 The definition of transnational used here is that of Nye and Keohane, via P.Clavin: ' "contracts, coalitions and interactions across state boundaries" that were not directly controlled by the central policy organs of government'; she describes the League as 'formally inter-governmental in control, highly multinational in the range of personnel

it employed and ... both international and transnational in its operations'; P.Clavin, 'Defining Transnationalism', *Contemporary European History*, 14, 4 (2005), 425-6.

10 Haswell, *The Doctor*, 4 – 5.

11 M.D. Mackenzie's 'Curriculum Vitae', TNA file MH 107/56.

12 I.Whitehead, 'The Training of Doctors for War' in R.Cooter, M.Harrison and S.Sturdy (eds), *Medicine and Modern Warfare* (Amsterdam: Rodopi, 1999), 163 – 9.

13 Haswell, *The Doctor*, 6.

14 Ibid., 39.

15 Ibid., 40.

16 Whitehead, 'The Training of Doctors', 166.

17 Mackenzie, *Medical Relief*, 8-9.

18 Haswell, *The Doctor*, 35.

19 Haswell, *The Doctor*, 17.

20 Haswell, *The Doctor*, 29.

21 J. Beinart, 'Darkly Through a Lens: Changing Perceptions of the African Child In Sickness and in Health, 1900-1945' in R. Cooter (ed.), *In The Name of the Child: Health and Welfare 1880 – 1940* (London: Routledge, 1992), 226 – 8.

22 Haswell, *The Doctor*, 35.

23 Mackenzie, 'Curriculum Vitae'.

24 L. Wilkinson and A. Hardy, *Prevention and Cure: The LSHTM*, (London: Regan Paul, 2001), 69.

25 Reference from H. Kerr for M.D. Mackenzie, 1 October 1924, TNA file MH 107/56.

26 Haswell, *The Doctor*, 39.

27 M.A. Balinska, 'Assistance and Not Mere Relief' in P.J. Weindling (ed.), *International Health Organisations and Movements 1918 – 1939* (Cambridge: CUP, 1995), 97.

28 'Day to Day in Liverpool' in the *Liverpool Daily Post*, 3 March 1922.

29 M.D. Mackenzie to mother and brother, 8 October 1922, Friends' House Archive (FHA) Mackenzie Papers, slide 272.

30 M.D. Mackenzie diary entry August 1922, FHA Mackenzie Papers, slide 230.

31 M. D. Mackenzie to mother and brother, 2 January 1923, FHA Mackenzie Papers (slide 301) said he would be Head of the Unit for a while, which included responsibility for feeding 100,000 people; M.D. Mackenzie, 'A New Scourge in Russia', *Huddersfield Daily Examiner*, 22 June 1922, said he was acting Chief Medical Officer of the International Nansen Relief Committee to cover absence; M.D. Mackenzie's 'Curriculum Vitae', 5, TNA file MH 107/56 said he was 'for a short time acting Senior Medical Officer to the Nansen Relief Administration in all of Russia'; Haswell, *The Doctor*, 50, reports M.D. Mackenzie's letter verbatim saying he would be acting Chief Medical Oficer and Haswell, *The Doctor*, 86, reports verbatim a letter from the Executive Secretary of the American Service Committee in Moscow and verbatim from M.D. Mackenzie's letter of 4 August 1922 which showed he was Senior Medical Officer of both the British and American units for a time.

32 Haswell, *The Doctor*, 87.

33 Mackenzie, *Medical Relief*, 65.

34 M.D.Mackenzie to mother and brother, 6 November 1922, FHA Mackenzie Papers, slide 277.

35 Haswell, *The Doctor*, 63.

36 M.D. Mackenzie to G. Dawson, 18 October 1923, FHA Mackenzie Papers, slide 2.

37 Unnamed newspaper article 21 March 1923 reports his 'brief visit' to England to raise awareness and funds for the Russian Famine Relief Mission. FHA Mackenzie Papers.

38 P.J. Weindling, *Epidemics and Genocide in Eastern Europe, 1890 – 1945* (Oxford: OUP, 2000), 146 – 8.
39 H. Mackay and M.D. Mackenzie, 'An Investigation into the Present Health of German Children', *Lancet* (22 March 1924), 615-17.
40 Reference from F.E. Fremantle for M.D. Mackenzie, 30 September 1924, TNA file MH 107/56.
41 F.E. Fremantle to G. Newman, 28 March 1924, TNA file MH 107/56.
42 H.A.L. to E.W.H. Millar, 19 January 1928, TNA File MH 107/56.
43 P. Weindling, 'The LNHO and the Rise of Latin American Participation, 1920-40', *História, Ciências, Saúde-Manguinhos*, 13:3 (2000), 3.
44 Handwritten note by Lord Lugard, West Africa. Liberia: Notes, 1931-3, Rhodes House Library (RHL) Lord Lugard Papers, MSS.Lugard Box 60 File 4.
45 M.D. Mackenzie, *Confidential Report on Public Health in Liberia*, C.H.1065 (Geneva: LN, 1931), 2 – 8.
46 F.J.D. Lugard and M.D. Mackenzie correspondence 1932 – 6, RHL Lord Lugard Papers, MSS.Lugard Box 60 File 3.
47 A. H. M. Kirk-Greene, 'Lugard, Frederick John Dealtry, Baron Lugard (1858–1945)', *Oxford Dictionary of National Biography* (Oxford: OUP, 2004).
48 M.D. Mackenzie to F.J.D. Lugard, 7 March 1934, RHL Lord Lugard Papers, MSS.Lugard Box 60 File 3; M.D. Mackenzie to F.J.D. Lugard, 9 March 1934, RHL Lord Lugard Papers, MSS. Lugard Box 60 File 3.
49 M.D. Mackenzie to F.J.D. Lugard, 20 November 1935, RHL Lord Lugard Papers, MSS. Lugard Box 60 File 4.
50 M.D. Mackenzie correspondence with mother, SOAS Mackenzie Collection, MS 380483, Box 1, File 2 & Box 2, File 6.
51 M.D. Mackenzie, 5 July 1932, SOAS Mackenzie Collection, MS 380483, Box 2, File 8.
52 Mackenzie, *Public Health in Liberia*, 9 – 14.
53 Haswell, *The Doctor*, 139.
54 'League Saves 12 000 Lives', *Daily Telegraph* (27 October 1932).
55 Unnamed newspaper cutting provided by Mary May, entitled 'Scotsman's Example to Europe: Disarmament this Way'.
56 Sasstown, Bollow, Dio and Wiseepo leaders to LN, 30 November 1936, LONA R 5662/50/10419/323
57 F.J.D. Lugard to M.D. Mackenzie, 5 November 1935, RHL Lord Lugard Papers, MSS.Lugard Box 60 File 3.
58 R. Gautier to Secretary-General and Treasurer, 13 February 1934, Geneva, LONA R 6088/8A/12884/3583.
59 'Review', *British Medical Journal* (8 September 1934), 479.
60 Ibid., 479.
61 M.D. Mackenzie, 'Recent Tendencies in the Development of General Hospitals in England', *Quarterly Bulletin of the Health Organisation*, Vol. III (1934), 220 – 288.
62 M.D. Mackenzie to C.L. Park, 30 May 1932, LONA R 5935/8A/36646/36646.
63 M.D. Mackenzie, 'Report on Dr Mackenzie's Visit to London', 27 March 1935, LONA R 6118/8A/37224/15197.
64 M.D. Mackenzie to Secretary-General, 16 February 1939, LONA R 5935/8A/37224/15197.
65 'Review', *British Medical Journal* (12 August 1939), 355.
66 M.D. Mackenzie to F.J.D. Lugard, 7 March 1934, RHL Lord Lugard Papers, MSS. Lugard Box 60 File 4.

67 M.D. Mackenzie, 'International Collaboration in Health', *International Affairs*, 26:4 (October 1950), 520.
68 Mackenzie, *Medical Relief*, 60.
69 'Unceasing War on Plague', *The Straits Times*, 31 March 1937.
70 I. Borowy, 'Manoeuvering for Space. International health work of the League of Nations during the Second World War', in S. Gross Solomon, P. Zylberman and L. Murard (eds), *On Shifting Ground:Health and Space in the Twentieth Century*, in press, p.1.
71 J. Osterhammel, 'Technical Co-Operation Between the League of Nations and China', *Modern Asian Studies*, 12:4 (1979), 664. Also Dubin, *LNHO*, 61 – 2.
72 J.A. Gillespie, 'Social Medicine, Social Security and International Health,1940-60' in E.Rodriguez-Ocanana (ed.), *The Politics of the Healthy Life: an International Perspective* (Sheffield: EAHMH Publication, 2002), 222.
73 M.A. Balinska, *For the Good of Humanity* (Budapest: Central European University Press,1998), 104.
74 Haswell, *The Doctor*, 250-1.
75 Ibid., 250.
76 Mackenzie, *Medical Relief*, 62.
77 Mackenzie, 'Potentialities of International Collaboration in the Field of Public Health', *American Journal of Public Health*, 35: 2 (Feb 1945), 102.
78 Dubin, *LNHO*, 70.
79 Rajchman to Flores, 25 October 1929 in LONA R 5911/8A/13967/13967, found by I. Borowy.
80 Newspaper (unknown title) 9 March 1939 reported in 'Eastern News in Brief' that Dr Mackenzie was going to China with £75 000 equivalent to 1.5m CHF; Times, 3 March 1939 reported that Dr Mackenzie was going to China with £15 000 equivalent to 1.5m CHF; Newspaper (unknown title) reported in 'Today's New's Name' that Dr Mackenzie was going to China with £75 000. Newspaper clippings provided by Mary May. Haswell, *The Doctor*, 250, states he was administering 2m CHF. The archival record is unclear, mentioning only that '500 000 Francs of the Chinese contribution will be lodged in Chinese money in China to the credit of the League and particularly in this connection you will be required to see that general arrangements are made with regard to the method and character of expenditure'. However, there is no mention of the entire amount allocated for the China effort. Smets or Lester to M.D. Mackenzie, 23 February 1939, letter outlining his duties and responsibilities whilst in China, LONA, R 5789/50/37258/30817.
81 For example: M.D. Mackenzie, Representative with the Chinese Government of the Secretary-General of the League of Nations, Kunming, 17 April 1939 to Dr Pollitzer. LONA R 5780/50/31861/30817; Ibid., Smets or Lester to M.D.Mackenzie, 23 February 1939.
82 M.D. Mackenzie to F.J.D. Lugard, 20 July 1938, Geneva, RHL Lord Lugard Papers, MSS.Lugard Box 8, File 4; and note by M.D.Mackenzie to be published in the *Lancet*, RHL Lord Lugard Papers, MSS.Lugard Box 95 File 3.
83 Smets to Treasurer, 4 April 1939, LONA R 5790/50/37503/30817, and see R 5776/50/31302/30817 whole file for development of debate.
84 M.D. Mackenzie, Acting Secretary of the Council Committee for Technical Collaboration with China, to Mr Lester, 26 August 1938, LONA R 5786/50/33625/30817; see also C. Smets, Secretary of the Council Committee for Technical Collaboration with China, to General Lasnet, 13 April 1939, Geneva, LONA Box R 5776/50/31302/30817.
85 Osterhammel, 'Technical Co-Operation', 680.

86 Mackenzie, Acting Director, LNHO to MacNalty, Chief Medical Officer, MoH, 26 September 1939 and MacNalty to Mackenzie 31 January 1940, TNA file MH 107/56.
87 Walters, *A History,* 814.
88 Sprigings, *LNHO to WHO*, Ch.3 for a discussion of 'epistemic community' in the post-1939 LNHO context.
89 Mackenzie, 'Potentialities of International Collaboration', 101 – 2.
90 Ibid., 102.
91 Siddiqui, *World Health*, 206 – 7.
92 M.D. Mackenzie, 'World Co-operation on Health' in *Problems of Peace,* 12th Series (London: Allen and Unwin, 938), 75.

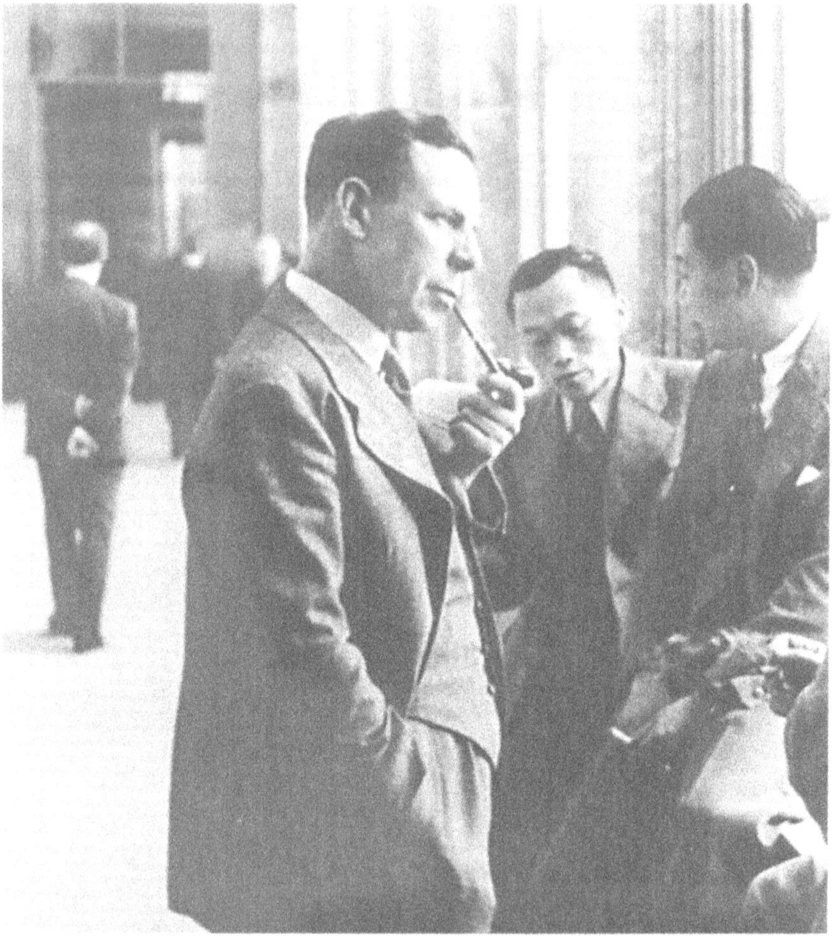

Melville Mackenzie

Actions not Words.
Thorvald Madsen, Denmark, and International Health. 1902-1939.

Anne Hardy[1]

The Danish physician Thorvald Madsen was born into a well-to-do Copenhagen family in 1870. Qualifying in medicine in 1894, Madsen is best known to posterity as the Director of the Danish State Serum Institute (DSSI) from 1907 to 1940, and as President of the League of Nations Health Committee from 1921 to 1937 (and Honorary president 1937-40). Both at the DSSI and at the LNHO, Madsen operated at the core of international humanitarian medical activity in the first forty years of the twentieth century. As a biographical subject, Madsen looks promising, since he left a voluminous archive, and he also features in LNHO related diaries, letters and other documents. Piecing together his official life and concerns from these records is not difficult, but penetrating the personal motives, principles and beliefs which determined his activities is more so. There is no explicit evidence of his political, religious and philosophical ideas or how these influenced his activities. He was not given to ruminations in print or at interview; his memoirs and reminiscences are largely factual and anecdotal. His parents were both said to have come of 'puritanical' Protestant stock, but there is no evidence of puritanism in Madsen's own life. On the contrary. He was something of a social snob. He enjoyed hob-nobbing with Royalty and staying in royal palaces (especially that of Jaegerspris, on the coast on Roskilde Fjord); he loved horse-riding, skating and large cars; and society, eating and dancing. His surviving correspondence is almost pathologically discreet in personal terms, and his portraiture shows a blandly smiling gentleman, the smooth contours of whose face give nothing away. Even his official biographer, who had known him personally, and talked to him about a biography some years before his death, seems to have had little insight into the convictions that drove him. He described Madsen as 'an alert, critical and constructive intelligence'.[2]

Educated in the days before psychology became fashionable, it seems probable that such an intelligence was not given to introspection and self-analysis. Madsen's social commitment is none the less apparent in the course of his career and into his retirement, when he worked in a voluntary capacity for UNICEF. It remains for the historian to examine the extent to which Madsen's career was influenced not just by a passion for science, but by a concern for the welfare of his fellow human beings; while influence and motivation may be difficult to ascertain, their effects at least may be examined. The biography was subtitled: "In the service of science and humankind". The historian may wish to challenge what was evidently a biased biographer's view, but the evidence suggests that there was indeed something in it.

Thorvald Madsen was born into a well-connected, well-to-do household, the only son in a family of four girls. He grew up in a privileged, politically and morally conscious world. His father, Vilhelm Hermann Oluf Madsen (1844-1917) was a military instructor from an army family, who crowned his career as Minster for War in Denmark's first liberal government, 1901-04. His mother, Albertine Petersen, (1838-1919) was the daughter of a country pastor, and a gentle, devout and devoted wife and mother. The young Madsen was, by his own account, inspired to seek a career in medicine as a result of the International Medical Congress held in Copenhagen in 1884. The eighth of its kind, the Congress attracted stellar medical personalities from across Europe, including Louis Pasteur, Joseph Lister and Queen Victoria's Physician, James Paget.[3] Modernising scientific medicine was present in force, and the Danish newspapers were filled with excited reportage. Copenhagen was then a small city of some 375,000 thousand souls.[4] It was still somewhat provincial, static in outlook, and with a volatile political culture.[5] The unfamiliar influx of international celebrities left the city seething with excitement, which deeply impressed the fourteen-year-old schoolboy, and, by his own account, determined him on a medical career.[6] He enrolled as a medical student at 16, and qualified aged 23 in 1893.

Late nineteenth-century Denmark was undergoing a period of rapid social and economic change. With the loss of Schleswig and Holstein to Prussia in 1864, Denmark had finally relinquished her past as a dominant Baltic power. The flood of American wheat into Europe had undermined her cereal-based farming economy after 1870, and the agricultural industry shifted emphasis, towards livestock and especially dairy farming. Although right-wing conservative governments continued to dominate parliament with the support of the Crown until 1901 (despite formidable opposition in the lower house of parliament), social legislation began to be implemented after 1880 following the German model, with the dual intention of benefiting the population and pre-empting socialist reformers. Traditionally, the Danish Crown exercised a benevolent autocracy, and Danes have tended to the conservative, viewing state activity and intervention as being directed to the public good. Indeed, the state's record in this respect was positive in the nineteenth century, including public education and a system of provincial district medical officers with preventive responsibilities, and later old age pensions, subsidies to the mutual sickness funds, and free treatment in infectious disease hospitals.[7] It is perhaps a testimony to the confidence, which the Danes invested in the state and in medicine that compulsory childhood vaccination against smallpox, implemented from 1810, was said to be viewed by the population with 'the greatest confidence'.[8]

The Danish medical world which Madsen entered was caught between the active stream of modernising scientific medicine and the broad, slow-moving river of established medical values and practices. In the course of his education, Madsen experienced this confluence from both sides. He was not an outstandingly diligent or brilliant student, although he was reportedly generally regarded as someone who would go far.[9] He certainly seems to have enjoyed his time as a medical student, following the traditional and rather unsystematic teaching available in the Copenhagen hospitals, and participating happily in student life and culture.[10] Part of his training was spent in Sweden, at the universities of Lund, where he practised dissection for a month in January 1891, and later, after he had qualified, at Uppsala, where he studied 'physiological chemistry' (biochemistry) for 3 months in 1896.[11] His Swedish experiences alerted him to differences in medical culture, not just between but also within national boundaries: social relations between staff and pupils were much more formal in Uppsala than in Lund; student life, however, was extremely lively in both.

Madsen's journey to Lund came about as the result of deficiencies in the provision for anatomical study within Danish medical education in the 1890s. The acquisition of corpses for dissection was still problematic in Copenhagen, and it was the practice for students to go to Lund where cadavers were easily obtained. Madsen described how the Danish students were taken down into the cadaver-cellar, where a great wooden chest held stacks of salted corpses. The laboratory assistant rummaged about among them, pulling up various arms, until he found one he considered suitable. He then hauled it out, threw it over his shoulder - it was frozen stiff - and hefted it to the dissecting room. As the Danish students did not have the time to use up the wealth of material made available to them, they were allowed to pack a chest to take home. Madsen never forgot the expression on the face of the Copenhagen customs official who insisted the box be opened: it was shut again in the greatest possible hurry.[12]

The deficiencies of medical education in Copenhagen, and the resistance of some medical staff to new ideas,[13] notwithstanding, the university did afford an opportunity to get to grips with bacteriological methods. Carl Julius Salomonson (1847-1924) had been professor of medical bacteriology in the university since setting up the University Medical Bacteriology Laboratory in 1886.[14] Operating in spartan conditions in a converted cellar in the Botanical Gardens, Salomonson offered the world's first taught course in bacteriology.[15] Salomonsen himself was an attractive character – Madsen described him then as young, happy and enthusiastic, and his laboratory as a hub.[16] In earlier years his course had attracted able students from all over Scandinavia, including the Danes Johannes Fibiger (1867-1928), who qualified as a doctor in 1890, and the distinguished veterinarian Bernhard Bang (1848-1932), but by the early 1890s something of a reaction to the early enthusiasm for bacteriology had set in. In Madsen's year, he was one of only two students enrolled for the course, and his contemporaries were bemused by his choice of option: 'What actually is it that you are messing about with?' they asked him. For themselves, they were only interested in getting into practice.[17]

The precocious intellectual attraction which Madsen himself highlighted as influencing his choice of career path may not have been the only factor at work. His interest may have been reinforced by personal experiences which he did not choose to publicise. Diphtheria was the scourge of Denmark's small population in the 1880s. It reached a peak in 1893, with a total of 23,695 notified cases, and a case-fatality rate of 12%.[18] In the summer of 1889, during one of the epidemic waves of the disease, Madsen contracted diphtheria, and was removed to Copenhagen's isolation hospital for treatment. His youngest sister also caught the infection. Too ill to be moved, she died at home, aged just 12 years old. His biographer remarks that the tragedy devastated the family, and surmises that the episode 'presumably first awoke his interest in diphtheria'.[19] Madsen himself nowhere refers to this experience; indeed his reminiscences are almost entirely free of family matters, but it seems probable that this episode taught him much about the physical and emotional suffering inflicted by infectious disease.[20]

Having recovered from his illness, Madsen went on to qualify as a doctor in 1893. That autumn, by long-standing arrangement, he journeyed to Hadsten in Jutland to work as assistant to a country practitioner, beginning on 1 November. Here he experienced the realities of medical practice in an age when medicine still had very limited therapeutic competence.[21] He had, however, already agreed to return to work with Salomonson, even though the latter at that time had no means of employing him.[22] Fortuitously, however, 1894 proved a seminal year in the history of diphtheria. That summer, Emile Roux announced the successful trials of diphtheria anti-toxin treatment at the *Hopital des Infants Malades* in Paris. Salomonsen made the trip to Paris in September 1894 to discover the miracle for himself.[23] On his return he sought, and was given, funding to establish a new serotherapeutic division within the department of medical bacteriology. Madsen was appointed its director. Although the new division was housed in two tiny rooms on university premises in Ny Vestergade, and consisted only of Madsen, a woman assistant and a lab technician, it was charged with producing diphtheria anti-toxin to meet the needs of Denmark and it dependencies – southern Jutland, Iceland, Greenland, the Faeroe Islands and Denmark's south Asian colonies.[24] Salomonson believed that there would be a rapid expansion in the diagnosis and treatment of infectious diseases, and he intended the SSI to foster the development of Danish expertise and research into serum treatments, microbiology and immunology. Early experience of expensive and poor quality products delivered by German pharmaceutical companies made him determined to improve the available diphtheria antitoxin and to develop new products rather than passively finance foreign firms.[25]

From 1894, Madsen's burgeoning research career was therefore focused on diphtheria and its treatment. Discrepancies in and doubts over the efficacy of anti-toxin surfaced very early. Robert Koch's German version of the magic serum reached Copenhagen in the autumn of 1894, and proved a disappointment in trials at *Blegdamshospitalet* (the city's infectious disease hospital); given the recent mishap with Koch's claims for tuberculin, scepticism began to spread. At much the same time, clinicians at the hospital noted a change in the virulence of natural diphtheria – a phenomenon already observed in Sweden.[26] As a result, clinical trials were instituted over the period from 13 May 1896 to 13 May 1897. The serum used was produced by Madsen, but the trials were conducted by S.T.Sorenson, director of the hospital, Salomonson, and Johannes Fibiger, who had completed an MD thesis on diphtheria in 1895. The results, calculated by Fibiger, vindicated the new treatment, but Madsen was not convinced: the statistics did not tally with what he had himself observed in the hospital wards.[27]

Madsen's research in the 1890s focused on the diphtheria anti-toxin, more especially on the question of how its strength should be measured. Charged with the production of antitoxin in Ny Vestergade, he quickly discovered that it was no easy task. to deliver a product with a sufficiently high antiserum content. The first diphtheria strains he used produced a very modest antitoxin response; the horses proved variably sensitive to the toxin, and there were big differences in the levels of antitoxin production in individual animals.[28] Madsen initiated a series of experiments to clarify the optimum methods for antitoxin production, and in 1896 defended his MD thesis, 'Experimental researches on diphtheria toxin'. Here Madsen compared the rival German and French production techniques, and concluded that the former was undoubtedly superior. 'It would be a great advantage', he wrote, 'if international agreement could be reached on the determination of diphtheria antitoxin's strength'.[29] This was the first appearance in his work of the concept of the international standardisation of biological products which was to feature largely in his subsequent career, and became the field in which he made his major contribution to international health.[30] The nature of the relationship between diphtheria toxin and anti-toxin was clearly a crucial element in resolving the issues around anti-toxin production, and Madsen turned his attention in this direction. It was a problem that also concerned Paul Ehrlich (1854-1915), and in 1899 Madsen visited Ehrlich in Berlin with a view to improving his understanding of the problems associated with toxin production. It was not, intellectually, a satisfactory visit. Madsen found Ehrlich much preoccupied with his side-chain receptor theory, but was himself unconvinced about the side-chains, and also by Ehrlich's ideas on the diphtheria toxin/antitoxin question.[31]

Meanwhile, public enthusiasm in Denmark for the new therapeutic agent, and pressure from provincial doctors for the distribution of anti-toxin free to all medical practitioners, set political wheels moving. Both Salomonsen and Madsen were well connected politically and they manoeuvred for a new serum institute attached to Copenhagen University. The University, however, felt it to be beyond its responsibility to enter pharmaceutical production, and a bill sponsored by the Ministry of Justice established the new institute as part of the health service. The law directing the creation of a state serum institute for the manufacture of diphtheria anti-toxin was passed in March 1901, and on 9 September 1902 the new institute, Statens Seruminstitut (SSI), opened its doors under Salomonson's direction. From the first, it was an institution with a mission: Salomonson believed that there would be a rapid expansion in the diagnosis and treatment of infectious diseases, and he intended the SSI to foster the development of Danish expertise and research into serum treatments, microbiology and immunology. Here again the early experience of expensive and poor quality products delivered by German pharmaceutical companies determined efforts to improve the available diphtheria antitoxin and to develop new products rather than passively finance foreign firms through purchases from abroad.[32]

The law establishing the institute was one of the very last acts of the right wing government, which later in 1901 gave way to Denmark's first liberal government, formed on the basis of a majority in the lower house of parliament. Following some turbulent years, the existing health board resigned, to be replaced by a new 'Health Commission'- a mixed cross-party board of health professionals and politicians. The commission's proposals for the re-organisation of the central and local health administration were accepted, as was a proposal to extend the remit of the SSI. It was now to research all infectious diseases as well as methods of alleviating their consequences. Moreover, the Health Commission set out its views on the utility of the SSI very explicitly. The institute was, it vouchsafed, 'established as a human and socially useful institution'. It further expressed the view that: 'by reducing hospital costs, and the costs of epidemics, and the consequent losses in trade and commerce which the infectious diseases bring about, [the Institute] will more than compensate the State for the costs of maintaining it'.[33] The idea that public health measures would result in savings to the public purse was, of course, not a new one, having motivated Edwin Chadwick, for example, in jump-starting the English public health reform movement in the 1830s.[34] None the less, its re-emergence in the context of the modernising Danish state reflects an enduring influence as a motive power for state involvement in matters of health. If the founding of the State Serum Institute was in itself a testament to Danish faith in medical research and the therapeutic promise of the new bacteriology, it was also part of the state's wider determination to limit the damage inflicted on its people and economy by infectious disease.

The amended act came into force in 1910. At this point Salomonson moved on to become Rector of Copenhagen University, and to focus his energies on his latest project - the new university Pathology Institute.[35] Madsen replaced him as director of the newly re-constituted State Serum Institute, and in the years that followed developed and elaborated the institution's role not only as a national facility but as a research establishment with an international reputation and international responsibilities. In part these developments came about as unforeseen consequences of the First World War and post-war international collaborative efforts towards peace, but their roots can also be traced in the SSI's pre-war operations and in the role which, under Madsen's leadership, it came to play in international welfare efforts during the war itself. Between 1910 and 1940, the SSI continued to play a central role in Denmark's own public health system but this core role was soon enveloped by a wide-ranging series of responsibilities for the international supply and monitoring of vaccines and sera, and the typing of strains of infectious disease. When the SSI was founded, Denmark already had a network of infectious disease hospitals providing free accommodation and treatment. The local administration of contagious disease prevention was vested in local Epidemic Committees composed of the chief of police, the local medical officer, and three elected lay representatives. In other words, the key to preventive action – and consequently the financial responsibility - rested with the lay members of the local community, although the active force in the committee was usually the medical officer. The system produced a remarkable degree of co-operation and compliance among patients and their families; by the 1930s it was generally assumed that the infectious disease hospitals were the natural locus of care for infectious patients.[36] From its earliest days, the Serum Institute fed into this preventive network by providing a central diagnostic facility for the country as a whole, and acting as epidemiological surveillance agent. It was also active in researching and trialling new products that might assist in the prevention of specific diseases; by 1930, for example, it was using its own whooping cough vaccine with a notable degree of success.[37]

It had been Salomonsen's vision that the SSI would not only provide anti-toxin to all Denmark, its colonies and dependencies, so freeing it from an expensive dependence on imported products, but also contribute to a dramatic extension in the diagnosis and treatment of infections generally. On both these counts, Madsen, first as director of research and then as Salomonsen's successor was to extend this aim – the SSI was to make best quality biologicals available as widely and as cheaply as possible. Already in 1903, the SSI was producing 8,800 four-unit doses of anti-toxin, at the cost of 25 ore (3 old pence) each; a comparable German serum was priced at 6.23 kroner (6 shillings and 3 pence).[38] The responsibility of serum production at the SSI resulted in a surge of associated research activity, as Madsen sought to refine antitoxin production methods and develop the understanding of immunological processes. International visits and visitors quickly became an integral part of the SSI's institutional life: as Madsen's biographer noted, 'the network of bacteriology became very tightly woven in these years'.[39] Even before the SSI was established, Madsen had embarked on travels to make contact with a range of leading researchers. Besides visiting Ehrlich and making friends with his assistant Julius Morgenroth and various other German researchers, he also visited von Behring, whom Ehrlich regarded as an arch-rival, and the Pasteur Institute; in 1901 made his first journey to the United States.[40] In the first decade of its existence, the SSI extended its research interests to the prevention and treatment of plague, cholera, syphilis and tetanus. In 1908, Madsen journeyed to St Petersburg to observe a severe outbreak of cholera. It was perhaps the second transforming experience of his life – he certainly recalled it in his last years as one of his greatest.[41] The account which he published on his return vividly conveys the horror of conditions in the wards, the anguish of the patients, the fear of their attendants, the pitiful ignominy of the dead. Denmark even in 1900 was a well-organised, hygiene conscious small country with high medical standards. The experience of Russia opened Madsen's eyes to extremes of poverty, disease and wretchedness.[42] If the International Congress of 1884 had committed him to the science of therapeutics, the Russian cholera of 1908 may have given him an awareness of broader social and medical issues.

With the outbreak of World War I, we can see Madsen's policies at the SSI taking a directly practical turn. The rapid evolution of trench warfare in the first months of the conflict resulted in an unforeseen explosion of tetanus infection among the wounded on both sides. While anti-tetanus serum had been developed a few years previously, none of the combatant countries had anything like sufficient supplies to meet the demand. By October 1914, tetanus infections were afflicting 34 per thousand wounded, with a case-fatality of 50 percent. Both British and German commanders were vociferous in their calls for supplies.[43] Denmark found herself in something of a tricky position at this point. She was a neutral state, but her peacetime economy was heavily dependent on trade with both England and Germany – and she too received the call for anti-tetanus serum. The SSI was initially in no position to help: it had only 2 horses devoted to production of the vital antiserum (enough to meet national need); the Danish economy had been destabilised by the outbreak of hostilities; and horses were a disappearing commodity commanding premium prices as German dealers swept the local markets to supply their military. The Ministry of Health refused to sanction funds for increased serum production. It did, however, agree that Madsen could take action entirely at his own financial risk. He borrowed money on his personal account and sent the stable manager out to buy horses, while the Institute's handyman improvised stabling. 46 horses were acquired and brought into production; by the end of the war the tetanus stud numbered around a hundred animals. And while the Danish supplies formed only part of a larger international effort, tetanus infection rates were down to 2 per thousand wounded by December 1914. Madsen, supplying serum to both combatants, cleared his debt, paid the SSI's running costs, and made a handsome profit for his political masters besides: in 1915, 29,000 kroner were handed over to the Danish Treasury.[44] A successful commercial enterprise perhaps, but Madsen also ensured that tetanus antiserum and a range of other sera and vaccines were being supplied free of charge to prisoner of war camps at the same time.[45] Here, already, we can see the importance of humanitarian impulses in the shaping of medical internationalism.

The plight of prisoners of war was very immediate to the educated Danish community. Already in October 1914, the Danish Red Cross had been instructed by the International Red Cross headquarters in Geneva to set up a prisoner-of-war department. Within months this had become a considerable enterprise, with a staff of 400 in offices by the waterfront in Copenhagen. By the end of the war, this operation held record cards for 3.5 million individuals.[46] Denmark's responsibilities were designated as German, Austrian and Hungarian prisoners held in camps in Russia, Siberia and Turkestan. Conditions across the region were appalling, and disease, hunger, cold and exhaustion rife. Hundreds of deaths were recorded daily. Of 25,000 POWs held in the Totzhoele camp, 17,000 died.[47] (The exaction location of this camp is uncertain; 'Totzhoele' brings up no hits on Google.) As an eminent scientist and director of an institutional benefactor, Madsen was called upon by the Red Cross to join its teams of observers on expeditions to camps across the vast expanse of Russia. He made three such journeys over the course of the war, acting both as observer and advisor on hygienic issues. In 1916, under pressure from his own government, he reluctantly agreed to dispense German supplied medicines and medical equipment to the camps, but only on condition that he was fronted by a Russian Red Cross nurse, and allowed to distribute his goods impartially to both Russians and POWs. His journey on that occasion took him from St Petersburg as far as the Chinese border.[48] On his last visit, as the Russian Revolution was breaking in March 1917, he negotiated the transfer of 2,400 Austro-German POWs to camps in Denmark. This was not an easy task, since the Russians had understood that Denmark would take 10,000 – a number that would have overwhelmed the resources of that small country.[49]

Madsen's humanitarian concerns and diplomatic skills were evidently noted elsewhere. When after the war the League of Nations set up its Health Committee in 1921, Madsen was one of the 24 selected members. At the first meeting of the Committee, in August that year, Madsen was elected unanimously to the powerful post of President. This was something of a surprise, as it had been expected, not least by himself, that the post would go to George Seton Buchanan, senior Medical Officer at the English Ministry of Health, who had been deeply involved in the setting up of the Health Committee.[50] But Buchanan was neither an internationally noted medical scientist, nor much of a diplomat. Indeed one English obituarist noted specifically that, 'superficially (he) did not compare favourably with scientific workers of his standing. His general scientific culture was not deep ... he was an unattractive public speaker'. And, perhaps more fatally in regard to the Health Committee, Buchanan was 'never able to forget that Great Britain was a different place from the Continent of Europe, inhabited by different people. He may even have sunk so low, in the apprehension of our younger intellectuals, as to think of the inhabitants of other countries as "foreigners"'.[51] Moreover, Buchanan belonged to the victors. Madsen came from a neutral state and had established good relations with both the French and especially the German medical research communities before the outbreak of war. [52] (Buchanan had visited the Middle East during the war on a health commission, but Madsen had been actively engaged with the work of the Red Cross.) If the Health Committee was to succeed, it had to make erst-while enemies and scientific rivals work together. In these circumstances, it was perhaps not surprising that the smooth, cosmopolitan Dane, very much a part of Europe's scientific and humanitarian communities, was elected over the arrogant, difficult Englishman. None the less, the appointment rankled with the English. Buchanan's obituarist was quite possibly jibing at Madsen when he emphasised Buchanan's insistence that the Health Committee's schemes be proven practicable:

> "Foreigners" of the most seductive kind, officially important, scientifically eminent, might draw up plans for a new international hygienic heaven and earth ... [Buchanan] would take pains to learn whether we could do so... he earned the steady hatred of all facile orators...[53]

Yet it seems a measure of Madsen's quality - or at least of the respect in which he was held, that, although the Presidency of the Health Committee was for a three year term, he was repeatedly re-elected until 1937, and then made honorary President. On the other hand, Denmark had been a neutral state during World War I, and post-war international tensions, only escalating during the 1930s, may have helped to keep him in this position of power. Together with Ludwik Rajchman, appointed as the League of Nations Health Section's Medical Director (with day-to-day responsibility for running business from the Geneva headquarters), Madsen determined to focus the Committee's energies on practical, feasible and realistic projects.[54] If the epidemics raging through eastern Europe were a first priority, the question of international standards for biological and pharmaceutical products stood high on the list.[55] This is not the place to track Madsen's contribution to the many and various initiatives developed by the LNHO in the interwar period, but the project of biological standardisation was peculiarly Madsen's own. The problem of how to measure the strength of the diphtheria antiserum had concerned him and others since the 1890s. the introduction of the 'unit' measurement had been an immediate answer to the problem, but it had soon become apparent that different national units had very different strengths, resulting from differences in national strains of laboratory mice: the German mice were very sensitive; the French ones tough and difficult to kill, while the English mice were hopelessly feeble. Thus French units were much stronger than German ones, which in turn were stronger than the English.[56] There was much accompanying medical confusion and anxiety as a result of the differing strengths of commercially-produced sera delivered by different companies trading internationally. The situation with tetanus antitoxin in World War I was very similar. One German unit of tetanus antitoxin was the equivalent of 67 American units, and 3,000 French ones, adding to the stress of war on medical personnel.[57]

In terms of post-war international co-operation, the standardisation of the new biologicals was of paramount importance for both research and clinical practice. The direct relevance of this project to international health was evident in, for example, the public health problem of Constantinople. The city acted as an entrepot for trade between Russia and Europe, but being awash with sailors and prostitutes, it was also the VD capital of the Mediterranean. The achievement of a sure and agreed technique of serum diagnosis for syphilis was one of the early and urgent objectives of the LNHO Standardisation Committee which was set up under Madsen's direction in November 1921.[58] In the immediate aftermath of World War I, international co-operation was not always an easy task. The Nordic countries joined the new League of Nations with enthusiasm, and many of their nationals involved themselves in the work of the new organisation.[59] Neutrality during the war may have given Scandinavian nationals some edge in easing the re-establishment of collaborative European ventures. The first meeting on biological standardisation was organised in London in 1921, but only after Madsen had exercised his diplomatic skills to the full, since both French and German scientists initially refused to attend. As Madsen later recalled, the prospect of shaking hands with the Germans had Albert Calmette and Emile Roux exclaiming in dramatic chorus, 'Jamais! Jamais!'[60] Madsen's preventive interests were not confined to standardisation, however. He had an active interest in the practical application of biologicals. Moreover he had, in Denmark, what was in effect a 'human field laboratory' for the testing of such products. Madsen seems to have seen the country as an experimental station in which measures of more general benefit could be tried and tested. In 1933, for example, he wrote:

> It is not always easy to be a small nation. But, although the difficulties of being a small nation are numerous, there are areas where they have advantages over the big ones when it comes to contributing to world progress. So Denmark can almost be compared to a laboratory where it is possible to conduct social and hygienic experiments and researches, I might almost say: of all kinds.[61]

His confidence in this respect was drawn from his personal observation and knowledge of his countrymen. He liked travel, preferably in a large, open-topped car, and had acquired an intimate knowledge of his country, its health personnel, and popular attitudes.[62] The concept of Denmark as an epidemiological laboratory appealed to him, and to others: as noted in one anonymous review of Madsen's Flexner Lectures, the country was compact and surveyable, it had a comprehensive system of infectious disease notification and death registration, good hospitals, a conscientious medical profession and a homogeneous population with a 'high degree of culture'.[63] Madsen discussed the nature of Denmark's political and intellectual culture for a French audience in 1933. He drew special attention to the Danes' innate sense of goodness and natural duty, a pronounced sense of social solidarity, and a marked aptitude and liking for collaborative action for the collective good. The latter was well illustrated, he observed, by the country's co-operative agricultural movement. Shrewdly, however, he had also observed that this co-operative willingness was maintained only for as long as there was no attempt to force co-operation. Anything of a coercive character was regarded with suspicion by his countrymen, and met with defiance.[64] While Madsen may have drawn more general lessons from this observation, on the best means for developing radical reform programmes medical or otherwise, he also emphasised another Danish trait which he regarded as particularly significant for the establishment of Denmark as a pioneering hygienic state. The country had been one of the first, he argued, to adopt the teachings of Louis Pasteur. Pasteurian principles had been applied with such success at the great Carlsberg brewery in the late 1870s that its founder, J C Jacobsen, in setting up a charitable foundation to safeguard the future of the Carlsberg Laboratory, also charged it with supporting scientific research.[65] Denmark's declining death rates for respiratory tuberculosis from circa 1890 also suggested a receptivity to notions of infectiousness, while the campaigns against bovine tuberculosis from around that date had contributed widely to educate the rural population in the significance of bacteria and their role in infections.[66] In respect of the latter, the significance of bovine tuberculosis and the impact of bacterial contamination on the qualities of butter were issues central to the success of Denmark's nascent dairy industry, and acted as powerful educative forces in the countryside.[67] Yet Denmark's pioneering stance on bovine tuberculosis was not widely followed by other nations at this period.[68] It was perhaps another instance of a small country where public health interventions were respected being able to achieve what larger countries with more diverse public and private interests found impractical.

The ways in which Madsen's understanding of his country and countrymen informed his work as a promoter of public health were demonstrated by his use of the Danish 'human field laboratory' in the national anti-tuberculosis project of the 1930s. As elsewhere in Europe, tuberculosis had become a central public health concern in Denmark at the turn of the nineteenth century, but because of the dairy industry, and veterinarian Bernhard Bang's concern for bovine tuberculosis, the links between human and animal disease were of greater interest, and assumed a greater practical importance, than in most other European states.[69] Although, the campaign against bovine tuberculosis encountered opposition from the farming community, and was slow to make an impact before the 1930s, Denmark in 1952 became the first country in the world to succeed in eradicating the disease.[70] Meanwhile the Danish government began implementing a state-funded tuberculosis prevention and treatment programme from 1905.[71] By 1935, Denmark had recorded the most striking fall in tuberculosis mortality in all Europe: from a peak of nearly 300 deaths per100,000 population (the highest in Europe) in 1885 to below 50 per 100,000.[72] An important element in this campaign was the BCG immunisation programme implemented on the island of Bornholm between 1932 and 1945. Here a careful diagnostic population survey was followed by a graduated introduction of BCG vaccination – a model that was subsequently adopted and utilised by UNICEF across Europe in the wake of World War II.[73] According to local record, Madsen was the initiator of this project.[74] In the light of his convictions on the value of biologicals, and of Denmark as a field laboratory, this exercise can be seen as an extended trial first, of the value and reliability of diagnostic tuberculin testing, and secondly of the value and efficacy of BCG vaccination.

The Bornholm BCG initiative suggests the ways in which Madsen's domestic activities could establish models for preventive action to be followed elsewhere. It was one of the defining characteristics of his life that from a cultural and geographic base in a small northern country, and from a scientific base in the highly specialised discipline of serology, he forged a double career as a key figure in the national public health programme but also as a prime mover in the international movement to develop programmes for improving health across the world. It was not a career path that could have been foreseen, and owed much to circumstance, especially the circumstances generated by the First World War. Madsen's sociability and diplomatic skills, his integration into the pre-war international bacteriological community, and the opportunities offered by his work for the Red Cross during the war combined with his (and Denmark's) political neutrality to make him available – and clearly valued – player on the international interwar stage. He was a close friend and associate of Ludwik Rajchman over nearly two decades of co-operation at the League of Nations Health Organisation between the world wars, and this connection supposedly paved the way for his voluntary service after World War II with UNICEF, which Rajchman founded and headed for several years.[75] Madsen, however, seems never to have provoked the enmity often associated with Rajchman. The repeated renewal of his tenure as president of the Health Committee suggests that his political adroitness and personal charm were qualities fundamental to his success.

1 An earlier version of this paper, jointly written with Nils Rosdhal, was given to the European Association for the History of Medicine and Health, Paris, 2005. A related paper, 'Questions of Quality: The Danish State Serum Institute, Thorvald Madsen and Biological Standardization', will be published in C. Gradmann and J. Simon (eds.), *Evaluation: Standardising Therapeutic Agents 1890*-1950, to be published by Palgrave/Macmillan 2009.

2 E. Schelde-Moller, *Thorvald Madsen. I videnskabens og menneskelihedens tjeneste* (Copenhagen: Nyt Nordisk Forlag Arnold Busk, 1970), 19.

3 See *Eighth International Medical Congress* (Copenhagen, 1884).

4 J. Lehmann, J. Carlson and A. Ulrik (eds.), *Denmark:Its medical organisation, hygiene and demography* (Copenhagen: Julius Gjellerup, and London: J & A Churchill, 1891), 368.

5 Schelde-Moller, *Madsen*, p. 24.

6 E. Gotfredson, 'Dr Thorvald Madsen fortaeller', *Medicinsk Forum*, 6 (1953), 197-217

7 See Lehmann et al, *Denmark*, esp. 36-40 and 326-331; also A. Rothery, *Denmark: Kingdom of Reason* (London: Faber and Faber, 1937), chapter 2.

8 Ibid., 337.

9 Schelde-Moller, *Madsen*, 22.

10 Ibid., 37; T. Madsen, 'Kandidattid', *Medicinsk Forum*, 15 (1962), 54-56; on Danish medical education at this time, see Lehmann et al, *Denmark*, 22-28. It is here noted (p. 23) that. apart from certain exam and proficiency certificate regulations, 'the study of medicine is perfectly untrammelled: thse students are not obliged to attend any lectures or exercises, much less to do so in a certain rotation'.

11 T. Madsen, 'Lund', *Medicinsk Forum* 14 (1961), 181-83.

12 Ibid, 181.

13 E. Gotfredson, 'Dr Thorvald Madsen fortaeller. II', *Medicinsk Forum* 9 (1956), 161-177: 165.

14 K. Jensen, *Bekaempelse af infektionssygdomme: Statens Serum Institut 1902*-2002 (Copenhagen: Nyt Nordisk Forlag Arnold Busk, 2002), 29.

15 Gotfredson, 'Madsen I', 198.

16 Ibid.

17 Ibid., 201.

18 J. Carlson, 'Diphtheria', in Lehmann et al (eds.), *Denmark*, 319-20.

19 Schelde-Moller, *Madsen*, 29.

20 The single exception is the pride which he evidently took in the shine which Elie Metchnikoff (1845-1916) took to his wife: T. Madsen, 'Forskere omkring arhundredskiftet: Koch, Ehrlich og Metchnikoff', *Medicinsk Forum* 18 (1965), 140-144.

21 T. Madsen, 'Landlaege', *Medicinsk Forum*, 14 (1961): 28-32

22 Gotfredson, 'Madsen I', 199

23 Jensen, *Bekaempelse*, 22

24 Ibid., 31.

25 Ibid.

26 Schelde-Moller, *Madsen*, 14. See also T. Madsen and S, Madsen, 'Diphtheria in Denmark', *Danish Medical Bulletin* 3 (1956), 112-121: 113.

27 Schelde-Moller, *Madsen*. 15-16; the doubts over Fibiger's results are briefly reviewed in Jensen, *Bekaempelse*, 25-6.

28 Jensen, *Bekaempelse*, 23-4

29 Schelde-Moller, *Madsen*, 41.

30 Ibid., 42

31 Ibid., 46.
32 Ibid.
33 Cited in Jensen, *Bekaempelse*, 36-7.
34 See C. Hamlin, *Public health and social justice in the age of Chadwick* ((Cambridge: Cambridge University Press, 1998), especially chapter 3.
35 Ibid., 36.
36 T. Madsen, 'Le Danemark, pays d'hygiene', *Revue d'hygiene* 55 (1933), 666-681: 669.
37 Ibid., 672.
38 Jensen, *Bekaempelse*, 34.
39 Schelde-Moller, *Madsen*, 65.
40 Ibid., 56; see also ibid, 42-52 and 54-9; T. Madsen, Forskerer omkring arhundredskiftet', *Medicinsk forum* 18 (1965), 140-44; idem, ''Rejse i Amerika ved arhundredskiftet', ibid, 19 (1966), 26-32.
41 Ibid, 76.
42 T. Madsen, 'Andet besog I Rusland. Koleraen i St. Petersborg 1908', *Medicinsk forum* (1965), 143-146, reprinted from *Hospitalstidene* 46-47 (1908).
43 Schelde-Moller, *Madsen*, 86.
44 Ibid.
45 Ibid.
46 Ibid., 88.
47 Ibid., 87.
48 T. Madsen, 'Tredie besog i Rusland', *Medicinsk forum* 15 (1962), 170-176: 172
49 Ibid., 100. See also T. Madsen, 'Fjerde besog I Rusland', *Med For. 17 (1964), 73-80*
50 Schelde-Moller, *Madsen*, 108-9;
51 M. Greenwood, 'Sir George S Buchanan', *B M J* ii (1936), 788-89: 789
52 Gotfredson, 'Madsen' II'; Schelde-Moller, *Madsen*, 42-52.
53 Greenwood, 'Buchanan', 789
54 Schelde-Moller, *Madsen*, 110; see also R. Gautier, 'The Health Organisation and biological standards', *Quarterly Bulletin of the Health Organisation*, 4 (1935), 499-554; 499.
55 Ibid.
56 Jensen, *Bekaempelse*, 66.
57 Schelde-Moller, *Madsen*, 110; see also Gautier, 'The Health Organisation', 499.
58 Schelde-Moller, *Madsen*, 122.
59 P. Munch, 'De nordiske stats indsats I Folkenes Forbund', *Nordisk Tidscrift* (1926), 261.
60 Schelde-Moller, *Madsen*, 112
61 Greenwood, 'Buchanan', 789
62 Jensen, *Bekaempelse*, 81
63 Anon, 'Notes and comments. Danish epidemiology', *Medical Officer* 59 (1938), 52
64 Madsen, 'Le Danemark', 677.
65 Ibid., 681
66 Ibid., 672- 674.
67 Ibid., 681.
68 See, for example, S.D. Jones, 'Mapping a zoonotic disease: Anglo-American efforts to control bovine tuberculosis before World War I', *Osiris* 19 (2004), 133-148; K. Waddington, *The bovine scourge: Meat, tuberculosis and public health, 1850-1914* (Woodbridge: The Boydell Press, 2006).
69 See F. Levison, 'Tuberculosis' in Lehmann et al (eds.), *Denmark*, 349-50.

70 Jensen, *Bekaempelse*, 104-5.

71 J. Ostenfeld, N. Heitmann and G. Neander, *Tuberculosis in Denmark, Norway and Sweden* (Geneva: League of Nations Health Organisation, 1931), 89-97.

72 M. Daniels, 'Tuberculosis in Europe during and after the Second World War', *B.M.J.* ii (1949), 1065-1072: 1066.

73 Schelde-Moller, *Madsen*, 166.

74 H.C.Olsen, 'Tuberculosis in Bornholm after B.C.G. vaccination', *Acta tuberculosea Scandinavica* 28 (1953), 1-30: 4.

75 See M. Balinska, *Une vie pour l'humanitaire* (Paris: Editions la Découverte, 1995), 335-40; see also Schelde-Moller, *Madsen*, 181-2.

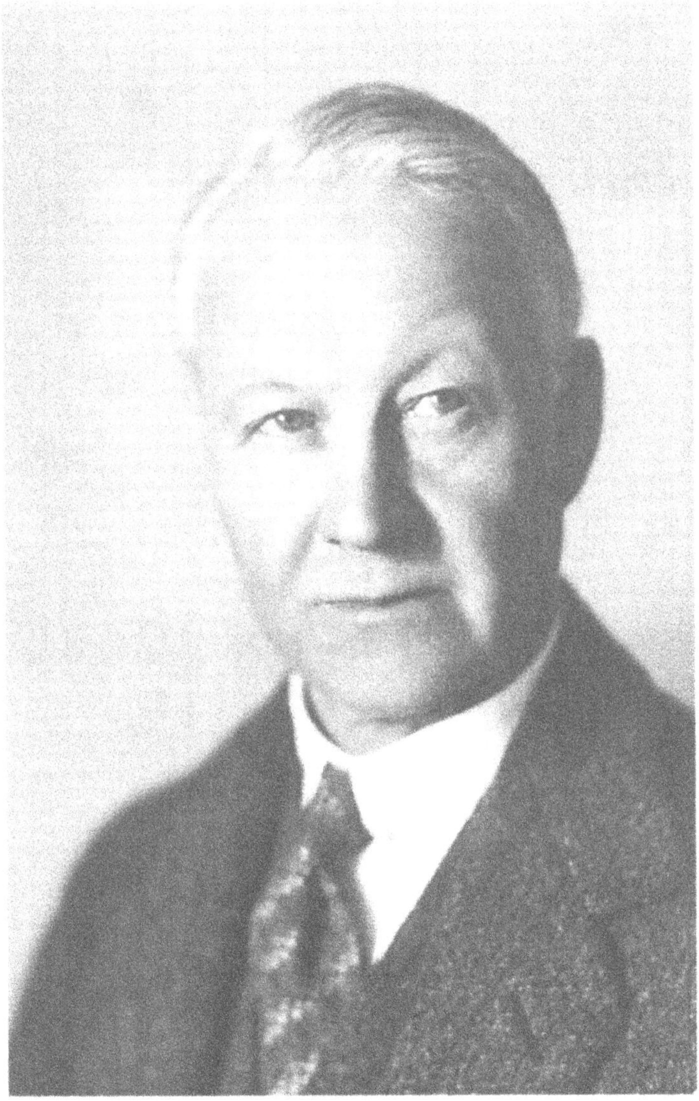

Thorvald Madsen

In the Shadow of Grotjahn German Social Hygienists in the International Health Scene

Iris Borowy

Social hygiene in Germany carried different, sometimes contradictory connotations. It had its roots in part in the nineteenth century sanitary movement. Beginning with demands by Virchow, sanitary concepts of disease prevention were connected with calls for social reform, which would result in more healthful living and working conditions. Later, hygienists such as Alfred Grotjahn, Ludwig Teleky, Alfons Fischer, Gustav Tugendreich, Adolf Gottstein or Ignatz Kaup, provided influential theoretical groundwork for a social medicine movement. After approximately 1920, theoretical discussions in Germany gave way to the institutionalisation of social hygienic teachings through the establishment of a chair for social hygiene at the University of Berlin, the integration of social hygiene into medical curricula and the foundation of several social hygienic academies in Berlin-Charlottenburg, Breslau and Düsseldorf.[1]

These developments tied into several overlapping layers of conflict. As in other countries, there was a natural tension between physicians working as public health officers and those acting as general practitioners or medical specialists. While the former were interested in preventive work, routinely reaching out to as many people as possible at public expense, the latter feared that these activities would encroach on their professional territory, and that a rival medical force would lure away patients with unfair advantages. At the same time, both groups were divided between a larger conservative group and a smaller faction which favoured progressive reform. Thus, associations of often elderly doctors tried to defend their status against upcoming rivals: the young, the - usually Social Democratic - representatives of insurance funds and health centres, the large group of Jewish physicians and the small but increasing number of women doctors.[2] Meanwhile, traditional public health based on state control was challenged by a lively social hygiene movement, which sought to safeguard the welfare of underprivileged groups rather than state authority. The various forms of conflict were intertwined and intensified after the economic depression narrowed the financial room for manoeuvre and potential compromise. And they were increasingly framed in confrontations between left-wing versus right-wing ideology: social reform versus conservative endogenous rationalisation of physical well-being, separation between prevention and therapy versus comprehensive public health efforts, national solution versus international cooperation.

Inexorably, the conservative side gained ground. In 1930, the medical associations prevailed in ensuring a strict separation between preventive and curative medical work by issuing binding guidelines.[3] Meanwhile, social hygiene shifted towards an understanding of prevention not through measures towards social progress but through the suppression of social groups that, through their genetic disposition, their behaviour or their "race," were perceived as dangerous to the population. In other words, the perception of health shifted from a social good, to which public health was supposed to provide general access, to a biological good, which public health measures were now meant to preserve for the benefit of society rather than the individual.

This turn towards a biologistic perception of health did not happen abruptly. There was a clear dividing line between the Weimar Republic and National-Socialist Reich in legislative terms, but the underlying conceptual development was much more gradual. It was a subtle development, in which proponents of different schools mixed various elements of the discourse until racialised medical arguments eventually gained a majority over interdisciplinary socio-medical concerns.[4] This ambivalent nature of social hygiene in Germany, even during Weimar times, was manifest in the eugenic leanings coupled with reformist instincts of Alfred Grotjahn, the doyen of social hygiene in Germany. Grotjahn assumed the first chair for social hygiene at the University of Berlin and was a formative force in the – limited – integration of social hygiene into medical curricula.[5] Thus, he was a natural centre of social hygienic training and attracted a new generation of experts interested in this field.

Social hygiene was one field that brought German experts into contact with the League of Nations Health Organisation (LNHO). The cooperation between Germany and the LNHO was short and fruitful, but always overshadowed by the political climate. After World War I German scientists were excluded from the international meetings of several scientific societies, and in Germany the League of Nations as integral part of the Treaty of Versailles was the object of intense animosity.[6] The LNHO's holistic approach to health led to its increasing focus on social hygiene, albeit in its reformist, inclusionary form, devoid of eugenic elements.[7] German expertise was most welcome. In 1927, Alfred Grotjahn cooperated in conceptual preparations for a centre of public health documentation, whose establishment was planned at the LNHO. Pertinent material, notably "documents, minutes of meetings, memoranda, printed and unprinted annual reports, the texts, decrees and regulations" were to be "collected, classified and analysed."[8] However, the project encountered financial difficulties, and when, eventually, the Rockefeller Foundation provided sufficient funds, Grotjahn apparently had become disenchanted with the project and was no longer part of it.[9] Grotjahn's real influence on LNHO work was indirect, via former students and colleagues who unwittingly came to personify the various facets of the field. German-LNHO cooperation in social hygiene temporarily united a group of German public health experts, whose fate during the following years would drive them far apart, geographically, politically and personally: Fritz Rott, Emil Roesle, Otto Olsen and Franz Goldmann.

The oldest of the group was Emil Eugen Roesle (1875-1962). Born in Augsburg in 1875 he studied medicine at Leipzig and Erlangen and soon developed an interest in medical statistics. The field was of relatively recent origin. Efforts to collect, systematise and interpret mortality data had only begun in the nineteenth century with pioneers like William Farr and Edwin Chadwick. Medical issues spurred the development of statistics as a discipline and cause of death classification was a central agenda item at the First International Statistical Congress as early as 1853.[10] Increasingly, medical statistics became an essential element of the medical discourse. Specifically, they provided the background information needed to decide on public welfare policies. By revealing correlations between living conditions and health, medical statistics soon formed an essential tool for social medicine.

Roesle's career took a decisive turn through the activities of the Saxon industrialist Karl August Lingner (1861 – 1915), whose interest in bio-medicine was partly motivated by the fact that it helped market his brand of mouthwash. After 1900, Lingner financed exhibitions of a new type, whose aim was to educate the public about the basics of medicine and hygiene. Roesle assumed the task of visualizing recent developments in public health, such as the prevalence of specific diseases, mortality rates and expectations of life, through an intelligent and innovative use of statistics. Fighting the stereotype of statistics as a lifeless and complicated discipline, Roesle developed audience-friendly strategies to familiarise the scientific and lay world with the rationale for public health policies through graphs and numbers.[11] His career quickly built on these beginnings. In 1903 he became director of Lingner's medical-statistical bureau. Here, Roesle created the first national and international data base with material relevant for evaluating the state of public health. In 1911 he co-organised the first International Hygiene Exhibition in Dresden, which reached millions of people. When the Berlin Imperial Health Bureau established a department for medical statistics, he was the natural candidate for the post of director and moved to Berlin. In 1914 he became co-editor of the the leading German journal for social medicine, the *Archiv for Soziale Hygiene,* then renamed *Archiv for Soziale Hygiene und Demographie.* Under his guidance, demography became a central part of the journal. During the following years, eugenics and racial hygiene were among the frequently discussed topics, albeit balanced by positive presentations of internationalism and pacifism.[12] He was the quintessential humanitarian scientist, clearly fascinated by his numbers and their scientifically correct management but similarly intent to make them serve the purpose of educating the public and administrations. His statistics, particularly their graphic presentation, drew attention to continuing high infant mortality and its relatively more benign state in areas with effective infant welfare activities.[13] Thus, he supplied the data that justified infant welfare initiatives, preparing the ground for those who were willing to implement them – among them Fritz Rott.

Fritz Rott (1878 – 1959), came from Gleiwitz in Upper Silesia. After medical studies in Halle he specialised in infant health and moved to Berlin, working at the children's ward at Charité hospital from 1906 to 1911.[14] Thereby, he entered one of the oldest and ideologically most contested areas of public health. Infant welfare dominated early concerns about the sanitary conditions in industrialising urban life. The spectre of innocent dying children had a powerful emotional appeal, and the first two decades of the twentieth century in particular "witnessed a virtual explosion of public concern over infant mortality and the consequent emergence of an international infant welfare movement of truly immense dimensions."[15] Increasingly, this humanitarian approach mixed with pro-natalist worries about falling birth-rates, feared to weaken affected nations relative to their potentially more fertile neighbours. Everywhere in Europe, governments took measures aimed at ensuring that more children would be born and that more of them would survive infancy.[16] Thus, Rott soon became part of a lively debate over reasons for, and implications of, the continuing high infant mortality rate in Prussia. While some statisticians and paediatricians observed that infant mortality rates were inversely correlated to family income, others blamed working class mothers, who increasingly worked outside the home, leaving their children in other people's care and who allegedly lacked hygienic understanding. Some observers welcomed infant mortality as a eugenic corrective that cleansed the nation of the weak, but during World War I it was a minority view, which Rott explicitly denounced as obsolete in 1917.[17] At that time, he had already established himself as a leading authority in the field: he was a senior member of the *Kaiserin Auguste Victoria-Haus* (KAVH), created in 1909 as a central institution to investigate questions of infant health and welfare. It included a laboratory and an experimental kitchen, wards for newborns and children, a birthing clinic and a visiting midwife service. After 1911, its infant welfare activities were placed in a separate department (*Organisationsamt für Säuglingsschutz*) with Rott as director. Energetically developing its archive, a scientific library and a collection of data, he made it the central place of reference for questions of infant welfare, for scientists as well as for public institutions, charities or private individuals.[18] In addition, Rott took a leading role in the German Association for the Protection of Infants (*Deutsche Vereinigung für Säuglingsschutz*), founded in 1909 as the central association for all institutions in charge of infant welfare. It served as a platform for discussion on numerous issues, ranging from breast-feeding to falling birth rates and regulations for day-care.[19]

Heart problems freed Rott from military service, so that he continued his career during World War I. His work was well recognised in government and conservative circles, whose attitudes he copied. By 1919, he had received several awards, and in 1917 he was accepted into the *Berliner Gesellschaft für Natur- und Heilkunde*, a select, nationalist association, open only to Protestant scientists and physicians.[20] He readily adopted the nationalist rhetoric that perceived falling birth rates and high infant mortality rates in terms of losses to the nation, and he compared efforts for better hygiene in infant day-care centres to the work of soldiers on the battlefield.[21] These measures, including long-time demands of social reformers, now met easy acceptance as perceived means to substitute for – temporarily or permanently – absent fathers.[22] After the war, Rott further broadened his range of activities. He was involved in public advisory bodies, notably the Imperial Commission for Population Issues (*Reichsausschuss für Bevölkerungsfragen*) where he warned of the dangers of a declining population and offered suggestions for reducing perinatal and infant mortality. Foreshadowing later ideological shifts, he recommended, among other welfare measures, safeguarding primarily the "valuable" parts of the population.[23] Rott also became actively involved, as writer or editor, in several journals of social hygiene. In 1925, he became co-editor of the re-launched prestigious *Archiv für Soziale Hygiene und Demographie*, which Roesle had created some ten years earlier. Here, Rott was responsible for the sections on social hygiene, international correspondence and – after 1933 – race hygiene.[24] He tried to broaden the base of social hygienists but failed in 1927 to convince the association of practicing physicians of the benefits they and their status would reap by getting involved in public health measures.[25] Nevertheless, by the mid 1920s he had worked his way into a well-connected position from where he was obviously willing to help shape the face of social hygiene in Germany. He profited from the climate of the Weimar Republic, which expanded its social welfare programme, particularly regarding child health, despite financial restrictions.[26] His options were further enhanced when he began teaching as one of the first lecturers at the newly established Academy of Social Hygiene in Charlottenburg.[27] In 1927, he became head of the German Welfare School (*Deutsche Fürsorgeschule*), which was affiliated with the KAVH and served 4000 students between 1927 and 1930. Other lecturers included virtually everyone active in social hygiene in Germany, including Franz Goldmann.[28]

Some twenty years younger than Roesle and Rott and of assimilated Jewish background, Franz Goldmann (1895 – 1970) began his studies in medicine at Heidelberg in 1913. After participating in World War I as a paramedic, he continued medical training in Berlin and qualified as a doctor in 1920.[29] Around that time he met Alfred Grojahn, who made a deep impression on him and convinced him to turn his back on practical medicine for a career in public health. Grotjahn also helped Goldmann gain a position in the Municipal Health Bureau of Berlin in 1922, one of the new institutions that were being established as part of the post-war re-structuring process, following heated economic and ideological discussions about the desired health system. In Berlin, the authorities implemented a mixture of demands by Grotjahn, who called for coordination of public health activities at district level, and a more centralised system.[30] Thus, Goldmann found himself at the heart of issues that would become central to his professional life. But initially his work at the social hygiene department was concerned with various other public health issues, ranging from venereal diseases to rheumatism. He soon focused on hospitals, working out ideas on how hospitals might achieve their shifting function from providing social welfare to scientific therapy at a time of limited financial means. Invariably, this issue took him to larger questions of how adequate health services (including welfare, prevention and therapy) could be organised and financed by coordinating existing public and private services, and through different concepts of health insurance. In 1929 he transferred to the Medical Department of the Ministry of the Interior. Continuing his academic studies he qualified for a professorship in social hygiene in 1932 and immediately began teaching at the University of Berlin.[31] His studies in the field brought him to the attention of the LNHO when the latter began a project on the role of health insurance in public health around 1926. He thereby came into contact with Otto Olsen, the German member of the LNHO Section.

Initially, Otto Olsen (1892 - ?) had a successful though relatively unfocused career. Of Danish background in Northern Germany, he studied at the universities of Heidelberg, Munich and Freiburg and worked at the St. Georg Hospital in Hamburg. In Freiburg, he was an assistant to Martin Hahn, whom he followed to Berlin when Hahn became director of the Berlin Hygienic Institute.[32] Olsen worked in the serological department at the hospital, and after 1922 as lecturer both for bacteriology and hygiene and so combined a sound background in both disciplines. A special interest in social hygiene was not obvious from his cv, though it might be guessed from his long connection to Martin Hahn, who was active, among other fields, in occupational health.[33]

By the mid 1920s, the four men were in Berlin and presumably knew one another. Though of different generations and cultural background, they moved in the circle of social hygienists around Grotjahn. Rott, Goldmann and Roesle presumably met while working at the Welfare School, the *Archiv für Soziale Hygiene und Demographie* and in Berlin health administration offices. To what extent Olsen was in contact with them at that time is less clear. He was certainly known to Grotjahn, and he would soon provide a connection for further efforts towards common goals through his position at the LNHO.

In Geneva, the Medical Director of the Health Section, Ludwik Rajchman, and long-time President of the Health Committee, Thorvald Madsen, were keen on strengthening LNHO cooperation with Germany and had for some time been looking for a suitable German scientist for the LNHO Section staff. Olsen was only their second choice after negotiations with the original candidate, bacteriologist and German nationalist Heinrich Zeiss, failed.[34] According to Paul Weindling, Olsen was recommended to the LNHO by Grotjahn, possibly in order to strengthen the hygienist part of LNHO work.[35] The contact may also have been through Olsen's mentor Martin Hahn, whom Madsen knew and had briefly considered as German member of the Health Committee (a post later taken by Bernhard Nocht).[36] Olsen was employed by the LNHO Section in 1925 and gave outstanding service to the organisation for the next fifteen years, regularly earning excellent internal evaluations.[37] He became the natural connection between the LNHO and German scientists.

When Olsen came to Geneva, Roesle had already been in contact with the LNHO for some years due to his expertise in medical statistics. In this context, the LNHO also appears to have been instrumental in arranging a tour to the Soviet Union, where he was supposed to conduct classes on demographic and sanitary statistics. He used this opportunity to visit the country, including hospitals and universities, and sent back enthusiastic reports on phantastic successes of the Soviet health system. In glowing terms he praised the egalitarian access to healthcare facilities and the decline in mortality rates. His reports were considered naïve and embarrassing by the Germany embassy in Moscow and the Ministry of the Interior in Berlin, and the LNHO never made use of them either. And although Roesle insisted that his views on health administrations were non-political and he was not Communist, this experience evidently spurred his fondness for Soviet health policies.[38] While this attitude would prove difficult later, it was remarkably unproblematic at the time as long as Roesle stuck to his statistical expertise. He was among the group of medical statisticians who cooperated in LNHO efforts to revise the pre-war List of Causes of Death, and when the LNHO formed an expert commission for the preparation of nomenclature revisions in 1926, he became one of its most important members.[39] In this context, he forcefully supported the idea of a fundamentally new classification for the systematic collection of morbidity data that would allow a more accurate assessment – or really any assessment at all – of the state of the health of the population.[40] Being granted leave of absence by the Imperial Health Bureau, Roesle spent some weeks in Geneva in early 1927 and took enthusiastic charge of collecting and categorizing LNHO morbidity material, as it was supplied by individual states.[41] A year later, he summarised his findings in a lengthy report, in which he recommended ways of preparing the statistical information, urged the need for a uniform list of sickness in order to allow international comparison and proposed one such list, based on the list of causes of death.[42] By mid November 1928, the report had been translated into English, French, Czech and Hungarian, and Japanese and Serbo-Croatian versions were planned, all part of a drive to get physicians everywhere interested in morbidity statistics.[43] Roesle saw increased standardization not merely as a means to increase the comparability of data, but also to generate data in the first place. He assumed that obvious lacunae in the statistics of individual states would motivate their authorities to fill the gaps and gain data not previously collected, thus improving their understanding of the public health status of their own countries.[44] Lending his expertise to the LNHO statistical service brought Roesle into contact with the international activities both of Olsen, who had started his work at the Health Section, and of his colleague Fritz Rott.

Although the four men worked in distinctly different fields, they shared the underlying ambition to reform the character of public health work: Rott wished to improve the status of social hygiene in general – and child health in particular - and integrate it into mainstream medicine; Goldmann tried to improve the organisation of public health administration; Roesle aimed to improve the knowledge of the true state of the health of the population, a knowledge he deemed essential both for physicians and health administrators; and Olsen tried to connect these efforts to the international world. In a sense, the way their paths crossed at Geneva was an expression of their separate but intertwined perspectives. Individually, they were engaged in specific projects which, collectively, had the potential to complement one another into a coherent effort of public health improvement in Germany and elsewhere. And for a while, chances looked promising.

In October 1925, the LNHO began preparations for a survey project on infant mortality and child welfare and asked Rott to act as German expert on their Advisory Committee.[45] Rott was a natural choice, both for his domestic expertise in the field and because of his prior contact to international associations of child welfare.[46] The survey aimed at securing "precise information in regard to the exact causes of infant deaths." Twenty-nine districts, both rural and urban, in seven countries (Germany, France, Great Britain, Norway, the Netherlands, Austria and Italy) were selected for the study.[47] Rott coordinated surveys in several regions of Germany (Augsburg, Kassel, Lippe and Strelitz), that soon produced detailed reports.[48] Rott himself contributed a lengthy paper on historical developments in Germany, which he published immediately, and which remains one of his most important papers.[49] Analyses of the international data in September 1927 and July 1928 showed a wide divergence of still-births and infant deaths. The proportion of deaths under one year of age per 100 births ranged from 3.94 in the Dutch city of Leyden to 19.5 in Engelhartszell in rural Austria. Although detailed studies were still needed, the data clearly indicated the central importance of qualified midwifery services or maternity welfare agencies. Their existence mitigated the effects of illegitimacy almost to vanishing point, and their absence severely exacerbated the risks of prematurity. The leading causes of infant death were universally found to be still-births and prematurity, respiratory diseases, and gastro-intestinal affections, though their relative significance varied. Digestive disturbances were most important in groups with high infant mortality rates, while perinatal problems dominated in groups with low infant mortality.[50] Rott's contribution to these results was substantial, supported by Roesle, who was in Geneva at the time. Indeed, in view of later developments, it is noteworthy how well Rott and Roesle complemented one another. Both tried to broaden the study and to strengthen the statistical character of the project. Rott sought funding to extend the survey into 1928 and to all live births. Citing Roesle, he argued that the specifics of a single year could obscure the picture and that it seemed a shame not to use the infrastructure, now in place, for a larger, more informative survey.[51] However, he could not convince the rest of the group, who were more interested in the clinical aspects of the study and did not believe that the results of an extension would justify the effort.[52] Despite this setback Rott was eager to strengthen ties with the LNHO. When he – erroneously – believed that the *Archiv für Soziale Hygiene und Demographie* was unknown in Geneva, Rott urged Olsen to subscribe to it. He pointed out that the journal frequently reported on LNHO activities, and offered to send back issues.[53] In 1929, he offered his services for a new LNHO Commission on Social Hygiene whose formation he had read about, reminding Olsen that he had just received his post-Ph.D. degree (*Habilitation*) in social hygiene.[54] While this degree did not open up membership in the commission, which focused on health insurance, the habilitation, supervised by Grotjahn, enabled Rott to lecture on the social hygiene of infancy at the University of Berlin, where he would continue teaching until 1944.[55]

Meanwhile, inexorably, mainstream perspectives in Germany and within the LNHO began to diverge. When the LNHO summed up the findings of the survey in March 1929, the report recommended a series of specific measures, including an increase in perinatal care, improved financial and legislative regulations protecting pregnant women, better training for midwives, effective vaccination and a series of social measures such as better housing, improved hygienic conditions and public education about the danger of infection from adults to children. No compulsory arrangements were envisaged. The report surmised that given suitable consultation and maternity leave, mothers would voluntarily make use of childcare services.[56] The recommendations aimed at providing optimal care while safeguarding freedom of choice for all mothers and their children. By contrast, in Germany, Rott's interpretation of the comprehensive German data betrayed a shift to biological thinking. De-emphasising living conditions, he blamed infant mortality mainly on biological weaknesses.[57] However, at the time, Rott appeared unaware of developing incompatibilities but continued to propagate the LNHO's work in Germany. In 1932, when Olsen and the head of the Imperial Health Bureau, Carl Hamel, looked for a medium to publish LNHO findings in German, he readily agreed that the *Archiv für Soziale Hygiene und Demographie* would regularly carry reports on LNHO work, usually translations of contributions to the LNHO Bulletin.[58] In late 1930 the LNHO instituted a *Reporting Committee on maternal welfare and the Hygiene of Infants and Children of preschool Age*, designed to provide tangible guidance to administrations and the public, and once again invited Rott.[59] Thus, he was one of five international experts who co-authored a long, detailed paper on maternal, infant and child welfare.[60] It was probably the most controversial LNHO paper ever published, widely criticised for its endorsement of birth control measures in cases where they served maternal health.[61] Work within the group appears to have unfolded smoothly, however, without evidence of ideological disagreements. For a while, work continued for a report on the health of school children in which Rott, again, participated. Whether he ever submitted his contribution is unclear. In January 1933, Olsen reminded him – strangely enough in French – to send his text, and by 1934, work on the project had stalled.[62]

Meanwhile, LNHO work on social hygiene and health insurance, undertaken in cooperation with the International Labour Organisation (ILO) attracted the participation of other German experts. Germany was particularly interesting to LNHO observers in the field: it had a relatively large number of insured and long experience with health insurance in various functions, including some with a social medical character. Germany also served as a prime example of how a variety of institutions, federal, state, municipal, public, private and corporate, needed to be coordinated to achieve satisfactory results. Thus, Rajchman was happy to get the cooperation of the heads of large insurance associations and other key German experts. Once again, Roesle proved essential in organising statistical data.

Strangely enough Goldmann, whose work would centre on this issue later, was not asked to cooperate in this commission, possibly because the German section was already taken by the very active Walter Pryll, head physician at the main insurance fund (*Allgemeine Ortskrankenkasse*), who had inspired the very formation of the joint ILO-LNHO Commission. But Pryll used, among other material, a study by Goldmann and Grotjahn, which he received from the LNHO Section.[63] This book-length text, *The Performance of the German Health Insurance from a Social Hygiene Perspective,* analysed how health insurance funds could be put to preventive use by financing various prophylactic and welfare measures.[64] The latter's' effectiveness, they found, was difficult to quantify, since by definition it would only show in the long term so that in most cases there were no suitable data. The relatively most convincing case was that of maternal and infant welfare. A variety of benefits for pregnant women and in perinatal care had formed part of insurance services for some thirty years, and their usefulness appeared to be underscored by falling infant mortality rates. While Grotjahn seems to have contributed the section on the need to coordinate and systematise insurance in a narrow sense, Goldmann called for a more efficient cooperation and coordination of insurance and social welfare institutions. For this purpose, he recommended the extensive formation of joint committees, *Arbeitsgemeinschaften*, which were successfully used in some German cities already.[65] This idea was taken up by the Sub-Committee on Preventive Medicine formed in Geneva shortly afterwards. After a study tour in April 1929 of health institutions and insurance organization in several German cities, the Sub-Committee stressed the importance of cooperation between social insurance and health and welfare organisations, both public and private, in order to prevent duplication of effort and to ensure efficient and satisfying efforts. It specifically recommended "Councils of co-operative action for social medicine," explicitly modelled after the German *Arbeitsgemeinschaften*.[66]

Co-operative councils were not the only item of the Goldmann/Grotjahn text that featured prominently in further LNHO work. Neither Goldmann nor Grotjahn had invented the concept of health centres, institutions that offered first aid and simple medical care in addition to a variety of welfare and sanitary services. But they emphatically recommended them. They regretted that the existing health centre in Berlin had been established against the wishes of physicians' associations, but made no effort to ease tensions when they commented that integrating social hygiene and medicine, i.e. therapy and prevention was not compatible with the existing structure of medicine as a free profession. Predictably, this part of the paper aroused most criticism in Germany.[67] Confidently – or naively - Goldmann and Grotjahn argued that in view of the obvious professional and financial advantages of such centres, in which a large number of patients could be served by general and specialist doctors sharing modern diagnostic and therapeutic equipment, surely patients, doctors and insurances would soon embrace the concept.[68] In the short run, this prediction proved erroneous, but the idea kept resonating in public health circles. Two years later an LNHO expert commission on rural hygiene declared health centres "the best method of organizing the health services in rural districts."[69] In various forms, the concept left traces in deliberations and decisions of European administrators.[70]

Goldmann had hoped to be able to translate some of his ideas into practical policy when, in 1929, he was promoted to the post of *Oberregierungsrat* in the Medical Department of the Ministry of the Interior. But he soon found that he could achieve little in the face of polite but determined opposition from his conservative and senior colleagues.[71] Forced to keep concentrating on theory, he submitted his *Habilitation* thesis in 1932 on the public health dimension of hospitals. Analysing their function in relation to therapeutic centres, welfare institutions and insurance funds he listed a range of their essential public health activities: generating crucial epidemiological data, isolating infectious patients, negotiating the economics of medicine between therapy and insurance calculations and providing a place of contact and cooperation between medicine and social hygiene, i.e. between the doctor and the welfare worker.[72] Goldmann's work gained unforeseen urgency when the economic crisis reached Germany in 1930, throwing the country into mass misery. The government of Chancellor Brüning reacted with drastic cuts in social services, including those of the health insurance funds, and by curtailing their negotiating powers with doctors. Goldmann was adamant that this strategy would not save money but, on the contrary, would eventually necessitate more costly measures. His lobbying activities resulted in a program of alternative proposals in which welfare institutions, charitable organisations, governmental departments and medical associations submitted their suggestions for cost-reduction measures. He also participated in Prussian Health Council negotiations about crisis management policies for hospitals. These activities failed to prevent serious and – he felt – unsystematic reductions in various parts of the German health budget. But they did draw international attention to his views, while health experts and administrations everywhere in Europe looked for ways to cope with the depression.[73]

LNHO officials in Geneva were among those trying to understand the health repercussions of the depression. In August 1932, Olsen summed up the state of knowledge in a paper titled *The Economic Depression and Public Health.* He depicted the enormous scope of unemployment and poverty, reaching 50 to 60 million people, but had to admit that at present "no appreciable effect on the aggregate mortality rates" was evident.[74] Indeed, a comparison of 1931 death rates in several European and US-American countries and cities with the average figures of the preceding years, showed that rates everywhere had remained constant or, indeed, even fallen. Nevertheless, the report insisted that this finding did not allow the conclusion "that there was no correlation between the economic crisis and mortality."[75] Clearly, more information was needed. In October 1932, the Health Committee specified that further work should discuss five points, among them statistical methods to study the effects of depression on public health and ways to safeguard health by the co-ordination of the work of all available public health institutions.[76] As it turned out, work on these two items largely evolved around central contributions from Roesle and Goldmann, respectively.

The mystery of how to trace the effects of the depression in public health data was an outstanding challenge for Roesle, both scientifically and in view of its obvious relevance to the public health problems of the moment. As suitable method of measuring the health of the unemployed he proposed a longitudinal health index.[77] His approach cautioned against the superficial interpretation of data. The health effects of unemployment would most probably be the result of a slow, gradual deterioration of nutrition and living conditions and consequently would only be visible in long-term observations. Meaningful results required careful comparisons between individuals or specific stable groups at different points before and during a prolonged period of unemployment. Roesle's paper provoked only limited response, respectful but critical. Corrado Gini, Roesle's Italian colleague, felt that morbidity statistics were in principle unsuited to the task. Instead, he advocated detailed studies of nutritional status.[78] The representative of the association of German insurance companies, Eduard Mosbacher, criticised Roesle's postulate of stable groups as unrealistic for insurance funds, which people tended to join and leave as circumstances changed.[79] Similarly, the renowned English statistician, Major Greenwood, commented that the method was scientifically accurate but entirely impractical and also, in the last resort, irrelevant. The most likely outcome of such complicated research would be to establish that unemployment was bad for you, a "truism" for which new evidence was unnecessary.[80] These comments appear to have discouraged any scientific study along the lines suggested by Roesle, according to Rajchman, "the Greenwood of Germany." [81] His response to the depression failed the test of international acceptability.

Goldmann's contribution was more successful. His lengthy paper on the money saving potential of better coordination of the public health structure served as initial point of reference for all discussions of the working group on this topic. His text emphatically argued against across-the-board cuts in health budgets at times of financial crisis. Instead, savings should be made by intelligent and considered choices regarding priorities for specific programmes and societal groups (e.g. children). In addition, Goldmann recommended an improved coordination of existing services offered by private and public medical, economic and social institutions, to avoid cost-intensive duplication, ideally by one central coordinating body. Preventive measures should be prioritised as money-saving devices.[82] As his colleagues were quick to point out, these considerations addressed general long-term structural questions rather than acute crisis management. But in reality the two points proved difficult to separate, because, as a hand-written note on the edge of his paper remarked, obviously "any rational method" would be "permanently applicable."[83] For a moment, this fact irritated some of Goldmann's colleagues, but Rajchman explicitly welcomed the general relevance of his recommendations.[84]

During a conference in mid-February 1933, Goldmann's paper served as a basis for discussions and for an international call for further comments. The results provided the material for a report, which appeared in the LNHO Bulletin.[85] The basic tenor had changed remarkably little since Goldmann's original paper half a year earlier. Citing examples from numerous countries the text showed that the amounts spent on prevention everywhere were a mere fraction of the amounts spent for curative purposes, a policy the report denounced as "anti-economic." Likewise, it characterised as "neither rational nor complete nor economical" healthcare services for the poorer classes that relied on confusing combinations of sickness and invalidity insurance, public medical assistance and health services, private associations, and voluntary organizations, resulting in "overlapping and waste."[86] Echoing Goldmann's views, the report postulated that any system must be based on a coherent, comprehensive plan and that an efficient public health system pre-supposed extensive participation of a large number of institutions, connected in "horizontal and vertical integration."[87] Goldmann would never come closer to having a receptive, international audience for his ideas as well as authoritative backing.

Ironically, it was also the moment when his career and – indeed – his life were in jeopardy. The rise of Nazi power in Germany did not create completely new ideas, but it altered the political framework in which the concepts of the Weimar Republic continued. The social-reform strand of social hygiene evoked pure hatred among National-socialist authorities and gave way to an increasingly eugenic format.[88] This ideological change was fast and profound, as doctors were ahead of all other professions in joining the National-Socialist party. Jewish and politically unwanted doctors were systematically removed from the German medical scene and while their "Aryan" colleagues, many of whom had found it difficult to open their own practices under the insurance system during the Economic Crisis, were eager to take over.[89] Goldmann was Jewish and a Social Democrat, both of which soon put him into danger. Rumours of his imminent arrest forced him to leave Germany in a hasty overnight flight.[90] He spent the summer of 1933 in Geneva and Paris, finishing the report on the February conference and, at Rajchman's suggestion, making studies of public health systems in several Western European countries.[91] In addition, he sought Rajchman's assistance in getting a position in China. The idea was not farfetched, since the LNHO was involved in reforming the Chinese public health system. Rajchman promised to help, and in September, Goldmann and his wife embarked for China. Accounts on circumstances and subsequent developments differ. Goldmann and his wife moved to Nanking but, gaining no employment, left the country again. Later, Goldmann and particularly his wife, a qualified physician, sent enraged complaints to the Secretary-General, claiming that Rajchman had given them formal promises of specific positions, which, as they then learned, he had no way of arranging.[92] They demanded compensation for the costs of passage to and from China and an official reprimand for Rajchman. However, the Secretary-General accepted Rajchman's explanation that he had merely promised help in case a position opened up in China, but had then found that chances were slim as Nanking was filling up with German refugees.[93] Indeed, Goldmann later apologised to Rajchman explaining that his desperate situation and his wife's nagging had prompted his behaviour.

In October and November 1933 the German Foreign Office ordered all Germans to terminate cooperation with the League of Nations.[94] Virtually all complied and swiftly distanced themselves.[95] By early 1934, the Health Committee and all commissions were without German members. Initially, LNHO reports continued to be published in the *Archiv für Soziale Hygiene und Demographie*, but Rott indicated upcoming difficulties and urged Olsen to come to Berlin.[96] Shortly afterwards the journal ended. The German authorities appeared unclear exactly what they wanted Olsen to do, but apparently the long-term plan was to have him return to Germany in some, as yet unclear, capacity.[97] But Olsen remained in Geneva. The scarce sources about his fate during the following years suggest personal stress as well as continued loyalty to his institution. In mid 1935 he was diagnosed as suffering from depression, which his doctor attributed to his son's death.[98] At that time he was in full charge of the large-scale LNHO project on housing, which he continued to supervise. In 1936 he declined the offer of a highly lucrative position as Director of the Institute of Hygiene at the University of Zurich in order to continue his work at the Health Section, a decision that much impressed Rajchman.[99] Simultaneously, he refused to return to his former position at the Friedrich-Wilhelm University Berlin, adding the snub that he had turned down more attractive offers at international universities, so that his former position was no longer an option.[100] In the following years, Olsen consistently received outstanding evaluations for his work at the Health Section. Expressions used included 'brilliant service to the Section and to the League', 'consummate ability to initiate investigations', 'brilliant study', 'particularly valuable services'. In particular, his studies on housing and nutrition received favourable comment.[101] At that time, he had every reason to believe that he faced a secure future at one of the safest places in Europe.

Meanwhile, Rott found his place in National-Socialist medicine. Initially, his career suffered a temporary setback when he was dropped from the list of lecturers at the Academy of Social Hygiene in Charlottenburg in 1934, and the *Archiv für Soziale Hygiene und Demographie* was discontinued.[102] But apparently these changes, though doubtlessly painful to Rott, merely reflected financial considerations unrelated to him as a person. At any rate, Rott was teaching again in 1936 and participated in a conceptual shift in child welfare in Germany, which increasingly adopted eugenic principles. Moreover, he actively supported the direction of the new government, ostracising former colleagues and friends.[103] In May 1933, Rott joined the NSDAP, and soon designed a strategy for the Ministry of the Interior for re-structuring the welfare system according to racial-hygienic and demographic considerations. He used the occasion to portray his former work at the various institutions and associations as pivotal efforts in this field. He was rewarded with the position of deputy director of the new Imperial Centre for Health Matters (*Reichszentrale für Gesundheitsführung*). The new Centre coordinated activities across the entire spectrum of welfare work through eleven sub-divisions. In this context, Rott actively participated in the process of bringing all strands of public activity under Nazi control (*Gleichschaltung*), including "cleansing" institutions of Jewish members.[104] In 1939 he was recommended for promotion to full professor for his achievements during the restructuring of the medical-scientific associations.[105]

In this new context, Rott continued working towards his former goals. Thus he laid great stress on medical statistics, notably the detailed analysis of the recent LNHO survey data on infant mortality.[106] Later, he was employed at the Imperial Health Office. This institution had, until 1933, remained largely untouched by eugenic and biologistic attitudes. Now, under the leadership of its new director, Hans Reiter, the Office changed character, dismissing Jewish and non-conformist staff members, among them medical-statistician Roesle, a man of avowed leftist sympathies.[107] He was forced to retire early, officially because of "professional unreliability," whereby presumably his positive views on Soviet medicine played a role.[108] His dismissal is noteworthy, since his undoubted expertise must have been in great demand by a regime that was obsessed with categorizing population and health in numbers. His whereabouts during the years of National-Socialism remain unclear. He appears to have been silenced but otherwise unharmed. By contrast, Rott, with whom Roesle had cooperated both in Berlin and in Geneva, prospered at the *Reichsgesundheitsamt.* He was responsible for the entire field of maternal, infant and child welfare, for school health, health passes, baths, hospitals and exhibitions, for the training of auxiliary staff and midwives, and eventually for scientific associations and congresses. He was also editor or co-editor of a series of pertinent journals.[109]

Meanwhile, Goldmann, after a short and misguided return to Berlin, had left Germany again for the USA and was trying to rebuild his career as a social hygienist and scholar. Prospects were not promising. Numerous German refugees with medical training were looking for work, while the country was still affected by the depression. But Goldmann was fortunate in that Roosevelt's New Deal policy demanded expertise in social medicine and provided more opportunities for experts in that field than ever before, or afterwards.[110] In addition, he received extensive assistance from Charles Winslow, Professor for Public Health at Yale University, who knew him through his LNHO work and who recommended him to a series of prestigious institutions.[111] From late 1937 to late 1938 he held a fellowship in Winslow's Department, which he used primarily to become acquainted with the US public health scene and with the English language, two crucial preconditions for teaching and doing research in the new country. Trying to reconnect to his earlier work with Grotjahn, he wrote a concept for mandatory health insurance in the USA. An enthusiastic Winslow put Goldmann into contact with some members of the small group of public health experts lobbying for health insurance. It was a mixed blessing. The paper helped Goldmann get noticed but also exposed him to the criticism of writing about a health system he did not sufficiently understand. He never found a publisher.[112]

The outbreak of the Second World War re-shuffled the cards once more. In Geneva, it caused the near disintegration of the League, politically and financially. Olsen was forced to resign from his post in December 1939, although he clearly would have preferred to stay, or at least a suspension of his contract with assurances of rehiring when possible.[113] Although he was in a more fortunate position than many of his colleagues, who were by then engaged in active warfare, his situation was by no means easy. At the age of 48, after 15 years of service with the League of Nations for which he had turned down other attractive positions, he found himself unemployed and with a problematic nationality. By the spring of 1940 he was planning to leave Europe.[114] But there were financial difficulties. He was entitled to an indemnity of more than one year's salary, which amounted to over 21,000 Swiss Francs. However, the League was more underfinanced than ever and Olsen's request to be paid in full was turned down.[115] Changing plans, he engaged in free-lance work for the League of Red Cross Societies. Apparently this was not enough, and he sought to re-establish contact with the German authorities, receiving support from the Overseas Organisation of the NSDAP and from Reiter.[116] In January 1941, negotiations began about his services to the Imperial Health Office on issues of international health.[117] During the following years Olsen received payment for sending LNHO information to Berlin, and he apparently joined the NSDAP.[118]

Olsen's activities were strangely ambivalent. He openly worked for the German Consulate, which enabled him to keep his residence in Geneva. He had the official permission of the League General Secretary to use the League library.[119] He sent material to Berlin after consultation with Yves Biraud, his former colleague, who remained virtually the only professional at the LNHO Section in Geneva. Apparently, Olsen listed LNHO documents, which Biraud found for him and occasionally provided with friendly notes to Hans Reiter, head of the German Health Office. The documents covered a broad range of topics, including biological standardisation, epidemiological intelligence, institutes of hygiene and general information about the LNHO. Whether the choice of topics came from Berlin or was his own, remains unclear, as does the quantitative extent of these activities.[120] By January 1942, he appears to have sent thirty-eight packages.[121] LNHO staff apparently welcomed Olsen's activities as a means of maintaining some, though limited, contact with the German authorities, on whose epidemiological data they depended. The German government hoped to get useful information about disease incidence in Europe. Remarkably, the British government knew about this flow of information and also welcomed it as a means to keep a channel of information open for more valuable data coming from the German-occupied territory (they were confident that their own data going out to Geneva were useless). [122] Thus, Olsen's activities may have ensured continued international communication by organising an exchange of superfluous information. For him personally, the project served as a way of avoiding combat and of remaining in contact with international health work, possibly also of keeping his options open in case of a German victory. In the complicated wartime world, separating survival instinct, ambition, idealism and opportunism may sometimes have been academic. By autumn 1943, the Director of the German Health Office, Reiter, urged Olsen to come to Berlin for consultations, which Olsen claimed to be physically unfit to do.[123] He diligently sent documents and signed his letters with "Heil Hitler," but he did not come to Berlin. As of autumn 1944, the language of the correspondence became less friendly. When Olsen explained that he considered his activities for the German Government "provisional" and returned to signing his letters "mit freundlichen Grüßen" (with best wishes), Reiter reluctantly ended their working relationship.[124]

By that time, Goldmann's life had consolidated into a calmer framework. With Winslow's help and after several fruitless attempts to gain employment, he was eventually hired at Yale University as associate professor in 1939. Until 1947, he taught classes on various aspects of public health policy, measures of disease prevention, general health insurance, health education, poverty relief measures and related themes. He was a dedicated teacher, creating new and innovative formats that connected the theory of the classroom with public discussions about ongoing real world issues of public health policy. Thus, he integrated field studies, and particularly his own research, into classes in which he compared different systems of medical care, notably the British tax-funded system with voluntary or mandatory health insurance schemes used in other countries. Apparently his classes were popular among students, and his ideas were noted, though not necessarily approved, by colleagues. Like all lecturers in public health, he faced strong reservations from the medical department with its built-in belief in the supremacy of medical studies. Nevertheless, he had established himself. After 1941, he taught additional classes at the New York School of Public Health at Columbia University and at the Department of Social Science at Connecticut College in New London.[125]

By 1945 the four former colleagues were worlds apart. In what was more than mere geographic separation, Rott and Roesle were in Berlin, Goldmann in Boston and Olsen in Geneva. All looked back on shattered dreams of past lives. The relatively best off was Goldmann. He had a last fleeting contact with public health affairs in Germany when, in 1944, he agreed to place his expertise at the service of the OSS. He wrote a 283-page Manual of German Health Services, a description of the German health system and the most important administrative and social welfare organisations.[126] This initiative appears exceptional and one of few examples of German public health specialists in exile supplying advice for US occupation forces.[127] But it is highly questionable whether his description had any tangible impact on US government planning in Germany.[128] Goldmann may not have been overly concerned. He wrote his report in support of US policies, and the idea of returning to Germany never seems to have crossed his mind. His real ambition by that time was to work towards the introduction of general health insurance in the USA. After his earlier, somewhat hastily drafted paper, he now approached the issue more systematically with a carefully researched volume on the state of *Public Medical Care*, which he published in 1945.[129] In this detailed analysis of the present US system, he once more reached familiar conclusions: the co-existence of various overlapping private and public, municipal, state and federal institutions and programs wasted resources and made it difficult for providers as well as patients to keep track of services. Echoing decade-old recommendations, Goldmann called for a careful determination of specific needs, based on statistical analysis, and for better cooperation and coordination.[130] Three years later, Goldmann added a volume in which he considered the US experience with various insurance models. He explained that the present system was wasteful and expensive because it excluded the lower classes, whose needs, on a costly emergency basis, had to be assumed by the state. He called for general voluntary medical care insurance in the United States. However, although the publication of his book coincided with an initiative for general health insurance by President Truman, his ideas had little chance in the face of aggressive anti-insurance lobbying by the American Medical Association. His university career continued at Harvard, where he taught from 1947 to 1958, but his teaching also suffered from the changing climate in the USA. Under the spectre of the Cold War, views like his were increasingly discredited as "socialist medicine." Disillusioned, Goldmann vacillated between demoralisation and efforts towards increasingly modest goals.[131]

Meanwhile, Roesle regained a respected place in academia. Between 1946 and 1951 he worked at the central department for health (*Zentralverwaltung für das Gesundheitswesen*) in the Soviet occupation administration and later in the newly established East German ministry of health, apparently acting mostly as instructor for epidemiological statistics. Rott, who chose the other Germany, left public service and obviously had to give up all ambitions of influencing the public health system. But his Nazi past did not prevent him from working in medicine. He practiced as private doctor in Baden-Baden, where he died in 1959.[132]

Olsen was less successful in regaining a position in international health. In November 1945, he wrote to the head of the personnel department of the now barely surviving League, and asked to have his name added to a list of former League servants who wished to continue service at the United Nations. He pointed out that he had given up his nationality due to serious difficulties with the National-Socialist government, and was now stateless.[133] There was little hope that this move would gain employment for him. At that time, plans for postwar health organisations had long moved to the USA, and League bureaucracy hardly possessed the clout to place former members. In October 1946, Olsen was still in Geneva but apparently planned to move elsewhere.[134] His fate in the following eleven years is unclear. In 1955, he was noted at the Rockefeller Foundation for his extraordinarily free translations when he accompanied the West German Minister of Health as translator.[135] Between 1957 and 1965, he appears to have had some affiliation with the WHO on temporary assignments.[136]

Conclusions

In a nutshell, the experience of these German social hygienists reflects the fate of social medicine in Europe at large. For a while Roesle, Goldmann, Rott and Olsen were colleagues, in heart and mind, sharing key ideas. They all favoured, and worked towards, an active public health policy, based on carefully established data, an intelligent and efficient health system, general insurance and a strong emphasis on prevention, notably in maternal and infant health care. In various degrees influenced by Grotjahn, they belonged to what Antoni has called the "second generation" of social hygienists, who no longer discussed theory but implemented different concepts.[137] Although they specialised in different aspects, it would not have been difficult to design a coherent concept on the basis of their collective ideas, involving careful statistical evidence, an efficient, well coordinated administration, special emphasis on infant welfare and fruitful international cooperation. In fact, between 1925 and 1933 they did all work together towards such a scheme in their collaboration with the LNHO. A decade later found them on different sides of geographical and political divides.

One wonders to what extent their different paths were inherent in their idiosyncratic ideas and to what extent they were forced upon them by circumstance. Rott's affinity to conservative, eugenic concerns showed early on. Such tendencies were not evident in either Olsen or Roesle, but hints could be found in Goldmann,[138] By the same token, Rott's early writings betray similar concerns over welfare as a means to public health and well-being as those of Roesle or Goldmann. It was certainly not coincidental that Rott integrated into Nazi ideology, that Roesle chose his post-1945 home in communist East Berlin and that Goldmann ended up in McCarthyite USA, but nor was it pre-determined. A plausible case can be made that, given more benign political development, they would have continued to work along quite similar lines. As it was, their ways parted, and inexorably they became, in varying degrees, participants in or victims of the ideologies of their time. Their lives are active proof of the multifaceted nature of social hygiene.

So how did they and their ideas fare in the various paths they took? The place that came closest to adopting their concept as a package, at least in theory, was probably East Germany: here health care centred on *Polikliniken*, similar to health centres albeit with a stronger curative function, and the system proclaimed equal access to healthcare for all members of society. Also, it strongly emphasized disease prevention and infant and maternal welfare as key tasks of public health policies.[139] Above all, public health was officially conceived as a task that was not merely a responsibility of the medical profession but involved society as a whole. These ideas did not necessarily reflect reality, but they formed the basis of the East German health system and, despite official Soviet control, they showed substantial continuity to Weimar Socialist plans.[140] Interestingly, the concept reads like a carbon copy of ideas discussed at LNHO conferences during the 1930s. However, Roesle's contribution was probably minimal. The GDR concept for a general social insurance system was substantially designed by Helmut Lehmann, who did not form part of the inner circle of German LNHO collaborators, though he had taken part in the original Geneva conference on methods of safeguarding public health during the depression in February 1933 as an ILO representative.[141] West Germany adopted a system of mandatory health insurance but otherwise based on private choices of individual healthcare, therapy rather than prevention and much reduced public involvement.[142] The system had little discernible similarity to LNHO discussions during the early 1930s, but nor did it follow Rott's schemes of racial hygiene. Goldmann was only marginally more successful. In the USA, the 1940s saw a series of initiatives for general health insurance, coming soon after Goldmann's early, unpublished concept but in discussions of which Goldmann took no active part. These schemes remained unsuccessful. Some of Goldmann's ideas regarding the coordination of public health measures resonated in the National Hospital Survey and Construction Act (Hill Burton Act) in 1946, but the Act was a feeble reflection with few consequences.[143] Medicare only became law in 1965, and it was a far cry from the comprehensive Goldmann plan. The goal of general health insurance remains unfulfilled in the USA even today.

Thus, none of the men was outstandingly successful, though the picture becomes more nuanced when mirrored against the men's specific goals. Roesle stands as a pioneer of medical statistics and their innovative use in both science and public health propaganda. The use of medical statistics as a basis for public health politics has been widely adopted. In this sense, Roesle's efforts left an imprint on medicine, and his legacy is acknowledged.[144] Goldmann, though less well known, can be considered one of the significant personalities of social in the twentieth century. His activities spanned fifty years, included research, teaching and contribution to the formulation of policy and left some 150 publications. He never succeeded in installing a rational health system, based on an intelligent coordination of public and private preventive and curative services. But he contributed substantially to a body of scholarship on the issue, part of which fed into various European welfare systems. Rott did for some years see the integration of his ideas on infant welfare policies into the mainstream medical discourse and gained a position of influence over this system in general. This status collapsed along with the Third Reich, and though he could end his life as a practicing physician, he is now mainly remembered as an example of how social hygiene could become corrupted into an inhumane ideology. The most forgotten and most ambivalent case concerns Olsen. In hindsight, it seems ironic that the only one of the men who was lucky enough to spend the time of dictatorship and warfare in the safe haven of Geneva was unable to re-connect to his pre-war career. His own efforts at connecting national and international experiences lay in shambles after 1945. But during fifteen years he contributed to processes of in-

ternational interaction which have since become daily routine. Besides, his effort at coordinating international cooperation is key to the real significance of the men's work. For while individually their impact has been decidedly limited, collectively they helped bring forward a concept which formed part of twentieth century civilisation. It is difficult to imagine how major improvements in public health could have been achieved without the intensive, international discourse of interwar social hygiene, to which the four men contributed. Their central success may have been the widespread acceptance of the citizens' entitlement to public concern about a broad range of issues including housing, nutrition, childcare and access to medical care, but also more far-reaching considerations about the social determinants of health, i.e. the interaction of social status and social inequality with health. These are key issues for how man as a social being organises society, and in as much as they contributed to a multi-voiced international effort to define a comprehensive concept for a healthier and better society, their activities during those years of cooperation were of lasting significance.
For some – or all – it may have been their finest moment.

Acknowledgments
I would like to thank Udo Schagen and Anne Hardy for most helpful comments on an earlier draft of the paper.

---

1 C. Antoni, *Sozialhygiene und Public Health. Franz Goldmann (1895-1970,* (Husum: Matthiesen Verlag, 1997), 37-41;

2 M.H. Kater, 'Die soziale Lage der Ärzte im NS-Staat,' in A. Ebbinghaus and K. Dörner (eds.), *Vernichten und Heilen. Der Nürnberger Ärzteprozess und seine Folgen* (Berlin: ATV 2002), 51-67.

3 G. Moser, '"Die Zukunft gehört der prophylaktischen Medizin" – Sozialhygiene, medizinisches Präventionsverständnis und Gesundheitsbegriff Ende der 1920er Jahre,' in U. Schagen and S. Schleiermacher (eds.), *Sozialmedizin, Sozialhygiene, Public Health* (Berlin: Charité, 2004), 15-20

4 For the entire context see G. Moser, *'Im Interesse der Volksgesundheit...' Sozialhygiene und öffentliches Gesundheitswesen in der Weimarer Republik und der frühen SBZ/DDR* (Frankfurt a.M.: VAS, 2002), 42-57; R. Winau, ‚Biologismus in der Medizin seit dem 19. Jahrhundert, Von der Eugenik zur Präimplantationsdiagnostik,' in U. Schagen and S. Schleiermacher (eds.) *100 Jahre Sozialhygiene, Sozialmedizin und Public Health in Deutschland*, (Berlin: Charité e-publication, 2005); W. Woelk and J. Vögele, Introduction in W. Woelk and Jörg Vögele (eds.), *Geschichte der Gesundheitspolitik in Deutschland* (Berlin: Duncker & Humblot, 2002), 11-48, relevant pages 11-28;S. Stöckel, 'Gesundheitsfürsorge – von der Armenpflege zur Profession,' in Sigrid Stöckel and Ulla Walter (eds.), *Prävention im 20.Jahrhundert. Historische Grundlagen und aktuelle Entwicklungen in Deutschland,*(Weinheim / München: Juventa, 2002), 65-77; A. Labisch, 'Die ‚hygienische Revolution' im medizinischen Denken. Medizinisches Wissen und ärztliches Handeln,' in Ebbinghaus / Dörner, *Vernichten und Heilen*, 68-89, esp.

77-87; P. Weindling, *Health race and German politics between national unification and Nazism, 1870-1945* (Cambridge: Cambridge University Press, 1993).

5 K.H. Roth, 'Schein-Alternativen im Gesundheitswesen: Alfred Grotjahn (1869-1931) – Integrationsfigur etablierter Sozialmedizin und national-sozialistischer 'Rassenhygiene', in: K.H. Roth (ed.), *Erfassung zur Vernichtung. Von der Sozialhygiene zum 'Gesetz über Sterbehilfe'* (Berlin: Verlagsgesellschaft Gesundheit, 1984), 31-56.

6 I. Borowy, 'Wissenschaft, Gesundheit, Politik. Das Verhältnis der Weimarer Republik zur Hygieneorganisation des Völkerbundes,' *Sozial.Geschichte, Zeitschrift für historische Analyse des 20. und 21. Jahrhunderts*, 20:1 (2005), 30-56.; S. Wulf, *Das Hamburger Tropeninstitut 1919 bis 1945* (Berlin: Dietrich: Reimer Verlag, 1994), 5; E. Crawford, *Nationalism and Internationalism in Science, 1880-1939* (Cambridge, CUP, 1992), 49-56; P. Weindling, 'The Divisions in Weimar Medicine: German Public Health and the League of Nations Health Organization,' in S. Stöckel and U. Walter (eds.), *Prävention im 20.Jahrhundert. Historische Grundlagen und aktuelle Entwicklungen in Deutschland* (Weinheim / München: Juventa, 2002), 110.

7 See I. Borowy, 'International Social Medicine between the Wars. Positioning a Volatile Concept,' *Hygiea Internationalis*, 6:2 (2007), 13–35.

8 Minutes of the Rockefeller Foundation, 25 May 1927, RF, RG 1.1, Series 100, Box 20, Folder 164, 27162; Minutes of the International Health Board, 22 May 1929, RF, RG 1.1, Series 100, Box 20, Folder 164, 29303-4.

9 Gunn to Russell, 23 April 1927, RF, RG 1.1, Series 100, Box 20, Folder 17; Minutes of the Rockefeller Foundation, 25 May 1927, RF, RG 1.1, Series 100, Box 20, Folder 164, 27163-5. Antoni claims Grotjahn received insufficient support from the LNHO. Antoni, *Sozialhygiene und Public Health,* 67.

10 See the special issue of *Continuity and Change* 12:2 (1997), devoted to the history of classification of causes of death: G.B. Risse, 'Cause of death as a historical problem', 175-188; J. Duffin, 'Census versus medical daybooks: a comparison of two sources on mortality in nineteenth-century Ontario', 189-218; B. Leidinger, W.R. Lee and P. Marschalck, 'Enforced convergence: political change and cause-of-death registration in the Hansestadt Bremen, 1860-1914', 219-246; E. Rodriguez-Ocaña and J. Bernabeu-Mestre, 'Physicians and statisticians: two ways of creating demographic health statistics in Spain, 1841-1936,' 247-264. See also G.C. Alter and A.G. Carmichael, 'Classifying the Dead,' *Journal of the History of Medicine* 54 (1999), 114-132.

11 R. Münch and J. Lazardzig, 'Inszenierung von Einsicht und Überblick. Hygiene-Ausstellungen und Prävention,' in Stöckel / Walter, *Prävention*, 78-95, esp. p. 84.

12 S. Stöckel, 'Sozialmedizin im Spiegel ihrer Zeitschriftendiskurse. Von der Monatsschrift für soziale Medizin bis zum Öffentlichen Gesundheitsdienst, in Schagen / Schleiermacher, *100 Jahre Sozialhygiene,* 7-10.

13 S. Nikolow, 'Der statistische Blick auf Krankheit und Gesundheit,' in U. Gerhard, J. Link and E. Schulte-Holtey (eds.), *Infografiken, Medien, Normalisierung: Zur Kartografie politisch-sozialer Landschaften* (Heidelberg: Synchron, 2001), 223-241; see also E. Meier, 'Entwicklung der Medizinalstatistik unter Emil Eugen Roesle,' *Bundesgesundheitsblatt*, 5:21 (1962), 329–332.

14 See biographical sketch, G. Moser, „Im Interesse der Volksgesundheit...", 384.

15 R.A Meckel, *Save the Babies: American Public Health Reform and the Prevention of Infant Mortality 1850-1929* (Ann Arbor: University of Michigan Press, 1998), 101.

16 M. Mazower, *Der dunkle Kontinent.* (Frankfurt a.M.: Fischer Taschenbuch Verlag, 2000), 126-134; (Original: *Dark Continent: Europe's Twentieth Century.* London: Penguin Books, 1998.); Meckel, *Save the Babies*, 101-103.

17 E. Schabel, *Soziale Hygiene zwischen Sozialer Reform und Sozialer Biologie. Fritz Rott (1878-1959) und die Säuglingsfürsorge in Deutschlang* (Husum: Matthiesen Verlag, 1995), 24-35.
18 Ibid., 51-53.
19 Ibid., 44-48, 54-56..
20 Ibid., 50-51.
21 Ibid., 69-70.
22 J. Vossen, ‚Die Entwicklung des öffentlichen Gesundheitsdienstes in Preußen/Deutschland und seine Aufgaben in Sozialhygiene und Sozialmedizin 1899-1945, in Schagen / Schleiermacher, *100 Jahre Sozialhygiene*, 5-6.
23 Schabel, *Soziale Hygiene*, 101-106.
24 Schabel, *Soziale Hygiene*, 113-114.
25 Moser, 'Zukunft,' 17.
26 Vossen, ‚Entwicklung des öffentlichen Gesundheitsdienstes,' 5-8.
27 Schabel, *Soziale Hygiene*, 99.
28 Schabel, *Soziale Hygiene*, 94-95.
29 Antoni, *Sozialhygiene und Public Health*, 22-36.
30 Ibid., 42-45.
31 Ibid., 48-56.
32 Cf. biographical sketch in Moser, 'In Interesse der Volksgesundheit...', 368.
33 Curriculum Vitae, Personal File of Otto Olsen, League of Nations Archive (henceforth: LONA); regarding Hahn see biographical sketch, Moser, 'Im Interesse der Volksgesundheit...', 368.
34 Borowy, 'Wissenschaft, Gesundheit, Politik,' 40-42.
35 Weindling assumes as much. P. Weindling, 'The Divisions in Weimar Medicine: German Public Health and the League of Nations Health Organization,' in Stöckel / Walter, *Prävention im 20.Jahrhundert*, 116; cf. P. Weindling, *Epidemics and Genocide in Eastern Europe, 1890 – 1945* (Oxford: Oxford University Press, 2000), 211.
36 Madsen to Rajchman, 9 April 1922, LONA, R 820/12B/26213/11346.
37 Evaluation forms, Personal file, Otto Olsen, LONA.
38 C. Böttcher, *Das Bild der sowjetischen Medizin in der ärztlichen Publizistik und Wissenschaftspolitik der Weimarer Republik* (Pfaffenweiler: Centaurus-Verlagsgesellschaft 1998), 55-58.
39 Minutes of the eighth HC Session, held 13 to 19 Oct, 1926, C.610.M.238.1926.III., 27 Nov 1926, 32-33. See also I. Borowy, 'Counting Death and Disease - Classification of Death and Disease in the Interwar Years, 1919 – 1939', *Continuity and Change*, 18:3 (2003), 457 - 481.
40 Roesle, *Vorschläge zur Internationalisierung der Statistik der Morbidität* and Roesle *Morbiditätsstatistik im Deutschen Reiche*, both undated in: LONA, R 994/12B/60615/58590.
41 Roesle to Tománek, Health Section, 19 Nov 1927 and 23 Dec 1927, both: LONA, R 994/12B/59241/58590; *Präsident des Reichsgesundheitsamtes* to *Reichminister des Innern*, 22 Feb 1927, Politisches Archiv des Auswärtigen Amtes (henceforth: PAAA), Akten betreffend Verwaltungs- und technische Fragen. Deutsches Personal im Generalsekretariat, Bd. 1, R 96816.
42 *Essai d'une Statistique comparative de la Morbitidité devant servir à établir les Listes spéciales des causes de Morbidité,* C.H. 730, Oct 1928, LONA, R 5972/8D/409/408.
43 Tománek to Roesle, 14 Nov 1927, LONA, R 994/12B/59241/58590; Boudreau to Huston, 28 Jan 1927, and Rajchman to Hamel, 18 Feb 1927, LONA, Roesle Personal Files.

44 Roesle to Wasserberg, 9 June 1927 and 7 Dec 1927, LONA, R 988/12B/58466/54691.
45 Infant Mortality and Child Welfare, C.H./P.E./5, undated, and C.H. 420, April 1926, both LONA, R 972/12B/46927/46927; Rajchman to Rott, 26 May 1926, LONA, R 973/12B/51810/46927.
46 Schabel, *Soziale Hygiene,* 122-129.
47 Annual Report of the Health Organization for 1928, A.8.1929.III (C.H. 788), 18 April 1929, 46-47.
48 See reports in LONA, R 973/12B/52771/46927.
49 F. Rott, 'Die drei Senkungsperioden der Säuglingssterblichkeit im Deutschen Reiche,' *Gesundheit fürs. Kindesalter*, 2 (1926/27), 491-508, in Schabel, *Soziale Hygiene,* 131.
50 Annual Report of the Health Organization for 1928, A.8.1929.III (C.H. 788), 18 April 1929, 46-47.
51 Rott to Rajchman, 28 Jan 1928, and 1 March 1928, both LONA, R 6002/8F/1407/1092.
52 See Pirquet to Rajchman, 7 May 1928, LONA, R 6002/8F/1582/1092.
53 Rott to Olsen, 29 April 1927,and Olsen to Rott, 5 May 1927, LONA, R 973/12B/51810/46927.
54 Rott to Olsen; 3 Jan 1929, LONA, R 6002/8F/9760/1092.
55 Schabel, *Soziale Hygiene,* 117.
56 Annual Report of the Health Organization for 1929, A.9.1930.III, July 1930, 37-39.
57 Schabel, *Soziale Hygiene,* 135.
58 Publications Committee to Health Section, *Abmachungsniederschrift,* 20 Feb 1932, undated, LONA, R 5871 / 8A / 14009 / 1990.
59 Campbell to Rott, 4 Nov 1930, LONA, R 6002/8F/23354/1499.
60 *Report on Maternal Welfare and the Hygiene of Infants and Children of Pre-School Age*, C.H. 1060, Geneva, 15 Oct 1931.
61 See correspondence in LONA R 6225/8F/2363/895.
62 Olsen to Rott, 9 Jan 1933, LONA, R 6225/8F/895/895; cf. Report to the Council on the Work of the 21st Session of the Health Committee, C.233.M.97.III, 7 June 1934, 8.
63 Pryll to Rajchman, 8 June 1928, LONA, R 6007/8G/6096/1718.
64 'Leistungen der deutschen Krankenversicherung im Lichte der sozialen Hygiene.'
65 Antoni, *Sozialhygiene und Public Health,* 63-71.
66 Annual Report of the Health Organization for 1929, A.9.1930.III, July 1930, 35-36.
67 Antoni, *Sozialhygiene und Public Health,* 68 and 72-73.
68 F. Goldmann and A. Grotjahn, *Die Leistungen der deutschen Krankenversicherung im Lichte der sozialen Hygiene* (Berlin 1928), 30; cited in Antoni, Sozialhygiene und Public Health, 68-69.
69 Memo for the Second Session of the Preparatory Committee, C.H. 948, 29 Nov 1930, 3.
70 See the chapters on Stampar, Johan and Mackenzie in this volume.
71 Antoni, *Sozialhygiene und Public Health*, 90-97.
72 Ibid., 74-90.
73 Ibid., 97-109.
74 'The Economic Depression and Public Health," Memorandum prepared by the Health Section, *Bulletin* I (1932): 428 and 132; Rajchman to Madsen, 30 July 1932, Archive de l'Institut Pasteur (henceforth: AIP), Fonds Rajchman.
75 'The Economic Depression and Public Health," Memorandum by the Health Section, *Quarterly Bulletin of the League of Nations Health Organisation,* I (1932), 432.
76 Work of the Health Committee During its Nineteenth Session, held Oct 10-15, 1923, C.725.M.344.1932, *Official Journal of the League of Nations*, Feb 1933, 354-355.

77 E.E. Roesle, 'Der Längsschnitt-Gesundheitsindex und seine Anwendung für die Gesundheitsstatistik der Erwerbslosen,' *Zeitschrift für Gesundheitsverwaltung und Gesundheitsfürsorge*, 3:20 (1932), 461-5.
78 Gini to Olsen, 29 Dec 1932, LONA, R 6041/8A/884/549.
79 Mosbacher to Olsen, 30 Jan 1933, LONA, R 6041/8A/2242/549.
80 Greenwood to Buchanan, undated, LONA, R 6116/8A/13812/13812.
81 Rajchman to Newman, 10 Feb 1928, LONA, R 6007/8G/1718/1718.
82 Goldmann to Rajchman, 14 Dec 1932, LONA, R 5936/8A/39992/39992.
83 ILO Memo, *Crise economique et santé publique,* 27 Dec 1932, LONA, R 5936/8A/39992/39992.
84 Rajchman to Maurette, 16 Jan 1933, LONA, R 6041/8A/549/549.
85 'Report on the best methods of safeguarding the Public Health during the Depression." *Bulletin* II (1933), 286-332.
86 Ibid., 293-5.
87 Ibid., 316 and 320.
88 W. Eckart, *Geschichte der Medizin* (Berlin: Springer, 2000), 344.
89 J. Cornwell, *Forschen für den Führer* (Bergisch Gladbach: Bastei LübbeVerlag, 2006), 182; (English Original: *Hitler's Scientists: Science, War and the Devil's Pact,* London: Viking Press, 2003); W.F. Kümmel, ,'Die Ausschaltung'. - Wie die Nationalsozialisten die jüdischen und politisch mißliebigen Ärzte aus dem Beruf verdrängten,' in J. Bleker and N. Jachertz (eds.), *Medizin im 'Dritten Reich* (2nd ed, Cologne: Deutscher Ärzte-Verlag, 1993), 70-77; E. Seidler, *Jüdische Kinderärzte: Entrechtet - geflohen – ermordet* (Basel / Freiburg: S. Karger Verlag, 2007).
90 Antoni, *Sozialhygiene und Public Health*, 13.
91 Antoni, *Sozialhygiene und Public Health*, 123-126; Rajchman to Secretary General, 22 May 1934, LONA, R 5710/50/7262/6501.
92 Antoni, *Sozialhygiene und Public Health*, 127-134.
93 Alice Goldmann to Secretary General, 14 March 1934; Goldmann to Secretary General, 12 March 1934; Note by Nisot, 30 April 1934; Rajchman to Secretary General, 22 May 1934; Goldmann to Stampar, 18 Sept 1933; Goldmann to Rajchman, 24 March 1936, all LONA, R 5710/50/7262/6501. Rajchman's version was supported by a letter from Goldmann to Andrija Stampar, confirming that he had been unsure of employment before leaving for China. Antoni, the author of a Goldmann's biography, doubts the authenticity of this letter. Some awkward German phrases lead her to assume that it may have been forged by a non-native speaker of German as a cover-up for Rajchman. Antoni, *Sozialhygiene und Public Health*, 130-131, note 431. This accusation appears improbable, because in this case Goldmann's subsequent letter of apology to Rajchman makes no sense, apart from being totally out of character for Stampar.
94 Protokoll Kommhoevener, AA, *Besprechung zu Auswirkungen des deutschen. Austritt aus dem Völkerbund*, 27 Oct 1933; letter forms, 9 Nov.1933, both Bundesarchiv R 1501/ 12534.
95 Borowy, 'Medizin, Wissenschaft, Politik,' 54-55.
96 Report by Boudreau, January 1934, including annex 1, LONA, R 6110/8A/9088/9088.
97 RMI to Olsen, 9 Nov 1933 and Kamphoevener to Abt. IV, Legationsrat Oster, 10 Nov 1933, both PAAA, Akten betreffend Verwaltung und technische Fragen. Personal. Deutsches Personal im Gesundheitssekretariat, R 96816.
98 Medical Certificate, Dr. Albert Dubois, 15 July 1935, LONA, Olsen Personal File.
99 Note by Rajchman, 21 January 1936, LONA, Olsen Personnel File.

100 Olsen to Dean of Friedrich-Wilhelm Universität, Berlin, 19 Jan 1936, PAAA, Akten betreffend Verwaltung und technische Fragen. Personal. Deutsches Personal im Gesundheitssekretariat, R 96816.
101 Certificates as to grant of annual increment 1935-38, LONA, Olsen Personnel File.
102 Schabel, *Soziale Hygiene,* 100.
103 Ibid., 140-145.
104 Ibid., 146-152.
105 Ibid., 118.
106 Ibid., 152.
107 Ibid., 156-157.
108 E. Marcusson and Dietrich Tutzke, 'Die Bedeutung des Lebenswerkes von Emil Eugen Roesle (1875 – 1962) für die Entwicklung der medizinischen Statistik in Deutschland,' *Zeitschrift für die Gesamte Hygiene*, (1975), 649-652.
109 Schabel, *Soziale Hygiene*, 165-167.
110 See Antoni, *Sozialhygiene und Public Health,* 170.
111 Winslow knew Goldmann's work, but it is unclear if the two men ever personally met in Geneva. Antoni, *Sozialhygiene und Public Health,* 175- 178, 182-189; Regarding Winslow, see also G. Rosen, *A History of Public Health* (New York: MD Publications, 1958, reprinted Baltimore: Johns Hopkins University Press,1993), 515.
112 Antoni, *Sozialhygiene und Public Health,* 180-188, see also 193 and 250-255.
113 Olsen to personnel department, 22 December 1939, Olsen to Avenol, 10 February 1940, LONA, Olsen Personal File.
114 Olsen to Personnel Department, 22 December 1939, and Olsen to Treasury, 23 March 1940, both LONA, Olsen Personnel File.
115 Balance Sheet, handwritten note by Olsen, 23 May 1940, and Jacklin, Treasurer, to Olsen, 24 May 1940, LONA, Olsen Personal File.
116 See Weindling, *Epidemics and Genocide,* 221.
117 Krauel (Konsulat Genf) to Olsen, 10 Jan 1941, cf. Note by Krauel, 10 Jan 1941, K.Nr.59, *Bescheinigung für die Reise vom Generalkonsulat Genf,* 7 May 1941, both PAAA, Konsulat Genf, Bündel 25, Informationen des Reichsgesundheitsamtes, der Reichsärztekammer etc., Band I (Kult. 11 Nr. 4).
118 See Weindling, *Epidemics and Genocide,* 221 and 245.
119 Hamel to Reiter, 26 Sept 1941, Certificate of consulate, undated, Olsen to Reiter, 5 July 1943, all PAAA, Konsulat Genf, Bündel 25, Informationen des Reichsgesundheitsamtes, der Reichsärztekammer etc., Band I (Kult. 11 Nr. 4).
120 See Biraud to Olsen, 19 June 1941; Biraud to Reiter, 19 June 1941; Olsen to Biraud, 1 Sept 1941; Biraud to distribution department, 1 Sept 1941, alle LONA, R 6069 / 8A / 41083 / 1263.
121 Reiter to Olsen, 29 Jan 1942, PAAA, Konsulat Genf, Bündel 25, Informationen des Reichsgesundheitsamtes, der Reichsärztekammer etc., Band I (Kult. 11 Nr. 4).
122 Memo M.S. Williams, 8 Sept 1942, Public Record Office, FO 371 / 30991.
123 Reiter to Olsen, 21 Oct 1943; Reiter to Olsen, 11 Feb 1944; Olsen to Reiter, 28 Aug 1944, all PAAA, Konsulat Genf, Bündel 25, Informationen des Reichsgesundheitsamtes, der Reichsärztekammer etc., Band I (Kult. 11 Nr. 4).
124 Olsen to Reiter, 16 Oct 1944 and Reiter to Olsen, 11 Jan 1945, both PAAA, Konsulat Genf, Bündel 25, Informationen des Reichsgesundheitsamtes, der Reichsärztekammer etc., Band I (Kult. 11 Nr. 4).
125 Antoni, *Sozialhygiene und Public Health,* 188-216.
126 Antoni, *Sozialhygiene und Public Health,* 216-226.

127 D. Ellerbrock, 'Gesundheit und Krankheit im Spannungsfeld zwischen Tradition, Kultur und Politik - Gesundheitspolitik in der amerikanischen Besatzungszone 1945-1949,' in W. Woelk and J. Vögele, *Geschichte der Gesundheitspolitik in Deutschland* (Berlin: Duncker & Humblot, 2002), 313-346, see 332.

128 See Antoni, *Sozialhygiene und Public Health*, 223, 260-274.

129 F. Goldmann, *Public Medical Care, Principles and Problems* (New York, 1945); F. Goldmann, *Voluntary Medical Care Insurance in the United States* (New York, 1948), both cited in Antoni, *Sozialhygiene und Public Health*, 193.

130 Antoni, *Sozialhygiene und Public Health*, 226, 235

131 Ibid.., 259 and 274.

132 Marcusson / Tutzke, 'Emil Eugen Roesle,' 649-652; See also biographical sketches in Moser, *'Im Interesse der Volksgesundheit... "*, 384.

133 Olsen to Vilette, Personnel Department, 24 Nov 1945, LONA, Olsen Personal File.

134 Stencek, Personnel department, to Olsen, 9 Oct 1946, LONA, Olsen Personal File.

135 Excerpt JMW (John Weir, Associate Director for Medical Education and Public Health, Rockefeller Foundation) Diary, Germany, Oct 31 – Nov 6, 1955, Rockefeller Foundation Archive, RF, RG 2, Series 1955 General Correspondence, Box 59, Folder 373.

136 Information from Ineke Deserno, head archivist of the WHO, Telephone conversation 13 March 2003.

137 Antoni, *Sozialhygiene und Public Health*, 40.

138 In his *Habilitation* thesis, he insisted on the need to cleanse hospitals of homeless, the unemployed, the old and infirm, who abused the institution for a substitute shelter. Antoni, *Sozialhygiene und Public Health*, 89.

139 S. Schleiermacher, 'Prävention und Prophylaxe in BRD und DDR. Eine gesundheitspolitische Leitidee im Kontext verschiedener politischer Systeme,' in Schagen / Schleiermacher, *100 Jahre Sozialhygiene;* U. Schagen, 'Aufbau einer neuen Versorgungsstruktur: Gesundheitsschutz als Leitkonzept," in Stöckel / Walter, *Prävention im 20. Jahrhundert*, 168

140 U. Schagen, 'Kongruenz der Gesundheitspolitik von Arbeiterparteien, Militäradministration und der Zentralverwaltung für das Gesundheitswesen in der sowjetischen Besatzungszone,' in Woelk/Vögele, *Geschichte der Gesundheitspolitik*, 379-404.

141 See biographical sketches in Moser, *'Im Interesse der Volksgesundheit... "*, 359-390.

142 S. Schleiermacher, ''Prävention und Prophylaxe in BRD and DDR,' 4-7; N. Schmacke, 'Die Individualisierung der Prävention im Schatten der Medizin,' in Stöckel / Walter, *Prävention im 20. Jahrhundert*, 178-189.

143 Antoni, *Sozialhygiene und Public Health*, 237-238, and 256-258.

144 See Marcusson / Tutzke, 'Emil Eugen Roesle', 649-652.

Gustavo Pittaluga (1876 – 1956)
Science as a Weapon for Social Reform in a Time of Crisis

Esteban Rodríguez-Ocaña & Iris Borowy

Gustavo Pittaluga was a key mover in the development of public health, parasitology and haematology in Spain.[1] As chief parasitologist at the National Institute of Health, chair of Parasitology and Tropical Diseases and director of the outpatient clinic for blood diseases at the University of Madrid until the start of the Spanish Civil War in 1936, he played a paramount role in sustaining a laboratory-based approach to the problems of health and disease in Spain. He also played a connecting role with the international sphere of health experts through the League of Nations Health Organisation, where he sat as Spanish representative after 1924. By conviction, aims and strategy he belonged to the generation of concerned educated people that was energetically engaged in a comprehensive modernisation programme — or, as it was called at the time, the *Europeanisation of Spain* — which was ended by the Civil War and its aftermath. Already exiled in France in the fall of 1936, the German invasion drove him to Cuba, where he settled in 1942 to contribute to science and culture, as so many other Republican Spaniards were doing throughout Latin America. This paper will review Pittaluga's multilayered interests, his endeavours and contributions to the shared project of those liberal minds that shaped a formative component of the interwar scientific scene.

Pittaluga's career in Spain was the result of several personal decisions early in his adult life. He was born in Florence into an aristocratic but ruined Italian family. His father was a high officer of the Italian Army and became governor of Venice during the First World War. Pittaluga studied at Rome University, where he earned a doctoral degree in Medicine with a dissertation on the pathogeny of acromegaly (July 1901) while serving as resident physician at the Sancti Spiritu Hospital (January 1900 to July 1901) under Giusseppe Bastianelli (1862-1959), assistant in Psychiatry (January 1900- March 1902) with Prof. Enzo Sciamanna (1850-1905), and assistant in the Institute for Comparative Anatomy (1899-1902) with Prof. G. Batista Grassi (1854-1925). In this last position he contributed to two experimental field interventions against malaria, at Ostia, July-November 1901, and at Terracina, June-mid July 1902.[2] On the advice of Grassi, Pittaluga travelled to Spain from August 1902 to May 1903 to survey malarious regions there. On 27 May he presented a paper at a regular meeting of the Società Geografica Italiana on the methodology for creating a map of malaria.[3] Obviously this trip left a deep impression on him. A year later, he settled in Spain.

We can only speculate what exactly made him decide to leave his native Italy for Spain, a country in social turmoil and with insecure political prospects.

Was it a sense of adventure? Was he attracted to the professional opportunities offered by a country with heavily malarious regions and few malaria specialists? Or to the woman he would marry soon after? Possibly, it was a combination of these. With his new nationality, Pittaluga embarked on a brilliant professional career that merged early and permanently with a willingness to become involved in the political life of the country. It is this intertwined connection between science, politics and his private life that characterises his activities during the following decades and that forms the basis of the analysis presented here. In the complex world of interwar Europe, and in ways that were familiar to most scientists of the time, Pittaluga's activities were marked by overlapping commitments to the profession, academics and politics.

The Spain he moved to provided a fertile ground for making such connections. The country had only begun to recover from the shock of the humiliating defeat in the 1898 war against the United States of America, in which it lost its last colonies and pretensions for a world power. A deep concern about political and social development and a widespread belief that the country suffered from societal 'backwardness', gave rise to a broad 'regenerationist movement'. Uniting different interest groups, it developed a somewhat confused political profile that combined a variety of issues with little obvious connection. They ranged from demands for lower taxes and for political change — sometimes with antidemocratic aims — to increasing nationalist and regionalist sentiment. They also included a perceived need for education, population and health programmes, which derived from the positivistic pro-science discourse of the 19th century, exemplified by the *Institución Libre de Enseñanza* (ILE, Free Board for Education, a private though persuasive enterprise that prepared the way for changes in Spain's educational framework). The combined effect of three arguments, voiced repeatedly in the academic world, brought science and medicine to the forefront of the social agenda: 1. Spain had failed to take part in the imperialist division of the world; 2. this political weakness resulted in part from a lack of scientific expertise; 3. the realm of 'science' was a part of 'Europe'.[4] In 1898, mathematician and President of the Royal Academy of Sciences (and 1904 Nobel Prize laureate for literature) José de Echegaray (1832-1916), declared that 'Spain was defeated by science and riches.' A year earlier, Santiago Ramón y Cajal (1852-1934), on the occasion of his official reception at the same Academy had pointed out that 'the Spanish disease' was none other than its 'distance from Europe (i.e. from science)'.[5] Cajal, an histologist, was the foremost scientific figure in Spain at the time, who was to share the Nobel prize with Camilo Golgi, in 1906. He belonged to the 'generation of wise men' that, from the 1880s, conducted a sustained effort to introduce modern scientific criteria into universities and the technical industrial world. This reform became institutionalised after 1898, when the authorities realised the need to promote national role models as examples of the 'regenerating' nation. This idea paved the way for the creation, under Cajal's guidance, of the Laboratory of Biological Research in 1900, the same year that saw the Ministry of Education appear as a separate office in the cabinet.[6]

These developments reflected a coalition between, on the one hand, some sectors of the government *élite* (i.e., members of the traditional oligarchy) and, on the other, the bourgeoning *intelligentsia,* a growing scientific middle class including engineers, physicians, chemists, and teachers, etc. that expanded along with the booming industrial and economic development between 1890 and 1920. Many of its representatives joined the ranks of the 'spiritual community' around ILE, sharing its aims without formally belonging to the institution. What Thomas Glick has called an unwritten agreement in search of modernisation first found political support from the Count of Romanones' wing of the Liberal Party, that resulted in the 1907 founding of the Board for Advanced Studies and Scientific Research (*Junta para Ampliación de Estudios e Investigación Científica,* henceforth JAE, its Spanish acronym) — fully active by 1910, under the presidency of Cajal — and of the Society for the Advancement of Sciences (*Asociación Española para el Progreso de las Ciencias,* AEPC) in 1908.[7] The former organised travel grants for young scholars enabling them to gain practical expertise in foreign laboratories and also directly funded a number of centres for experimental biology and the humanities. The AEPC was active as a forum for scientific exchanges, through its annual meetings, each in a different city, which were used to popularize science throughout the country.

These developments were supported by a number of intellectuals, among them the philosopher José Ortega y Gasset (1883-1955), a staunch activist and promoter of reformist campaigns. His principal aim, introducing scientific competence into the political realm, was explained in a series of articles published in February 1913. There he declared that: 'A new Spain will only be possible when the merging of these two terms, democracy and competence, is fulfilled'. Reaching adequate (i.e. European) levels of scientific and technological competence would be 'a revolution' in itself. [8] The connection to science appeared particularly evident in public health problems (infant mortality, tuberculosis, the flu epidemic in 1918-19) that could easily be linked with existing conservative concerns about the supposed decline of the population and an allegedly gloomy future of the 'Spanish race'. Public health therefore became the object of many regenerationist proposals that provided a fertile ground for the flourishing scene of social medicine.[9] In this context, public health work gained important political and cultural connotations. The strong emphasis on the importance of expertise and science for national development combined with the idea that scientific competence would be tied to 'Europe', created an ambivalent mixture of meanings that included modifying the character of the nation and integrating it into the community of European countries. Thus, performing science in Spain was a political act, at the same time patriotic in the sense that it advanced the national agenda, and vaguely threatening in demanding fundamental social and political changes to the country. Obviously, being a scientist in Spain at this time had far-reaching implications.

The evidence suggests that in 1902, Pittaluga was mostly moved by tangible considerations about malaria, in which he possessed an expertise that facilitated his entry into the Spanish medical world. Malaria was an enduring and crippling condition in many rural areas of Spain, where death rates had increased temporarily in the wake of the 1898 war. In 1905, the number of cases of malaria was estimated in around 800.000 per annum.[10] Scientifically, malaria had been brought to the fore of medical and public health awareness thanks to the exciting discoveries made by Alphonse Laveran, Patrick Manson, Ronald Ross, Camilo Golgi, Battista Grassi and Robert Koch, among others, in the years around the turn of the century.[11] By Spanish standards, Pittaluga held exceptional expertise on anophelism, having done field work under Grassi, zoologist, parasitologist and frustrated competitor for Ronald Ross' Nobel Prize, awarded for discovering the malaria cycle.

In 1901, one of Pittaluga's first professional commitments had been a field experiment on malaria treatment and prevention at Ostia, near Rome, where he first encountered the vicious circle of disease, malarial environment and extreme poverty in rural families. Malaria, he wrote then in the socialist journal *Avanti!*, 'is a social phenomenon closely linked to *latifundia* (great rural properties)' – conditions similar to those in Spain. [12] He also encountered the discrepancy between newly won scientific understanding and continuing widespread popular beliefs about the disease, which persuaded him that the first duty of physicians active in the field was to convince target populations of the rationale behind necessary measures.[13] His subsequent travels around Spain and his search for help for intended future field trips brought him into contact with Francisco Huertas Barrero (1847-1933), a wealthy Madrid-based clinician, personal physician to Santiago Ramón y Cajal, and co-author of the first official study of Spanish malaria that accepted the mosquito doctrine. Huertas shared the chair with Pittaluga at the malaria session of the 14th International Medical Conference, held in Madrid and Barcolona (1903). It was he who introduced Pittaluga into the Spanish scientific community and its social circle, including Cajal and his future wife, Huertas' sister-in law. Pittaluga was valuable in this company, notably to Cajal. His excellent scientific credentials were attractive and his training in pathology gave him an expertise in microscopical methods in which Cajal was keenly interested. In addition, Pittaluga carried the sponsorship of the pharmaceutical firm, Bisleri, to test and promote a therapeutic drug against malaria. Last but not least, Cajal must have recognised in the young Italian the personal qualitites, such as the intellectual ambition and the hard-working ethos, he required of those seeking a scientific career.[14]

Scientifically, Pittaluga's move to Spain was an immediate success. Within three years, he had co-chaired a session of the 14th International Medical Conference, edited an epoch-making book on malaria in Spain, directed at least two field expeditions in heavily malaria stricken areas in Catalonia and Estremadura and been on an official mission to study malaria in the Canary Islands.[15] He also married into high-society, obtained anew his license as physician and, under Cajal's direction, a new doctoral degree in experimental biology.[16] Other endeavours were more disappointing. With characteristic ambition, Pittaluga set out, 1903, to establish a scientific journal, *Archivos latinos de medicina y de biología,* intended to publish selected contributions from Italy, France and Spain, under the umbrella of Bisleri. The chief editors were two outstanding members of the profession from each country, S. Ramón y Cajal and C. M. Cortezo from Spain, R. Blanchard and A. Robin from France and B. Grassi and E. Maragliano from Italy, while Pittaluga acted as managing editor. Unfortunately, this project only lasted three issues.[17] Pittaluga's early search for an academic position also proved difficult. He aimed at the chair of Public Hygiene, a second-rank specialised discipline, somewhat at the margin of the School of Medicine. He entered the public competitive examinations for this chair, in 1905 and again in 1907, without success. The first time, the position remained unfilled, in 1907 it was given to a well-known ear-nose- and throat specialist, with no knowledge whatsoever of laboratory procedures, needed for diagnosis and research.

In the ensuing scandal, the conditions of recruiting university staff came under scrutiny, and criticism was levelled at a procedure loaded with favouritism in which obscure conditions of influence or even bribery counted more than the scientific qualification of candidates.[18] Tellingly, Pittaluga's career only advanced when he, too, received the support of a highly placed individual: in 1906 Cajal appointed him to the disinfection team of the National Institute of Hygiene (NIH). In 1908, he entered the Permanent Council against Tuberculosis, by co-optation from the Ministry of Interior.[19] In 1909, also at Cajal's suggestion, he directed a scientific expedition to the Spanish colony in the Gulf of Guinea — a trip that emulated similar colonial missions by other countries, usually focussing on sleeping sickness.[20] There he found a new species of a hematophagous insect that he immediately named *Clemmys Africana Haemoproteus Cajali*, in honour of his patron.[21] This mission proved a career boost. In 1911 he was put in charge of a section of Parasitology within the NIH, and won the new chair of Parasitology and Tropical Diseases at the University of Madrid, which he kept until his exile in 1936. By 1915 he had made important contributions to cytology (he described the cellular structure of the filaria embryos, 1903, as well as the centrosome of leukocytes, 1909) and to the study of parasitic diseases. [22] Pittaluga thereby promoted a view of medicine as applied biology, using laboratory-based experiment as an integral part of his approach to human disease. He managed two university laboratories for pathology, bacteriology and parasitology at the School of Medicine, both in the department itself and at the Central Laboratory for Clinical Research (founded in 1912, under Pittaluga's direction after 1920), which produced generations of young scientists who adopted his concept. Thus, he strengthened the spread in Spain of the new understanding of scientific medicine that had already gained ground in other European countries and North America. The integration of the laboratory into medicine revolutionized the general understanding of disease, the role of doctors and their relation to their patients.[23] Pittaluga must have been aware of these consequences, because in addition to his post in academia, he maintained a successful private practice. Among other postings, he worked as head of pathology at the *Instituto Rubio de Terapéutica Operatoria*, a private centre that excelled in surgery, as physician to the Royal Music Theatre, and as personal physician to the heir to the throne of Spain.

For Pittaluga personally, laboratory work intensified his life-long fascination with blood. His training in pathology, i.e. microscopical imaging, and his familiarity with parasitological diseases, many of which produced blood and blood-related troubles, led him to turn toward haematology in his clinical practice. In 1916 he started teaching on blood diseases and, in 1918, established a specialty outpatient clinic at the University hospital. He departed from a mostly morphological understanding of haematology ['the study of normal and pathological blood morphology'] introducing the view of an interrelationship of histological, metabolic and endocrine aspects framed by constitutional typology. Pittaluga's approach thus served to promote the growth of Internal Medicine as a discipline.

Pittaluga's scientific achievements coexisted with a fruitful career in the domain of health administration. In 1915 he was chosen by the regional *Mancomunitat de Catalunya* to head the Catalonian health services, where he conducted the first publicly funded campaign against malaria.[24] Five years later, the Spanish central government decided to follow a similar path, and Pittaluga was entrusted with its organisation as president of the first national commission against malaria, where he remained as a regular member after 1924. According to the testimony of one of his students, he resigned from the National Hygiene Institute following the military putsch by General Primo de Rivera.[25] We have not found any further proof of Pittaluga's resignation; but in February 1924 the position of chief of Section of Parasitology at the National Hygiene Institute was open to internal competition. It went to Sadí de Buen Lozano (1893-1936), Pittaluga's direct disciple and right hand in the malaria business.[26] In 1930 Pittaluga became Director of the new School of Public Health (*Escuela Nacional de Sanidad*), a position that he kept with the Socialist-Republican coalition under the Republic until the end of 1932, and a Conservative government named him head of the National Institute of Public Health (*Instituto Nacional de Sanidad*) that was reorganized in 1934. Until the outbreak of the Civil War in 1936, he also maintained several positions granted to him in 1932 by the first Republican government —a place on the board of directors of the Permanent Commission for Health Investigations (*Comisión permanente de Investigaciones Sanitarias*), and chief editor of the official journal of the Spanish health administration, *Revista de Sanidad e Higiene pública.*[27] In such posts, he was instrumental in broadening the concept of 'public health' from a narrow bacteriological perspective to a broader understanding that included concern over nutrition, engineering, architecture and industrial work.

Parallel to —and connected with— his professional activities, Pitttaluga threw himself into the mainstream of political life, supporting the reformist side.[28] By 1907 he had joined the *Ateneo de Madrid*, a cultural club. He participated as a teacher for philosophy of science and attended several *tertulias* — literary gatherings that served as social spaces for intellectuals, organised, among others, by José Ortega y Gasset. In 1917 he moved his Masonic membership from the Great Orient of Italy to the Hispanic American Lodge in Madrid, a fact that later in his life served as a charge against him by Francoist authorities.[29] Pittaluga also joined the *Junta Nacional*, the National Council of the Reformist Party, created in 1913 by Melquiades Álvarez in a failed attempt to attract the Monarchy to the side of liberal democratic middle-class. Pittaluga defended the party's official policy for health matters at the national assemblies of November 1918 and May 1921 and at the 1919 National Conference on Health Services (*Congreso de Sanidad civil*), where he delivered the closing speech.[30] Pittaluga's contribution to the health agenda of the Reformist Party, the only party with a coherent political programme on public health by that date, was expressed in a pamphlet he published in 1921.[31] This text echoes the belief of the democratic movement in the benefits of combining technical expertise with political reformist determination. At the moment of greatest social and medical unrest, scientific knowledge, administrative skills and political determination must merge into the discipline of Social Medicine, whose task should be entrusted to a coalition of social organisations, independent from the state. Accordingly, Pittaluga took part in the foundation of an Institute for Social Medicine (1919-1923) and, later, of a Spanish League for Social Medicine (1920-1923), an association that offered 'biological' counsel to the government.[32] The immediate goal of these institutions was to educate the people in matters of health, defined both as an individual right and as a civic duty, with a corresponding emphasis on the role of experts.

Between 1915 and 1923 Pittaluga also participated in other reformist initiatives, attending philosopher José Ortega y Gasset's political lectures, writing articles for *España* and supporting the Spanish Democratic Union, *Unión Democrática Española,* created in November 1918 by an illustrious group of democratic intellectuals, including Miguel de Unamuno, Ramón Menéndez Pidal, Luis Simarro, Américo Castro, Gregorio Marañón or Manuel Azaña.[33] This ephemeral Union wanted to forge ties to Europe and to strengthen a Spanish branch of the new international postwar institutions. In 1922, Pittaluga was also among the supporters of the League for Human Rights (*Liga Española de los Derechos del Hombre*), founded in 1913 in close collaboration with freemasons, with the aim of raising the democratic consciousness of Spanish society.[34]

Pittaluga's political convictions also tied into his concern about malaria. His appointment as president of the national campaign against malaria in August 1920 must be understood as part of the Reformist compromise policy package for social improvement.[35] The first Malaria Commission was designed by Pittaluga as an NGO that should unite a number of interested civil organisations, including the Red Cross, without interference from the government, a strategy that had been successfully tried in Italy. The work of the Commission was to be based exclusively on scientific considerations, free from all political influence. Its technical personnel was provided entirely by the Parasitological section of the National Institute of Health, which Pittaluga headed, an organisation he considered free from political taint. Thus, in addition to improving the malaria situation in the country, the Malaria Commission was meant to serve as an example of how mobilisation of the educated members of society could achieve public health aims, which, in turn, could provide a model for further social goals.[36] However, his ideas soon turned out to be somewhat removed from reality. Philanthropy was totally absent from public concern on malaria and the presence of civil society was wishful thinking. Instead, malaria campaigns developed thanks to the active involvement of local and provincial administrations while the technical structure generated merged with the National Health Department.

This experience of widespread lack of interest and empathy among the public may have been disappointing, but it was not inexplicable, given the social context of the disease. Malaria in Spain was mainly a rural problem, very much linked to the peasants' poverty and social destitution that characterised most of the southern Iberian Peninsula. Long ignored, it became an explicit state concern only when extensive rural strikes and riots broke out in between 1917 and 1920. Increased attention to those rural regions revealed the extent of the disease burden, particularly in southern and eastern rural and mining areas. In the early 1920s, Pittaluga estimated that there were around 250,000 patients and more than 2,000 deaths per year, causing the loss of five million working days.[37] In 1924 a new regulation changed the structure of the National Malaria Commission, taking the executive tasks away from Pittaluga.

Ironically, as he distanced himself from the military government, Pittaluga began his active cooperation with the League of Nations Health Organisation

(LNHO), whose decision-making body, the Health Committee, he joined in 1924. This juxta-position is noteworthy. Though Health Committee members were officially appointed for their expertise and did not represent governments, in practice they usually did. Pittaluga's colleagues routinely considered the interests of their administrations during discussions on specific issues and reported back to their ministries.[38] The Health Committee minutes list him merely as member of the School of Medicine at the University of Madrid without administrative connection.[39] Whatever the political background, as a member of the LNHO Health Committee, Pittaluga travelled to Geneva once or twice a year and discussed the variety of public health issues that formed the broad work programme of the LNHO. He retained his seat until the end of 1936, serving as Vice President during the last years.

While reducing his involvement in the national malaria commission, Pittaluga became active in the LNHO Malaria Commission. This brought him into contact with colleagues from other, mostly European, countries, among them eminent international malariologists, including Émile Brumpt, Bernhard Nocht, James Hacket, Nicolaas Swellengrebel and his former supervisor, Giuseppe Bastianelli. Malaria was of considerable concern to the LNHO during the 1920s. The steady decline of the disease in Europe in the second half of the nineteenth century had been reversed in several regions by the effects of the First World War. The exact extent of this increase was a matter of controversy, but the fact as such was beyond doubt.[40] To LNHO Medical Director, Ludwik Rajchman, malaria appeared in 1923 'undoubtedly the most important epidemiological problem of Europe.'[41] The Malaria Commission grew to be one of the largest LNHO bodies, organizing surveys, cooperative studies, and international courses. Given the broad relevance of the disease, many countries were keenly interested in international counsel, and while Rajchman's view that Spain saw its 'only hope of real progress in international co-operation on practical lines' may have been an exaggeration, there certainly was an interest in sharing experiences with other countries.[42]

As the foremost expert on malaria in a malaria-ridden country, Pittaluga was invited to join the LNHO Malaria Commission in 1924.[43] In this capacity, he travelled to the Balkans and the USSR in 1924, a journey remembered in literary sketches — including a short depiction of Andrija Stampar with whom he was obviously impressed— that were published in Spain in 1926.[44] Also in 1926, Pittaluga participated in a study of malaria in the deltas of the Danube, Po and Ebro, allowing comparisons between different places with similar conditions In this context, he cooperated with his Romanian, Italian and Dutch colleagues, professors Jean Cantacuzène, Donato Ottolenghi and Nicolaas H. Swellengrebel.[45] He also went to Greece in 1929, with other members of the Committee, to prepare the LNHO scheme to reorganise the Greek public health system.[46] In addition, Pittaluga took part in international malaria courses, which the Malaria Commission organised in order to alleviate the lack of qualified malariologists. Courses consisted of two parts, a first period of theoretical lectures and laboratory work, and a second practical part of field work in malarious regions, among them areas in Spain, under the aegis there of the Institute for Malariology established at Navalmoral de la Mata. The classes were popular both among students and organizers. Doubtless, they offered another opportunity for colleagues from different countries to meet, though such meetings did not always create the desired effect of international camaraderie, as Pittaluga acknowledged when students from Romania and Yugoslavia got into a fist fight during field work in 1928.[47] The political agenda that sustained anti-malaria intervention in Spain was made clear by Pittaluga in a lecture at the Engineering School of the University of Madrid in 1927. He forcefully underscored the link between health and citizenship, explaining that a minimum level of physical comfort was needed by peasants 'so they could experience human dignity and achieve consciousness as citizens'.[48] It was this exclusion from citizenship that made rural unrest a political challenge, threatening the integrity of society. These factors had an ethical as well as a tangible political perspective, as Pittaluga made clear when he discussed similar issues on an international level while opening the European Conference on Rural Health in 1931. In what was only superficially a conservative remark, he argued that World War I had demonstrated how neglecting the health of rural people, the backbone of all populations, compromised the security of nations.[49]

Indeed, during those latter years of the 1920s, Pittaluga was in a paradoxical situation. Internationally, he was becoming a recognized public health expert, while domestically his position was locked in political limbo: He was part of the public scene on issues of health, but not part of the inner circle of power. This ambivalence showed in his relations with the Rockefeller Foundation. Pittaluga was in regular contact with Rockefeller officials, as they strove first to negotiate and then to implement an agreement with Spain. Rockefeller fellow Selskar Gunn recognized that Pittaluga's distance from the actual group in power discredited him in some quarters.[50] He considered it 'a cloud', which did not, however, prevent him from considering Pittaluga the best trained Spanish expert in public health and most in line with the goals of the Foundation.[51] Gunn's colleague, Charles Bailey, who worked in Spain from December 1924 to June 1926, agreed that Pittaluga probably would be the best Director of Public Health, were that politically possible.[52] At the time it was not. When the acting Director, Francisco Murillo Palacios left his post in the spring of 1928, Pittaluga was not even considered, owing, he was convinced, to political concerns.[53]
Pittaluga's working conditions improved when the political system changed. He actively contributed to this circumstance as a member of the directorate of the prominent *Ateneo de Madrid,* that between 1925 and 1930 led the intellectual

criticism of the dictatorship.[54] In this context he took part in the various activities, including protest campaigns, public pronouncements and growing disorder among artists, literary men and university professors, that contributed to the fall of Primo de Rivera in December 1929 and the end of the monarchy after the municipal election of April 1931.[55] The complex web of political forces complicated decisions and loyalties. This time Pittaluga did not accompany his old friends Ortega and Marañón, who formed a group intent on supporting the cause of liberal republicanism: instead he honoured his lasting commitment to Melquíades Alvarez and to the former Reformist Party, now called Liberal-democratic Republican Party in 1931. However, when, later in 1932, Álvarez moved further to the right, Pittaluga abandoned him. In 1935 he joined the Republican Left (*Izquierda Republicana*). For a while he was an influential, albeit controversial force in political developments. When the new republican constitution was being drafted, Pittaluga successfully argued against the need for a candidate to be born in Spain to become President of the Republic. His triumph brought scathing commentaries against him in the right wing press. Repeatedly he suffered attacks by philo-fascists journalists regarding his foreign origin, some of which were answered by public hommages as the one offered by his friends on 20th March, 1933.[56]

In September 1930, the national and the international arenas connected when the transitional government of Spain proposed that the League of Nations, in cooperation with the International Institute of Agriculture, organise a conference for the study of rural hygiene in Europe.[57] This initiative may have been an attempt to defuse an increasingly explosive national situation. In Spain the politically influential class of conservative *latifundistas* faced bitter demands from the landless poor, which were repeatedly vented in local uprisings and temporary occupations. Although the climax of these upheavals had already passed in 1920, the question continued to destabilize the fragile political order in the profoundly divided Spanish society.[58] For Pittaluga, the initiative was explicitly motivated by 'the effort to remodel her internal life undertaken by Spain.'[59] Honouring his pivotal position in the initiative, the LNHO Health Committee appointed Pittaluga president of a new Sub-Committee on Rural Hygiene, in charge of preparing a large European conference on Rural Health. The preparatory meetings of representatives of national health administrations, of the ILA and the International Labour Office during the following months revealed several principal difficulties. Indicative of the main problem of social medicine, discussions centered on the questions of how to balance medical with broader social and technical concerns at the upcoming interdisciplinary event. Some, such as the German representative Hamel, were concerned about a loss of weight of medical opinion, while others, including Pittaluga, feared the potentially influential opposition of physicians. The latter was indeed a delicate issue, in which principles of public welfare were frequently at odds with those of the liberal professions. Country doctors often had to scrape a difficult living among people of limited means and therefore disliked seemingly unfair competition from publicly funded health centres, while public health officials naturally aimed at reaching the entire population with preventive and curative services, regardless of whether they could pay for doctors. There was also a more fundamental question of whether public health was regarded primarily as a medical or a social issue. In this tension, Pittaluga clearly preferred the public health perspective, while trying to avoid antagonizing doctors' associations.[60] This was only one of several balancing acts he had to master while presiding over the European Conference on Rural Hygiene in Geneva between 29 June and 7 July, 1931. It was by any standard a major event for its time.[61] Collectively, more than fifty people from all over Europe had contributed to the planning, and twenty-four countries were represented at the conference. Delegations varied widely in size. Several countries sent only one person, while France, Italy and Spain had each authorized ten experts. They were joined by twenty-two observers from eight extra-European countries[62] and international organisations.[63] As hoped, the meeting was impressive not only for gathering people from different countries, but also from a variety of professions including public health administrators, agricultural experts, physicians, engineers, hygienists and insurance delegates. Nevertheless, there were conspicuous absences: The Spanish delegate of his country's General Workers' Association, Enrique Santiago, formally protested against being the only representative of the working classes.[64] His criticism revealed that it was a conference on the health of rural populations from which — with the notable exception of the Spanish contribution — these populations were largely excluded.

Pittaluga tried hard to turn the conference into a historical moment. Urging his colleagues to dare embrace ambitious goals, he declared in his opening address: '[...] we are not going to lay down rules and principles with a view to stabilising an existing state of things, but [...] we are going to change the existing state of things in so far as we are able to do so and to promote progress.'[65] At least on paper, this claim was borne out by a number of resolutions on medical assistance, health services and sanitation in rural areas, derived from months of meticulous preparation. Aiming at defining minimal standards for health services, the conference insisted on universal access to first aid as well as diagnostic services, laboratories and specialized treatment, financed either through health insurance or state systems of free medical assistance, All rural health should assume responsibility for infectious disease control, campaigns against social diseases, maternal and infant welfare, the sanitation and hygiene of milk and foods. Lending credence to the 'apolitical' nature of health, the Conference declared that these demands should be met everywhere in Europe, regardless of the political structure of different countries and their health administrations. At the same time, the conference betrayed its ties to reformist thinking in Spain —and elsewhere— by declaring improvement of the general level of education to be essential preconditions for these aims, and health authorities were urged to spread modern knowledge concerning hygiene among rural people by all available means.[66] In his closing remarks, Pittaluga emphasized its historical significance:

> I am sure that this first European Conference on Rural Hygiene will mark an epoch in the history of hygiene in agricultural and rural districts. For the first time on so large a scale and with so much authority, practicing physicians, health officers, administrators, agriculturists, engineers and organizers of agricultural associations have met together for the thorough study of those questions which are most important for the improvement of conditions of life in rural districts from the standpoint of hygiene and health. It will not be the last time. There is still a long road to be travelled, but this Geneva Conference, convened by the League of Nations, marks the starting-point on that road [...][67]

Though the conference was clearly considered a major event by contemporaries, its tangible effects are difficult to define. It gave rise to several follow-up studies, to which Pittaluga also contributed ideas and, apparently, data. But in relation to the ambitious original plans, the results appeared patchy and disappointing.[68] Clearly, in the face of the lingering economic crisis and increasing political tension the early enthusiasm could not be sustained. However, the concepts and ideas of the conference appear to have survived to a much greater extent. By 1939, Pittaluga commented that 'the directing principles for an efficient organisation of rural health services [sprung from the Conference of 1931] have been accepted and applied by many countries in Europe and have spread to other parts of the world'.[69] While this statement may have been the exaggeration of a man in exile who remembered one of his finest moments, it seems certain that in its aftermath, some impact of the Conference was felt in Eastern Europe as well as in Spain.[70] In Spain, the conference recommendations served as arguments in favor of the health reforms launched by the first Republican government.[71] Pittaluga himself seems to have valued the event and have taken pride in it, since he sometimes quoted his own words from his presidential address in varied contexts. Plausibly, he may have felt that the occasion added weight to arguments he held dear beyond malaria and rural hygiene, notably the integration of scientific, social and political knowledge as prerequisite for successful public health efforts.[72]

In terms of international exposure, this moment constituted the climax of Pittaluga's career, and it coincided with a highly productive phase in research, particularly as head of a team of young researchers in the field of haematology.

Between 1930 and 1936 twenty-four doctoral dissertations, prepared under his supervision, were defended at Madrid University, and probably around 100-120 scientific articles were published by people working at the laboratories and the clinic he directed. In 1934, his monograph on diseases of the reticuloendothelial system was published, full of practical data produced by the clinical work of his team.[73] A revised, updated version appeared after Pittaluga had settled in Havanna, and a treatise on the physiopathology of blood was found on his desk the day of his death.[74] At the same time, his presence in some French journals such as *Archives des maladies du coeur des vaisseaux et du sang* or *Le Sang. Biologie et pathologie*, increased. In 1933 Pittaluga joined the French Society of Haematology and was elected Foreign Vice-President in 1935. In addition, he multiplied his travels and contacts with Latin America and obtained membership of the Medical Academies of Rio de Janeiro, Mexico and Buenos Aires, as well as an honorary chair of histology at the National University in Mexico (1935).

The outbreak of the Civil War abruptly ended Pittaluga's life in Spain.[75] In the days of confusion that followed the reactionary military uprising, a workers' committee at the National Institute of Health removed Pittaluga from his office.[76] It seems that he was on his way to attend a meeting in Geneva, returned and then left Spain for good in October 1936, explaining: 'We are all asked to be either Red or Blue and I'm unable to turn into any such'.[77] He stayed in France during the whole of the Civil war, ignoring the Republican Government order for all civil servants to return to their offices and, as a result, being dismissed in December 1936.[78] Unlike his friends Ortega and Marañón, who also moved to France during the war, Pittaluga did not immediately accept Franco's victory. Instead, he engaged in anti-fascist resistance, founding the first civil organisation in exile, a Union of Spanish University Professors in Foreign Countries, (*Unión de Profesores Universitarios Españoles en el Extranjero*, later called *en el Exilio,* in exile) that met in Paris in 1939 under his presidency. In February 1939, two months before the end of the Spanish war, the victorious Fascist authorities expelled him from the rank of professorship, together with other fourteen other academics, citing 'their permanent anti-national and anti-Spanish convictions'.[79] Like others, Pittaluga was removed from public service by both Republican and Francoist governments!

We have but incomplete knowledge of the details of Pittaluga's endeavours in France. In the early autumn of 1937, his presence was noted at the second international conference on blood transfusion in Paris.[80] Having neither a government that could nominate him nor a scientific position, he was not re-elected into the LNHO Health Committee in 1936. Instead, he was hired as 'specialist expert' for six months ostensibly in order to draft the forth Report of the Malaria Commission.[81] His tasks included not only the original assignment, but the preparation of a further international conference on rural hygiene, this time to be held in the Americas. For this purpose, he travelled to Cuba and Mexico and produced a long scholarly review on the conditions for rural health in countries low-density populations.[82] However, the opposition of the Pan-American Sanitary Bureau and the general deterioration of the international situation in 1939 undermined these efforts, and the planned conference never materialised.[83] Otherwise, we have scant knowledge of Pittaluga during this period. . There is some evidence that he earned a living working as a private consultant on pathology, mainly but not exclusively concerned with blood diseases. He seems to have been linked to the hospitals Cochin and Saint Antoine, where Arnault Tzanck developed the first regular blood transfusion service in France.[84] Short research papers or clinical contributions signed by Pittaluga appeared regularly in the journal of the French Society for Haematology, *Le Sang*, during 1939 and 1941.[85] In October 1939 he contributed to the discussion on blood transfusions with a summary of experiences during the Spanish civil war.[86]

The fall of France drove Pittaluga from Paris to Marseilles. Travelling further was difficult and possible places of refuge unclear. The Rockefeller Foundation provided some protection but no help for his plans to go to the USA. For several months he and his family stayed in Casablanca, before he finally settled in Cuba in October 1942.[87] After the second meeting of the *Union of Spanish Professors in Exile*, which he organised in Havana in 1943, he felt his political task was fulfilled: he abandoned politics with a mixture of relief and resignation.[88] He concentrated on securing a living, renewing his qualifications for permission to work as a physician and as consultant in a variety of official settings on a temporary basis.[89] Up to his death, he remained remarkably productive as a scientific writer with papers on the physiology and pathology of blood, as well as on laboratory procedures. At the same time, he made numerous written and oral contributions to Cuban cultural life in books, journals, newspapers and even radio serials (he was elected a member of the Cuban Academy of History in 1948). And, finally, he kept a passionate correspondence with Maria Zambrano, a philosopher of the intellectual circle around Ortega y Gasset, who had settled in France after her first exile in Cuba.[90] Despite his active life and apparent assimilation into Cuban society, he longed for Spain and tried to return, once he was granted retirement as University professor in March 1955, although illness and economic shortage prevented him from travel.[91]

Conclusions

Considering his biographical road map, Pittaluga personified scientific internationalism. Born and educated in Italy, he lived in Spain from age twenty-five to sixty and spent the final 20 years of his life in France or Cuba. While this form of internationalism was partly forced on him, his international scientific outlook was a matter of choice and of a political agenda. Ironically, this agenda was both transnational and national. His ideas about social progress and the social and scientific nature of medicine defied borders in that he shared them with colleagues in other countries, but by applying them to specific Spanish needs he gave them a patriotic function. His active pursuits of scientific internationalism, which he shared with the elite of cultivated Spaniards, derived from the ideals of the movement for free education and the quest for national 'regeneration.' They also tied into a belief in the common values of European civilisation, including representative democracy as a political necessity. A man of multiple interests, he was a notable writer and convincing speaker, acclaimed scientist, public health officer and politician. A firm believer in progress, he argued that technical expertise had to be at the service of social improvement Thus, all his laboratory research was directly connected to practical applications. His work on malaria, where the connection between science, medicine and politics was particularly apparent, was a case in point: improving the general understanding of malaria served to improve the living conditions and consciousness of peasants, which, in turn, would enable them to contribute more self-confidently and meaningfully to society. In this context, he dreamt of a 'Madrid school of haematology', as he was a keen supporter of the Spanish school of malariology built around the Malariological Institute at Navalmoral de la Mata, and of the anti-malaria medical corps that he co-organised in the early 1920s.

Not all of his efforts were successful. Tragically, the project of modernising Spain, which he shared with many intellectuals, eventually crumbled under the onslaught of Franco's army. Nevertheless, important elements of his mission to transfer knowledge and ideas between Spain and the international arena had lasting effects. His involvement in rural hygiene demonstrated the bipolar effect of this activity. While the original plan was to use international pressure and expertise to reform rural conditions in Spain, the result can just as well be described in opposite terms: it was the Spanish impetus and reformist enthusiasm that turned rural hygiene into a high-profile international issue. More than anyone else, Pittaluga was responsible for upgrading rural hygiene on the international and a number of national agendas, and as a result of the development in Spain after 1936, his efforts were arguably more influential in other countries.

Sadly, after decades of acting within a clear understanding of the interdependence of politics, medicine and health, he eventually proved unable to reconcile these fields. Wars and exile turned him into a cultivated old man who had to rely heavily on writing to earn a living in progressively deteriorating private circumstances. Unlike colleagues such as Andrija Stampar or René Sand, who emerged from years of imprisonment to rise to new heights of acclaim and see their ideas of international and holistic health work rehabilitated and –

within the constraints of the post-war world – implemented, Pittaluga was forgotten. He was keenly aware of this impending fate when, in October 1943, he confessed to his confidant María Zambrano that he was likely 'to enter the eternal dark night of oblivion'.[92]

---

1 F. Vega Díaz, 'Recordatorio de un gran intelectual: Gustavo Pittaluga (1876-1956)', *Nuevo Índice*, 2:14 (1983), 1-11; S. Martín Gómez, *Vida y obra de D. Gustavo Pittaluga Fattorini* (Madrid: Universidad Complutense [Colección Tesis doctorales nº 395/88], 1988); E. Rodríguez-Ocaña, 'Pittaluga Fattorini, Gustavo', in W.F. Bynum and H. Bynum (eds.), *Dictionary of Medical Biography* (Westport,CT /London: Greenwood Press, 2007), vol. 4, 1018-1020.

2 Personal Files, *Relación de méritos y servicios del Dr. Gustavo Pittaluga Fattorini, 5 de Julio de 1913*, Real Academia Nacional de Medicina de Madrid; Martín Gómez, *Vida y obra*, 10-11; G. Pittaluga, 'Studi sulla patogenesi dell'acromegalia e sulla funzione dell'ipofisi,'*Annali dell'Istituto Pschiatrico delle R. Università di Roma*, 1902; anno 1 [offprint kept at Biblioteca de la RANM de Madrid]; B. Grassi et al., *Relazione dell'esperimento di profilassi chimica contro l'infezione malarica, fatto ad Ostia nel 1901* (Milano: tip. Rancati, 1902).

3 G. Pittaluga, 'Per la carta de la distribuzione geographica della malaria,' *Bolettino della Società Geografica Italiana*, (1903), fasc. VIII [offprint].

4 On the shifts in social representations of science and technology from 1875 to 1906, see L. López-Ocón, *Breve historia de la ciencia española* (Madrid: Alianza Editorial, 2003), 304-342; on the projets to overcome the feelings of scientific backwardness, see J.M. Sánchez Ron, *Cincel, martillo y piedra : historia de la ciencia en España (siglos XIX y XX)* (Madrid: Taurus, 1999), 171. A useful reader on the development of Spanish science and technology is J.M. Sánchez Ron and A. Lafuente (eds), *Un siglo de ciencia en España* (Madrid: Residencia de Estudiantes, 1998).

5 J.Fornieles Alcaraz, *Trayectoria de un intelectual de la Restauración, José Echegaray* (Almería : CECA, Monte de Piedad y Caja de Ahorros de Almería, 1989); S. Ramón y Cajal, *Reglas y consejos sobre investigación biológica. Reproducción del discurso de ingreso en la Academia de Ciencias exactas, físicas y naturales (sesión del 5 de diciembre de 1897)* (Madrid: Imprenta de T. Fortanet, 1899) [last reprint as *Reglas y consejos sobre la investigación científica*, Madrid, CSIC, 2005]; J.L. Barona, 'Ramón y Cajal, Santiago', in Bynum and Bynum (eds.), *Dictionary of Medical Biography*, 1049-1053.

6 A. Baratas, 'La investigación biológica en la España del primer tercio del siglo veinte', in Sánchez Ron and Lafuente (eds.), *Un siglo de ciencia en España*, 94-113; A. González de Pablo, 'El Noventayocho y las nuevas instituciones científicas. La creación del Laboratorio de Investigaciones Biológicas de Ramón y Cajal', *Dynamis*, 18 (1998), 51-79.

7 T.F. Glick, *Einstein y los españoles. Ciencia y sociedad en la España de entreguerras* (Madrid: Alianza Editorial, 1986);J.M. Sánchez Ron (ed.), *1907-1987. La Junta para Ampliación de Estudios e Investigaciones Científicas, ochenta años después* (Madrid: CSIC, 1988) (particularly, vol. I, 1-61); E. Ausejo, *Por la Ciencia y por la Patria: La institucionalización científica en España en el primer tercio del siglo XX. La Asociación Española para el Progreso de las Ciencias* (Zaragoza: Siglo XXI de España Editores, 1993); P. García Sierra, 'La evolución filosófica e ideológica de la Asociación Española

para el Progreso de las Ciencias (1908-1979),' *El Basilisco*, 15 (1993), 49-81. (http://www.filosofia.org/rev/bas/bas21504.htm). A useful catalogue of more than 600 pages accompanies the exhibition *El laboratorio de España. La Junta para Apliación de Estudios e Investigaciones Científicas, 1903-1939* (Madrid: Sociedad Estatal de Conmemoraciones Culturales, 2007).

8 Ortega's articles, reprinted in *ABC* [suplemento cultura], March 20, 1998; F. Villacorta, *Burguesía y cultura: Los intelectuales españoles en la sociedad liberal, 1808-1931* (Madrid: Siglo XXI, 1980); M. Tuñón de Lara, *Medio siglo de cultura española (1885-1936.*(Madrid: Tecnos, 1977); A. Elorza, *La razón y la sombra. Una lectura política de Ortega y Gasset* (Barcelona: Anagrama, 1984).

9 E. Rodríguez-Ocaña, 'Medicine as a Social Political Science: The Case of Spain c. 1920', *Hygiea Internationalis,* 6:2 (2007), 37–52.

10 R.O. 25 May 1905, endorsing the purchase of a poster against Malaria by the schools, *Gaceta de Madrid*, no. 154, 3 June 1905, 883.

11 M. Worboys, 'Tropical Diseases', in W.F. Bynum and R. Porter (eds.), *Companion Encyclopedia of the History of Medicine* (London: Routledge, 1993) 512-536; G. Corbellini, 'Paludisme', in D. Lecourt, (ed.), *Dictionnaire de la pensée médicale* (Paris: Presses Universitaires de France, 2004); E. Rodríguez-Ocaña, 'International Health Goals and Social Reform: The Fight against Malaria in Interwar Spain', in I. Borowy and W.D. Gruner (eds.), *Facing Illness in Troubled Times. Health in Europe in the Interwar Years, 1918-1939* (Frankfurt a.M.: Peter Lang; 2005), 247-276.

12 G. Pittaluga, 'Lettere sulla malaria. Ostia, Giugno-Novembre 1901', *Avanti*! [Roma, setiembre-novembre 1901], 49 [offprint].

13 '[...] *che il nostro primo dovere, il primo dovere d'un medico in questo tempo, sia quello di persuadere bene se stesso e di sapere bene persuadere gli altri, tutti gli altri, chela febre malarica è data dalla puntura di una speciale zanzara, l'Anopheles* [...]', ibid., 13.

14 The 'moral prerequisites' for those entering research were, in Cajal's terms, 'independence of judgement, perseverance, passion for glory, patriotism and a taste for originality'. *Reglas y consejos sobre la investigación científica* (Madrid: CSIC, 2005) [first published in 1897, as *Fundamentos racionales y condiciones técnicas de la investigación biológica*], 47-66.

15 G. Pittaluga (ed.), *Investigaciones y estudios sobre el paludismo en España. Études et recherches sur le paludisme en Espagne (1901-1903), à l'occasion du XIVe. Congrès International de Médecine Madrid-Barcelona, Avril 1903* (Barcelona: Tip. La Académica, 1903); Mission to the Canary islands by Royal Order issued on June 3rd, 1905 (according to his Personal Files, kept at the Royal Academy of Medicine in Madrid).

16 G. Pittaluga, *Sobre el mecanismo patogenético de los síndromes sueroterápico* (Madrid: Idamor Moreno, 1905).

17 Journals on the *Index catalogue of the Library of the Surgeon-General's Office. U.S. Army*, ID 21209341040: 'Archivos latinos de medicina y de biología. Revista mensual, publicada bajo la dirección de Carlos María Cortezo [et al.]. Redactor jefe: Gustavo Pittaluga. Madrid, Nos. 1-3, v. 1, October to December, 1903. Ended.'

18 G. Pittaluga, *Por la moralidad, El Sr. Forns y la Cátedra de higiene de la Facultad de Medicina de Madrid* (Madrid: impr. Fortanet, 1908).

19 R.O. 15 February 1908, *Gaceta* 16 February, 667.

20 Expeditions by the English Royal Society from 1903, by the German Commission to East Africa in 1906-07, and French expedition to Congo in 1906-1908.

21 G. Pittaluga, *Informe de la Comisión del Instituto Nacional de Higiene de Alfonso XIII enviada a las posesiones españolas del Golfo de Guinea para el estudio de la enfermedad del sueño y de las condiciones sanitarias de la colonia* (Madrid: Ministerio de Estado, 1910); G. Pittaluga, 'Ein neuer Blutparasit der afrikanischen Schildkröte, Clemmys Africana Haemoproteus Cajali', *Centralblatt für Bakteriologie, Parasitenkunde und Infektionskrankheiten*, 64 (1912), 241-243.

22 *Observaciones morfológicas sobre los embriones de las filarias de los perros* (Madrid: Imp. y lib. de Nicolás Moya, 1904); *Estudios acerca de los dípteros y de los parásitos que transmiten al hombre y a los animales domésticos* (Madrid: Impr. Gaceta de Madrid, 1905); *Sobre los caracteres morfológicos y la clasificación de los tripanosomas* (Madrid: Impr. Gaceta de Madrid, 1905); *La enfermedad del sueño (Tripanosomiasis humana) en la Colonia española del Golfo de Guinea* (Madrid: N. Moya, 1909), and J. Blass, 'Hallazgo de leishmania infantum, protozoo parásito del kala-azar infantil, en la costa de Levante de España', *Boletín de la Real Sociedad Española de Historia Natural*, Oct. 1912 and *Revista Clínica de Madrid* (1912), 283-289; *Elementos de Parasitología y nociones de Patología tropical*, (Madrid: Calpe, 1st. ed. 1913; 2nd ed.,1916-17).

23 J.M. López-Piñero, *La medicina en la historia* (Madrid: La Esfera de los Libros, 2002), 435 and ff.; A.M. Brandt and M.Gardner, 'The Golden Age of Medicine?', in: R. Cooter J. Pickstone (eds.), *Medicine in the 20th Century* (Amsterdam: Harwood Academic Publishers, 2000), 21-37.

24 J. Bernabeu-Mestre, 'Cultura, ciencia y política. La lucha antipalúdica de la Cataluña de la Mancomunidad, 1914-1925,' *Medicina e Historia*, 73 (1997).

25 C. Rico-Avelló, *Historia de la Sanidad española, 1900-1925* (Madrid: impr. Giménez, 1969), 328.

26 The official announcement was issued at the *Gaceta,*7 February 1924, and reproduced by *El Siglo Médico*, 3662 (1924), 180-181.

27 J. Bernabeu-Mestre, 'La utopía reformadora de la Segunda República: la labor de Marcelino Pascua al frente de la Dirección General de Sanidad, 1931-1933', *Revista Española de Salud Pública*, 74 (2000) (monograph issue), 1-13.

28 M. Suárez Cortina, *El reformismo en España. Republicanos y reformistas bajo la Monarquía de Alfonso XIII*, (Madrid: Siglo XXI; 1986), 114-125; N. Towson (ed.), *El republicanismo en España (1830-1977)* (Madrid: Alianza Editorial, 1994); S. Juliá, 'Los primeros intelectuales', *El País,* supl. *Babelia.* 25 April 1998.

29 M. Granjel, 'La represión de la masonería en las Facultades de Medicina españolas tras la guerra civil', in J. Castellanos et al., (eds.), *La medicina en el siglo XX. Estudios históricos sobre medicina, sociedad y estado* (Málaga: SEHM, 1998) 303-310: 305. Files of the intended trial against Pittaluga followed by the Special Tribunal Against Masonry and Communism, Exp. 13192, Archivo General de la Guerra Civil Española, Salamanca.

30 'Reuniones sanitarias. III Congreso Nacional de Sanidad Civil', *El Siglo Médico*, 66 (1919), 93-95; 'Sesión de clausura del III Congreso de Sanidad Civil', *El Siglo Médico*, 66 (1919), 120-121.

31 G. Pittaluga, *El problema político de la sanidad pública* (Madrid: Calpe, 1921).

32 'Liga Española de Medicina Social', *El Siglo Médico*, 70 (1923), 1050.

33 F. Villacorta, *Burguesía y cultura: Los intelectuales españoles en la sociedad liberal, 1808-1931* (Madrid: Siglo XXI, 1980); J. Tusell and G. Queipo de Llano, *Los intelectuales y la política* (Madrid: Nerea, 1990); V. Cacho, *Los intelectuales y la política : perfil público de Ortega y Gasset* (Madrid : Biblioteca Nueva, 2000).

34 L.P. Martín, 'Un instrumento de democracia: la Liga Española de los Derechos del Hombre (1913-1936)', *Derechos y libertades*, 6 (1998), 377-395.

35 E. Rodríguez-Ocaña, 'The birth of the anti-malaria campaign in Spain during the first 30 years of the 20th century: scientific and social aspects', *Parassitologia*, 47 (2005), 371-377, and 'Medicine as a Social Political Science', 37-52 .

36 G. Pittaluga, 'Trabajos de la Comisión para el Saneamiento de Comarcas Palúdicas.' *Anuario de la Dirección General de Sanidad, 1921* (Madrid: Ministerio de la Gobernación, 1922), 422-428.

37 E. Rodríguez-Ocaña, 'International Health Goals and Social Reform', 250.

38 I. Borowy, *Coming to Terms with World Health. The League of Nations Health Organisation* (Rochester: Rochester University Press, forthcoming).

39 Health Committee, Minutes of the Second Session, C 213.M.69.1924 III, 17 May 1924.

40 B. Fantini, 'Malaria and the First World War', in W.U. Eckart and C. Gradmann (eds.), *Die Medizin und der Erste Weltkrieg* (Pfaffenweiler: Centaurus, 1996), 241-272; L.J. Bruce-Chwatt, and J. de Zulueta, *The Rise and Fall of Malaria in Europe* (Oxford: OUP, 1980).

41 Rajchman to Madsen, 20 December 1923, LONA, R 820/12B/26213/11346.

42 Quote see Rajchman to James, 29 March 1924, LONA, R 870/12B/28002/28002. On the local/global relationship of the time concerning malaria in Spain, see E. Rodríguez-Ocaña, 'Foreign Expertise, Political Pragmatism and Professional Elite: The Rockefeller Foundation in Spain, 1919-39', *Studies in History and Philosophy of Biology and Biomedical Science*, 31:3 (2000), 447-461.

43 HC minutes of First Session, 11-21 February 1924, C.63.1924 (C.H.192), 3

44 The official report was signed by D. Ottolenghi, *Rapport sur le voyage de la Commission du Paludisme en Yougoslavie*. L.N. C.H./Malaria/19, 1924; G. Pittaluga, 'Pre-Oriente. Días de Yugoslavia, 1924', in G. Pittaluga, *La intuición de la verdad y otros ensayos* (Madrid: Caro Reggio, 1926), 215-230; Stampar's portrait 225: ' A vigorous, man, tytanic, simple and rude as a rock, Stampar, conducts Yugoslavian Public Health [...] His creative fever and energetic action spread to his subordinates, infect political actors, thrill in the organisation of services and demand formidable performances from his personnel".

45 Annual Report of the Health Organisation for 1926, 4 February 1927, A.9.1927.III (C.H. 529), 13-4. Societé des Nations, Organisation d'hygiène, *Paludisme dans les Deltas: delta de l'Ebre, delta du Danube* (Geneva, 1932). Pittaluga applied unsuccessfully for RF funding for this specific purpose. Three months report (third trimestre) from Bailey, 12 November 1926 [sent to Russell, 27 November] RAC, RF, RG 5, Series 1.2, Box 273, Folder 3464.

46 League of Nations Health Organisation, *Collaboration with the Greek Government in the Sanitary Reorganisation of Greece.* Geneva, May 1929, (Official N.C. 162.M.63 1929 III); T. Vassiliki and D. Carastani, 'Health policies in interwar Greece: the intervention by the League of Nations Health Organisation', *Dynamis*, 28 (2008) (forthcoming).

47 Pittaluga to Rajchman, 24 August 1928, LONA, R 5819/8A/149/131.

48. G. Pittaluga, *Médicos e ingenieros en la lucha contra el paludismo. Conferencia pronunciada el día 7 de abril de 1927 en la Escuela de Ingenieros de Caminos de Madrid*, (Madrid: Escuela Superior de Ingenieros, 1927), 32.

49 G. Pittaluga, 'Opening Address of the European Conference on Rural Health, 29 June 1931', in: *European Conference on Rural Hygiene*, Vol. II, Minutes, C.473.M.202.1931.III., 18, (henceforth: *European Conference)*

50 Gunn to Russell, 17 November 1925, RAC, RF, RG 5, Series 1.2, Box 238, Folder 3059.

51 Gunn to Russell, 25 November 1925, RAC, RF, RG 5, Series 1.2, Box 238, Folder 3059; Bailey to Gunn, 18 March 1926, RAC, RF, RG 5, Series 1.2, Box 273, Folder 3464. Maintaining contact with Pittaluga is recommended to Rolla B. Hill when preparing his journey to settle in Spain. G.K. Strode's Diary, October 27, 1930, Paris. RAC, RF, RG 1.1, Series 795, Box 2, Folder 16.

52 Bailey to Russell, letter 2 Juin 1926, RAC, RF, RG 5, Series 1.2, Box 273, Folder 3461.

53 Pittaluga to Rajchman, 2 May 1928, LONA, R 5819/8A/149/131.

54 M. Pérez Ferrero, *Tertulias y grupos literarios* (Madrid: Editorial Cultura Hispánica, 1974), 53-57.

55 Pittaluga, together with Marañón, Unamuno and Piñerúa, were the first to express opposition against the dictatorship. C. Rico Avelló, *Historia de la sanidad*, 312.

56 M. Gómez, *Vida y obra*, 258-259; 'Los discípulos del Profesor Pittaluga', *Revista de Sanidad e Higiene Pública*, 8:1 (1933), 321.

57 Proposal by the Spanish Government, C.H. 917, 16 September 1930, Annex 5 to Minutes of the Sixteenth HC Session, 29 September to 7 October 1930, C.527.M.248.1930.III, 106. Pittaluga had been in contact with the International Institute of Agriculture at least since 1927, and its inclusion into the LNHO initiative may very well go back to his influence. See Pittaluga to Rajchman, 12 November 1927, and Rajchman to Pittaluga, 25 November 1927, both LONA, R 998/12B/63320/82870.

58 The issue would eventually contribute to the outbreak of the Civil War. W.L Bernecker, *Europa zwischen den Weltkriegen 1914-1945* (Stuttgart: Eugen Ulmer, 2002); 190-193; E. Malefakis, *Agrarian reform and peasant revolution in Spain. Origins of the Civil War* (New Haven: Yale University Press, 1970) [translated into Spanish with a slightly different title: *Reforma agraria y revolución campesina en la España del siglo XX*, Barcelona: Ariel 1971]

59 Pittaluga, 'Opening address', 19. There is a Spanish translation that includes all Spanish official documents concerning this international meeting: G. Pittaluga, *La Conferencia Internacional de Higiene Rural convocada por la Sociedad de Naciones (29 de junio de 1931)* (Madrid: Publicaciones de la Escuela Nacional de Sanidad, 1931).

60 Minutes of the 16th HC Session, 29 Sept to 7 Oct 1930, C.527.M.248.1930.III, 9-10.

61 A comprehensive description of the procedures and achievements of the Conference, according to the Spanish participants, is given by J.L. Barona, 'The European Conference of Rural health (Geneva, 1931) and the Spanish Administration', in J.L. Barona and S. Cherry (eds.) *Health and Medicine in Rural Europe (1850-1945)* (València: Seminari d'estudis sobre la ciència, 2005), 127-146.

62 Bolivia, China, Colombia, Cuba, India, Japan, Mexico, USA.

63 IIA, LRCS, ILO, International Association of Medical Officers and the HC of the LNHO (represented by Madsen).

64 *European Conference,* 43-44.

65 G. Pittaluga, Opening Address, 19.

66 Technical Recommendations by the Preparatory Committee. Extracts from the Report of the Preparatory Committee, Document C.H. 1045, in *European Conference,* 142-161.

67 *European Conference,* 71.

68 Barona, 'The European Conference', 141-143; cf. Pittaluga to Olsen, 20 August 1931, LONA, R5932/30087/30078.

69 G. Pittaluga, 'Sur l'établissement des services de santé rurale dans certains pays d'Amérique et en général dans les pays à faible densité de population', *Revue d' Hygiène et Medicine Préventive*, 61 :1 (1939), 5-23: 5.

70 E. Ingebritsen, 'Right radicalism and rural health in Hungary 1933-1941', in A.Andersen, T. Grønlie and T. Ryymin (eds.), *European perspectives on medicine, sickness and health. Conference proceedings,* [Report, 4] (Bergen: Rokkansenteret 2006), 187-200; Barona, 'The European Conference', 146; M.A. Balinska, 'The National Institute of Hygiene and Public Health in Poland 1918-1939', *Social History of Medicine*, 3 (1996), 427-445.

71 E. Rodríguez-Ocaña, 'La Salud Pública en la España de la primera mitad del siglo XX', in E. Rodríguez-Ocaña, *Salud Pública en España: Ciencia, profesión, política, siglos XVIII-XX,* (Granada: Editorial Universidad de Granada [Serie Collectánea], 2005), 87-112.

72 See G. Pittaluga, 'La obra de la Organización de higiene de la Sociedad de las Naciones en los dominios del cáncer', in *Congreso Internacional de Lucha Científica y Social contra el Cáncer celebrado en Madrid del 25 al 30 de octubre de 1933* (Madrid: Blass, 1933), 199-208. Also in French, 189-198.

73 G. Pittaluga, *Las enfermedades del sistema retículo-endotelial* (Madrid: Espasa-Calpe, 1934).

74 G. Pittaluga, *La patología de la sangre y el sistema retículo-endotelial (Fisiología, Semiología y Terapéutica)* (La Habana: Editorial Cultural S.A.,1943); and *Tratado de fisiopatología de la sangre* (La Habana: Editorial Cultural S.A., 1956).

75 F. Giral, *Ciencia española en el exilio (1939-1989): el exilio de los científicos españoles* (Barcelona: Anthropos, 1994).

76 Memo n.º 102, R.M. Taylor to R.B. Hill, 5 October 1936, RAC, RF, RG 6.1, Series 1.1, Box 34, Folder 426.

77 '*Se han empeñado en que seamos rojos o azules y yo no puedo ser ni una cosa ni otra*". Testimony of Alonso Burón, collected by Martín Gómez, *Vida y obra,* 28.

78 Decreto del Ministerio de Sanidad y Asistencia Social, *Gaceta de la República*, n. 347, December 12, 1936, 969.

79 *Boletín Oficial del Estado*, n. 48, 17 February 1939, 932.

80 'Deuxième Congrès International de la Transfusion Sanguine. Paris, 29 sept au 2oct 1937'. *Gaz. Hôp.* 1937 ; 110 (nº 96): 1535-36; 1554-57 (signed by A.T.).

81 Rajchman to the Secretary General of the League of Nations, Dec 15, 1936, approved on February 17, 1937. Prof. Pittaluga. Société des Nations. Personnel Office. Health Section. File Temporary #2857. 1937. The Report appeared as the work of an editing committee formed by Sergent, Balfour, Pittaluga and Sinton [Nouvelles. Organisation d'Hygiène de la Société des Nations. Quatrième rapport général de la Commission du Paludisme, *Revue d'Hygiène et de Médecine Préventive*, 60 :197 (1938)].

82 Pittaluga to Rajchman, May 28, 1937. Prof. Pittaluga. Société des Nations. Personnel Office. Health Section. File Temporary #2857. 1937; G. Pittaluga, 'Sur l'établissement des services de santé rurale dans certains pays d'Amérique et en général dans les pays à faible densité de population', *Revue d' Hygiène et Medicine Préventive*, 61:1 (1939), 5-23 ; (2): 95-124 ; (3): 179-207.

83 Avenol to Rajchman, 30 November 1938, and Rajchman to Secretary General, Conférence de Mexico, 6 December 1938, both LONA, R 6098/8A/28028/8855; cf. Pruneda to Gautier, 2 September 1938 ; Olsen to Rajchman, 27 August 1938; Note of Conversation, Secretary-General, Lester, Podesta Costa, Rajchman, 7 September 1938, all LONA, R 6098/8A/28028/8855.

84 G. Pittaluga, 'Les infections à Bartonella', *Bull Inst. Pasteur* (31 Oct 1938), 961; A. Parturier, *Organisation de l'Oeuvre de la Transfusion Sanguine d'Urgene,* (Paris: Société Générale d'Imprimerie, 1933); C. Salmon, 'La transfusión sanguine est née à

Saint Antoine', *La Gazette du CHU. Gazete d'informations hospitalo-universitaires*, 8 (1991), 193-196.

85 G. Pittaluga, '[review of] Plum, *Clinical and experimental investigations in Agranulocytosis. With special reference to etiology* (Copenhagen & London: Lewis and Co., 1937)'; *Le Sang*, 13 (1939), 93-94; 'Célulles de Sternberg et Mégacaryocytes', *Le Sang*, 13 (1939), 833-852; 'Sur la pathogénèse des anémies érythroblatiques des adultes', 14 (1940-41), 129-159; 'Étude expérimentale er clinique sur le traitement des anémies par les extraits globulaires', [14 : 264-270]; 'Étude général de la leucémie aigüe', *Progrès médical*, 69 (1940), 94; G. Pittaluga, 'Les caractères de la maladie de Niemann-Pick', *Bull Mém Soc méd hôp Paris*, 55 (1940), 1356-1358.

86 'Académie de Chirurgie. Séance du 18 octobre 1939. Considérations sur la transfusion dans la guerre de Espagne ['M. Pittaluga expose...']', *Gazette des Hôpitaux*, 112: 87-88 (1939), [14 nov 1939]: 1357-1358.

87 J.L. Barona, 'El tortuoso camino hacia el exilio de Gustavo Pittaluga (1876-1955)', in M.F. Mancebo (ed.), *L'exili cultural de 1939. Seixanta anys després. Actas del I Congreso Internacional celebrado en Valencia del 1 al 4 de diciembre de 1999* (Valencia: Universitat de València-Biblioteca Valenciana, 2001), vol. 1, 425-434; S. Rodríguez and V. María, 'Perfil biográfico de dos paradigmas de la cultura médica exilados en Cuba: Gustavo Pittaluga y Pedro Domingo', *Congreso Internacional Guerra de España 1936-1939, Madrid, 27-29 noviembre 2006*, accesible at http://www.secc-es.com/media/docs/30_2_SUEIRO.pdf

88 '*Creo que he llevado a cabo una obra buena, de trascendencia para España. Creo que he cumplido honestamente [...] Creo que he conducido la labor colectiva con serenidad y firmeza y que he logrado encauzarla hacia soluciones de concordia [...] Me siento satisfecho de ello, dentro de una gran fatiga [...] Basta pues de vivir. Creo que el destino se ha cumplido y que hay que entrar en la negra noche eterna del olvido*', G. Pittaluga to M. Zambrano, 1 October 1943, reproduced by Blanco, Rogelio, 'Gustavo Pittaluga (1876-1956). Un renacentista que asume el destino', *Revista de Occidente*, nº. 307 (2006), 103-118:117.

89 R. Delgado, 'Evocación del profesor Gustavo Pittaluga en el vigésimo quinto aniversario de su fallecimiento,' *Cuadernos de la Historia de la Salud Pública*, 66 (1983), 149-164; A. Vigil, A. González and R. Martell, 'Científicos españoles exiliados en Cuba', *Revista de Indias*, 62: 224 (2002), 173-194.

90 R. Blanco, 'La relación epistolar de Gustavo Pittaluga y María Zambrano. Seguido de Cartas de Gustavo Pittaluga a María Zambrano', *Revista de Occidente*, nº. 313, (2007), 39-45 and 46-69.

91 *BOE*, March 31, 1955; 2076. A letter from Pittaluga informed Marañon, on 21 September 1955, about his and his wife's bad health (Archives of the Fundación Gregorio Marañón, Madrid). On their financial distress, Luis Amado Blanco recounted to Francisco Vega Díaz, how a collection made by friends and colleagues in Cuba ended with the misappropriation of the money by someone close to them, Recordatorio..., 10.

92 See note 89.

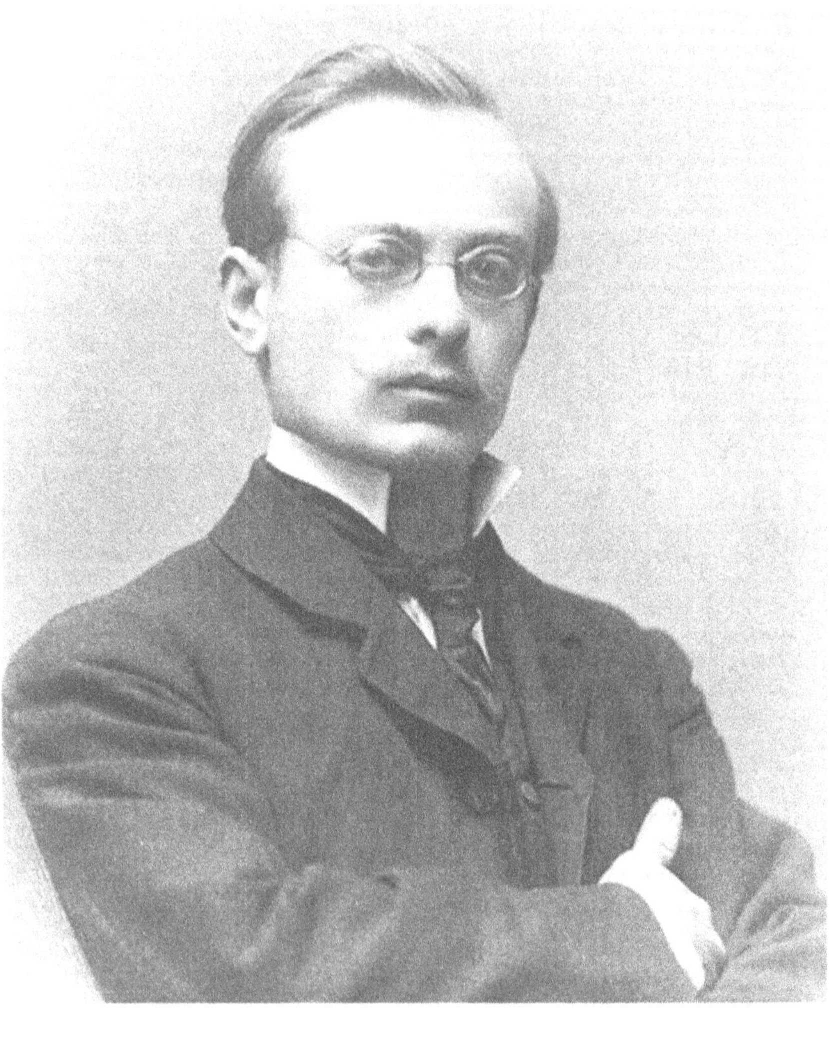

Gustavo Pittaluga

Photograph courtesy of the Real Academia Nacional de Medicina, Madrid

A Posthumous Audit
Medical Biography and the Social History of Medicine

Patrick Zylberman

> He was supposed, perhaps correctly, to be the greatest admiral since Nelson. But it did not add up to much. Nelson's domination of the seas lasted a hundred years; Fisher's about ten. Now he has only the wistful charm of yesterday's music-hall comedian.
>
> A.J.P. Taylor, Admiral Fisher: A Great Man?

The time is not very long past when general history tended to look down on biography, which scholars and academics were pleased to leave to journalists and (a mistake) to British historians.[1] For all that, 'history's lame cousin' (in Marc Ferro's phrase) continues to do quite well. For example, out of all the history and geography books published in France from 2002 to 2005, the percentage of biographies (of all kinds) rose from 39 to 48 per cent.[2] The social history of medicine should by rights have sounded the death knell of medical biography. The Society for the Social History of Medicine, founded in May 1970, certainly had the intention of dropping the 'great man' cult in favour of studies better attuned to formulating the main lines of health policy.[3] Yet this new emphasis on social and political considerations did not produce any fall-off in the number of medical biographies printed in the UK. In France, where biographical works had for a long time fared worse than anywhere else, the publication of medical biographies experienced a spectacular upsurge in the mid-1980s.[4] Nothing like the number of titles published in Britain, certainly, but, if the number of purchases by libraries can be taken as a guide to the tendencies at work in the ideas market, the trend was unmistakable (Fig.1).

If proof were needed of this thriving health, the editors of the new Dictionary of Medical Biography – intended to be comprehensive with its 1,140 entries – declare flatly that 'the biographical approach adopted in the five volumes reflects best contemporary historical practice.'[5] Alternative medicines, interaction between Western and traditional medicines, women's increasing role in the medical profession, recognition by historians of nursing as a practice, 'French doctors' – the individual has not lost his place and status in medical historiography. What is the explanation for this 'rising from the dead'[6] of a genre which the ascension of the social sciences and the decline of the narrative should ordinarily have completely eliminated?[7] What purpose is served by biographies? Leaving aside the individual's role in history, does a place still exist for 'great men' in the new social history of medicine? These are some of the questions we shall briefly

Fig.1: Cumulative numbers of medical biographies in the catalogues of the Wellcome Library (London) and the *Bibliothèque interuniversitaire de médecine* (Paris), 1950-1999

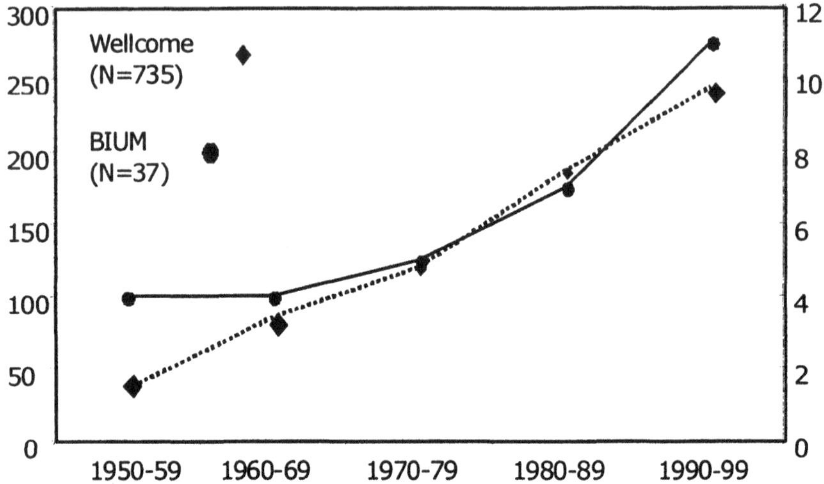

discuss in the following pages, taking our cue from two sets of academic encomia (Academy eulogies), one from the *Bulletin de l'Académie nationale de médecine*[8] and the other from the 1981 World Health Organization notes on the Léon Bernard European prize-winners, these being mere samplings of a time-honoured but still vigorous custom that, needless to say, transcends national frontiers and languages.[9]

It is unlikely that anyone today could write that 'biography is not, as has been claimed, history's handmaiden; it is history itself.'[10] Yet this view has a venerable tradition behind it, going back to Ibn Abi Usaybi'a (13th century) and Giovanni Tortelli (15th century), who made the distinction between biography and hagiography and used it for classifying books.[11] Despite strong condemnation under the *Aufklärung*,[12] biography continued to be an often-used tool in medical history. One of the most eminent examples was An Introduction to the History of Medicine published by Fielding Garrison in 1913.[13] Georges Daremberg was alone, in 1907, in separating 'history of great doctors' from 'didactic history of medicine'.[14] The enduring primacy of the author and his work in the history of medical thinking – the model for the history of social medicine being Erwin Ackerknecht's Rudolf Virchow[15] – owes much to the failure of 'externalist' theories. As Mirko Grmek writes, 'Psychologically-based explanations (in particular, tracing the birth and elaboration of scientific ideas to the "genius" of "great scientists") or epistemological ones (relying on the internal logic of the way ideas develop) are attractive, since it is difficult or impossible to derive the content of scientific theories from social conditions alone.'[16] The 'great man' approach obviously has its pitfalls. There are those who see this enduring fascination as a reflection of the concern with memory, heritage and identity that has influenced our societies since at least the 1980s.[17] Could there not, however, be a more down-to-earth reason for the interest in eminent personalities? Some of our heroes, without being illustrious scholars or artistic geniuses (we are referring especially to men and women engaged in public health), were in a sense minority figures, in medicine as in politics. A kind of compensatory mechanism appears to be at work. What makes these people interesting today from a post-modern point of view, which revalues the role of the misfit, the humble and the eccentric, is precisely their marginal status.[18] In doing this, the new historians are perhaps resurrecting unwittingly an old controversy pitting Johann Gustav Droysen against Jacob Burckhardt.[19]

Laudatio memoriae

It must be admitted then that learned history has not, despite its pretentions, repudiated the image of the 'great doctor'. It continues to inform both the profession's idea of itself and popular opinion. There may be a more structural cause for this persistence than the ones we have mentioned. In the case of France, biography as a form has gained its stature thanks to its association with a hallowed institution, namely the Académie française and its eulogies.[20]

We know that biographical narrative has its origin in the 4th century BC Greek panegyric. As a form, its successive stages were developed by the Socratist biography (Plato, Xenophon, the Aristotelians). Considered as the portrait of a public figure and not the account of a private life, it sought to express the possibilities latent in a character. It made unashamed use of the imagination, inventing or recreating as needed the words and acts it was ostensibly recounting. Fiction, as Arnaldo Momigliano observes, preceded, accompanied and inspired what would become real biography.[21] Plutarch made the distinction between 'history', the account of the grand events of military and political history, and 'biography', whose domain was rather the tiny fact, a word, a trifle, what Roland Barthes nineteen centuries later would call 'biographemes' – the 'signs that reveal the soul'.[22]

Is the scientist also a 'hero'? Is the 'great man' a 'hero'? The 'great man', we have been taught, came into being with Voltaire in 1735, on the dead body of the 'hero'. 'You understand that for me great men come first and heroes come last. What I call great men are all those who have excelled in the useful or the agreeable. Province ransackers are merely heroes.'[23] In France, his gestation time lasted a century, the century of Louis XIV, the 'century of eulogies'.[24] For sixty years, the Académie française was 'a temple dedicated to this cult',[25] a national sport verging on obsession. The Quarrel of the Ancients and the Moderns gave the ordinary man his day, on a footing with the intellectual and learned professions. Charles Perrault's contribution, a gallery of the *Hommes illustres qui ont paru en France pendant le siècle* (1696), did not escape from the panegyric mode. It nevertheless represented 'a decisive step towards the pantheon of modern Great Men which the Enlightenment would substitute for Plutarch's Lives and the Lives of the Saints.'[26] The victory of the Moderns was also that of the scholars: Descartes, Pascal, Mersenne.[27] Half-way through the century, a new secular and civic eulogy contest in praise of the 'nation's famous men' completed the transformation of the Académie française's solemn sessions into 'politico-socialite events'.[28] Fontenelle successfully did the same thing at the Academy of Sciences, which he headed for forty-two years, authoring seventy eulogies during that period.[29]

Fontenelle left a lasting imprint. From Condorcet to Louis de Broglie, all the Life Secretaries of the Academy of Sciences heeded his precepts. Appointed Life Secretary of the Academy of Sciences in 1697, Fontenelle had ten years earlier firmly taken sides with Perrault in publishing his *Digression sur les Anciens et les Modernes*. In 1699, he devised and established the rules for eulogising scientists. He added substance to what in Perrault had been no more than short notices and steered eulogies away from being simple panegyrics to draw them closer to biography, initiating thus the distinct conflation of eulogy and biography that prospered hereafter in the practice of scientific and medical academies.[30] Fontenelle's eulogies were 'concise and simple accounts, often epigrammatic, even when he was being serious'.[31] Their aim was to recount the Academician's life from the cradle to the grave. He was the first Secretary of the Academy of Sciences to deliver his speeches in French. He managed to prevent the eulogies of scientists from being overblown. Unlike Condorcet, he did not put himself in the picture, nor did he argue and discuss. His guiding principle was to avoid excess. This rule would be flouted by both Vicq d'Azyr, Life Secretary of the Royal Society of Medicine (1776) and elected to the Académie française in 1788, who was the first to devote eulogies to physicians, and Etienne Pariset, an alienist, appointed Life Secretary of the Academy of Medicine in 1823, who would become the corporation's 'first Academy biographer'.[32] The biographer-Secretary was the eulogy manager; he circulated the eulogies within the closed circuit of the Academicians under a strict protocol designed to accredit and protect their authors and their audience (families and associates). This has several implications for the study of medical biographies as well as the definition of greatness. The eulogy of a physician was the product of a 'discursive society', outside of which any manifestation of the form was unthinkable.[33] Without considering such an institution any interpretation would err, since what constituted greatness was contingent on what was or was not possible within a given 'discursive society'. Each biography begot a semantic persona; the biographer's subject was the paper doctor cloistered inside the Academy. The great man owed his existence solely to what was said of him on solemn occasions, and his greatness lay in being an institution. Sainte-Beuve, elected to the Académie française in 1844, thought that truth and reality – depicting the man behind the practitioner – 'should be introduced more and more' (a revealing phrase), but advised using them 'discreetly and tastefully'.[34]

The motivation and aim in every eulogy and biography is to impose an image. Biography, it has been said, is 'an active creation of images'[35] of the biographee, not a tale of her/his more or less heroic deeds. Every biography is a creation of a myth or a legend, to which contemporaries, forerunners and successors effectively contribute. For a person's life eventually makes sense only when compared to other person's deeds or misdeeds, to other people's failures and accomplishments. Authority and prestige are relative to colleagues' power and sway, and an ultimate function of one's rank in a distinct environment. We must keep this conceptual elaboration at the back of our minds as we proceed towards the description of a rather awkward issue for biographers: the problem of praise and blame. But does a historian choose his own great men? Below we examine how eulogies established a hierarchy of great men. Yet, other mechanisms are also at work – not only scientific self-congratulations such as the Nobel Prizes, but also political and media forces.[36] In 1895, the French Republic ordained a state funeral for Pasteur. Ten years later, the readers of a popular paper, the *Petit Parisien*, placed Pasteur at the head of a list of the 19th century's ten most illustrious French personalities.[37] It would have been difficult for any biographer at the time to accord less than heroic status to Pasteur.

Other great men in the field of public health, whose renown is not dependent on a public vote, are the product of a feature associated with the rising power of international organisations. We refer to the creation of 'epistemic communities', which are networks of recognised specialists having some claim to authority in their particular field. These experts, from widely differing subject areas, share common notions of scientific rationality (causal beliefs) and ethical standards (principled beliefs).[38] Two of these networks can be said to have laid the foundation for the international health hall of fame. The Rockefeller Foundation, which between the two world wars acted as a veritable head hunter, organised the talents so spotted – Jacques Parisot, Andrija Stampar, Bela Johan or Gustavo Pittaluga, regarded by the Foundation as their countries' most eminent public health personalities and the ones most in harmony with its aims – into networks. The other was the League of Nations' Health Committee, to which Thorvald Madsen, Parisot, Pittaluga and René Sand owed their reputation at home and abroad. After the Second World War, the Léon Bernard Foundation, set up in 1937, carried on the selection of social medicine's great men initiated by the League of Nations. Since 1951, the WHO General Assembly has awarded, in solemn session, the Foundation's prize to 'a person having accomplished outstanding service in the field of social medicine'.[39] The two networks dictate the historian's choice. The issue of how 'memory' was produced in the field of public health in the 20th century would merit more reflection and study. Sources might be unearthed or subjected to new evaluation, using the methods of cultural anthropology or narration theory. Might it not be worthwhile investigating, for instance, the way Andrija Stampar, whose bronze bust greets the visitor entering the WHO's hall, was 'canonised' by the Geneva organization? (This issue of the choice dictated to the historian by academies and professional bodies should not be confused with a distinct but practically related question, namely access to the departed's papers, where families and rights-holders obviously play a determining role.) Does this mean that, given these choices mostly foreordained by the academies, foundations and international committees, the historian has no room to move? Not necessarily. The renown attaching to the great figures in public health stems from their insertion in a kind of corporate myth fabricated by the medical historians themselves. George Rosen or Henry Sigerist set René Sand, Charles Winslow or Andrija Stampar, all of whom named as Rudolf Virchow as spiritual father, as exemplars for any candidate claiming to greatness in social medicine. It remains true, generally speaking, that the historian is not master of the 'historical greatness' ranking order. The institution does his thinking for him.

Jousting and bel canto

In the view of George Weisz, medical encomia fulfil three explicit purposes. They have a historical goal, which is to situate the subject's work in the recent evolution of his discipline. They are the memento of a life devoted to the greater glory of medicine. Last, the eulogy must present the deceased as a model for the profession and for humanity. The moral dimension is never far away.[40] The eulogy is a sort of grand funeral. As with military honours and state pomp, it elevates the 'honoured colleague' to the status of 'man of exception'.[41] To pass moral judgements: this classic purpose of history and biography has been widely recognized. More rarely acknowledged is that, besides their historical, sacramental or moral functions, eulogies had a rank-attributing goal. But what was the aim of ranking biographees? And which were the means?

It is no exaggeration to say that competition is the cornerstone of scientific progress. Science does not advance without rivalry and competition among researchers. Nietzsche reminds us of the Greeks' passion for contests and jousting. Disagreement was for them a legitimate sentiment. Covetousness, jealousy and envy were all good for men since they impelled them to work and act. All the same, jousting was incompatible with the lasting supremacy of any one person, the fear being that the contest would stop suddenly and never resume. It was the same for science. Excellence stifled competition; the great man was likely to bury research and the researchers under the weight of his genius.[42] Survivors as well as contemporaries had therefore a vested interest in making sure that competition would just go on. This cast some light on the thorny problem of praise and blame in Academy eulogies and biographies.

To praise or to blame? Polybius, in an oft-quoted passage, distinguishes between the biography or eulogy – in which the facts are the object of a sequential recounting open to embellishment – and history – a truthful account supported by evidence, in which praise and blame are equally at home.[43] It goes without saying that the panegyric as delivered at the Académie française glossed over faults and vices. This was not the case, however, at the Academies of Inscriptions, of Science and of Medicine. This is not to say that their subjects were systematically rubbished post mortem. Every eulogy was required to obey the three principles of caution, benevolence and judgement. To praise (without excess), to blame (as little as possible) – the biographer could disturb this delicate balance, only at the risk of disappointing 'the insatiable appetite for compliments' and arousing 'the quarrelsome ire' of the 'almost equally abusive' sons, sons-in-law and widows.[44] This was a not infrequent misstep, and one which befell Antoine Louis (1732-1792), Life Secretary of the Royal Academy of Surgery. He found himself telling an irate wife brusquely one day, 'I actually believe, Madam, that I could benefit from your approval were you to examine calmly what I said and be grateful for what I did not say.'[45] The author would do well, in other words, to refrain from mentioning anything in the life of the defunct that might hint at sex, sadism and snobbery. 'Great men should be approached from their grand side', remarks Sainte-Beuve, 'and any pettiness that may be noticed in them should be set only within the broader whole.'[46] D'Alembert had already said this, in his Encyclopedia entry on 'Eulogy'. The truth, he asserted, should be tempered and sometimes kept silent, but never disguised or deformed.[47]

The Academy biographies, which were amiable and serious fiction, scrupulously respected this conventional distance between a retouched image – a biography neither quite factual nor quite fictitious designed to wow the audience – and an unvarnished or intimate life, of which friends and family would take a very dim view. As we have noted, the audience at the solemn sessions extended well beyond the commissions of specialists, present to posthumously audit their departed fellow. Colleagues, families, friends, occasionally politicians, scholars and (high) society jostled together.[48] The inherent ritual of Academy eulogies set strict limits on what the biographer might or might not say. That being so, how much place was left for frankness? The boldness of Emile Littré, who, 'writing the life of a man whom he regarded as his mentor [Auguste Comte], was able to carry sincerity to the point of hiding nothing capable of making this man appear dislikeable,' completely stunned Ernest Renan. This was boldness in the service of science ; and science, as we know, considers life – here a life – from a very high altitude ![49] The image of the learned man was beginning to evolve. In the 1850's, scientism was taking the place of romanticism. The scholar, wrapped in goodness in the humanitarian age, became a neutral species in the age of positivism.[50] Just as biographies gradually moved away from eulogies as these had earlier moved away from panegyrics, opprobrium and criticism began in some cases to assume importance.[51] Yet Georges Cuvier had remarked, 'It is not when we speak leaning, so to speak, on the funeral urn of a master or friend that we may be expected to exercise the cold impassiveness of history.'[52] Littré, in lifting the 'delicate veil'[53] draped over certain areas of the truth, had doubtless shown bad taste. Objectivity was not and should not properly have been the tone of a eulogy, just as it should not have been that of a biographer. The biographic undertaking, despite its access to papers and witness accounts not available at the time of the person's death, retained the spirit of praise and admiration characteristic of the Academy eulogy.[54]

Right up to the 1980s, the Academy eulogy resembled a bel canto aria, a sometimes grandiloquent oration which bestowed on its hero the glittering helmet of the warriors of antiquity.[55] But since scholars 'love championships', as Paul Veyne aptly puts it, the clash of rival forces must never be allowed to abate. Encomia therefore strove to classify, order and rank personalities[56] for the pleasure of taking part in a never-ending joust. The measuring categories cast a rather broad net. 'Science, genius, beneficence [...] in this funereal but glorious list, Grancher, through his accomplishments and good works, holds an honourable place.'[57]

Hierarchy of fictions

The eulogy was thus inseparable from the competition or contest that underpinned it. In the Age of Enlightenment, 'the benchmark for choice depended on an opinion which was at once official and in tune with society'. This opinion, expressed by the Académie française, 'no longer coincided with the specialised knowledge of a tiny minority of learned men.'[58] The Academies, companies and coteries exercised a prescriptive function. With their quasi-monopoly over the evaluation of scholars and thinkers, they imposed a hierarchy of fictions. It could also be called a projection of the real and possible positions reserved unequally by these institutions for different individuals. They preselected the candidates for 'greatness', picking them unabashedly from within themselves. With the aid of a ritual *cursus honorum*, the academic institution composed an honours list of all its dear departed. This did not mean that outstanding talents were allowed to stand on the same steps of the podium as great men. Sainte-Beuve, for example, separately classified 'geniuses' (Diderot) and 'infinitely distinguished minds' (the physiologist Pierre Flourens, 1794-1867, Life Secretary of the Academy of Sciences).[59] Pariset set out 'to mark the rank which [every excellent mind he reviewed] ought to occupy in men's esteem'.[60] Beginning in 1837, shorter obituaries were read at the dead man's tomb. This gave the Life Secretary the opportunity to establish a new ranking system. 'There are', he said, 'the illustrious who aspire to the honour of an academic éloge; there are those who are more modest and who could be content with a simple notice.'[61] Pariset's recipe survived well after him.[62] Medical biographies sometimes reflected this ranking in their physical formats, presenting the minores, 'those who deserve mention but not too much space'[63] in smaller print. Another method involved the selective repetition of eulogies. The obituaries read at the time of death, a preliminary assessment of the deceased, were in some cases followed by a more substantial eulogy delivered in solemn session a few years later when the person's work and life appeared to have weathered the passage of time.[64]

Thomas Carlyle, in his 1840 lectures On Heroes, Hero Worship and the Heroic in History, 'identified the whole of historical life with the life of great men.'[65] A prophet, a god, a priest, a king, the great man was a Proteus, a universal man, that is, one unattached to any particular sphere of activity. Burckhardt also took a deep interest in 'historical greatness', the title of a lecture delivered at the Museum in Basle on 6 November 1870. Historical greatness expressed the universal in the typical as well as in the singular; it resulted from the intermeshing of an exceptional situation, a historical event, with the 'magical fascination' exerted by a personality. Just as the hero was for the Scotsman 'Heaven-Chosen', the great man was for the Swiss an exception (not a model), a charismatic emanation of the mythology generated by popular imagination. Places in the pantheon of great men were hard to come by: they required nothing less than entering into contact with the entire universe. Artists, poets, philosophers and a few scholars qualified; the hoi polloi of inventors and technicians did not. It was Goethe who said, 'Each biography is a universal story.'[66] It would appear that the romantic aesthetics of history correct the wise man of Weimar. Science hands out medals, which the philosophy of history regards as mere baubles. Each discipline 'attributes greatness to the scholar who has most contributed to that discipline's development' and not to what is universal. It is therefore more fitting to distinguish between the unique and irreplaceable great man, who represents novelty, and 'great talents' who exploit what exists already.[67] This distinction can be detected in the deliberations of the Léon Bernard Prize jury. It sets a small group of social medicine 'pioneers' on a different plane from that of the general run of 'administrators' who put the first group's principles into practice. Once again we are faced with a 'ranking', even though it can be difficult to situate certain personalities on one or other side of the fence. The jury considered, for example, that Karl Evang (1902-1981), who had long been Director-General of Health in Oslo, despite being co-founder of the WHO, was 'much more of an organiser than a theoretician' of social medicine.[68]

Doctors, generally speaking, have a hard time climbing to the top rung of the podium. Kant refused to grant the title of genius to scientists, since science was the product of intellectual faculties which controlled and sometimes fettered the other powers of the spirit (*Geist*).[69] Sainte-Beuve intimates that, in the Academy biographies of doctors, 'greatness, on the assumption that it is naturally present, enters into them on but rare occasions.'[70] For that reason, grandiloquence was out of place. 'It is time,' he added, 'especially in the field of science, to bring [the Academy form] more into line with truth and lower the tone.'[71] Even in the 1920s, Sigerist felt obliged to liken doctors to artists in order to accord them historical greatness. He took his inspiration from an idea advanced by art historian Heinrich Wölfflin. In 1915, Wölfflin had defined 'style as an "expression" of the state of mind of an age and a people, as well as of a personal temperament'.[72] Not long after he arrived in America, socio-economic determinism displaced aesthetics in his thinking. He came to believe that the history of medicine should stop being the history of great doctors and should tend towards being a history of civilisation. In this way, it would contribute to the understanding of society and culture. Up till that point, the young Sigerist had regarded the culture of a period, and its maladies, as the expression of a 'style' in the sense intended by Wölfflin, whose philosophy of history in turn owed much to Jacob Burckhardt.[73]

Greatness had no truck with inner feelings. Eulogies giving a physical description of their subject,[74] or the colours of their personal surroundings, were few and far between.[75] While friendship was a must, the necessary expression of the bond uniting the members of the medical profession – the community of doctors is a code of conduct not a sociology – the audience had little chance of glimpsing things of the heart.[76] Paediatrician Julien Marie (1899-1987) at the celebration of the centenary of Robert Debré's birth in 1982, was reluctant to reveal two lines of dedication ('from your old chief, your old friend') written for him by the man he called his spiritual father when that man had been elected to the Academy of Sciences in 1961, 'because they are part of our intimacy'.[77] Just as obituaries were 'essentially the summing-up of a public life',[78] or of a life in public view, eulogies, after a few biographical indications, went on about the deceased's 'writings and work'.[79] As the 20th century approached, all this began to seem less obvious. Where we find genuine analysis of the biographee's scientific and clinical achievements or the occasional outline of medical history, it is usually in subsequent éloges or sessions commemorating the person's centenary.[80] The ordinary eulogy did not have much room for discussing the person's work.[81] The occasion did not seem to lend itself to 'a full enumeration of the scientific work' of the departed.[82] The fact is that every eulogy ran into an 'almost insurmountable' barrier, as Sainte-Beuve tells us. Entering into the details of the person's work risked going over the head of the crowds attending the solemn sessions, even where they were educated and cultivated. (There was less of a problem, Sainte-Beuve comments, where the learned man had shone in the fields of physiology.) Fontenelle had no trouble skirting the difficulty. 'He was content to say just a word about scientific details and subjects; he did not discuss them. His main, indeed his single, purpose was to reveal the scientists' character, physiognomy and habits.'[83] Almost from the beginning, evaluation had tended to turn itself into a ritual celebration of the Academy's values. As George Weisz notes, 'evaluation had become a form of representation.'[84]

Public life, private life, the sources for these provided the biographer with means of a curious strategy.[85] The above-mentioned distantiation from the inner self sheds some light on the ambiguous ties linking the biographer to the biographee. The scientific milieu has produced, as a sort of outgrowth, an anti-scientific culture where 'pushiness and political skills are rewarded too much, and imaginative approaches, high-quality results and logical argument, too little.'[86] This culture has been called by some an 'audit society', since the performance indicators used to appraise researchers (number of articles published, position in the list of authors signing articles, impact factor of the journals publishing the articles) often count for more than the intrinsic interest of the work presented. Academy eulogies and biographies had their own sets of performance indicators –naturally quite different – enabling them to arrange their subjects in order of rank. Dorinda Outram has studied several of these indicators. The scientist's character, for example, was the clue to scientific style in the 18th century but, in the 19th century, it became the yardstick for measuring progress in a particular discipline. Natural history saw itself reflected in the mirror of Georges Cuvier's personality,[87] and bacteriology in that of the pasteurian bacteriologist Albert Calmette (1863-1933).[88] In our day, a scientific expert's legitimacy rests on not only his competence but also his personal ethics – honesty, sincerity, disinterestedness. The expert is both a brain and a conscience. For much of the time, the 'great man' had overshadowed the person, spotlighting the persona in the man. This duality has a long past. According to Jacob Burckhardt, when real biographies, and not just chronicles devoid of any feeling for the individual being portrayed, began to appear in the 15th century, it was not long before the new form itself split into two kinds. The first was interested in an individual's deeper being, his profound convictions, inner struggles, secrets; the second, on the other hand, restricted itself to tracing the steps in a career. The goal was no longer moral edification; it was to recount 'the life of a nondescript man when and because he had played a great role'.[89] We have here the early model of the balance between the person (ordinary) and the persona (mighty) strictly followed in the eulogies of scientists or doctors.[90]

The persona's portrayal left no place for improvisation. Since the 19th century in France, a writer's life had to 'comprise three chapters devoted to the noble activities of writing, women and politics.'[91] A biography worthy of the name was obliged to respect this pattern. The ideal life of a doctor had to conform with a quite different model: the Ciceronian one of senator, man of letters and philosopher. Pasteur Vallery-Radot (1886-1970), a nephrologist who followed a 'medical, scientific, teaching, literary and social career'[92] (he was member of the

Académie française as well as the Académie de médicine), also sat in parliament for the Rassemblement du Peuple français (RPF). He was acquainted with Paul Valéry and Claude Debussy. 'The medical career of Pasteur Vallery-Radot, for all its importance, was but a portion, and sometimes the smallest portion of his activity.'[93] Was not his prime achievement the publication of the complete works of his grandfather, Louis Pasteur? Robert Debré, his friend and companion on the Resistance's Medical Committee under the Occupation, was not only 'the unchallenged leader of French pediatrics'; he was also a writer.[94] When hematologist Jean Bernard (1907-2006), also an academician, called on him in his house in Touraine (Debré was then aged 94), he found him in his study. 'I have decided to write,' the old man told Bernard, showing him two manuscripts lying on the table. There follows a reference to the Loire riverside 'country lane' joining their two properties, the shades of a poet at the court of Henri III, Balzac's Femme de trente ans and Barnabooth, the aesthete and imaginary double of Valéry Larbaud. 'Robert Debré', concludes Jean Bernard, 'never separated his scientific research from his literary or philosophical preoccupations.'[95] The eulogy etched the portrait of the doctor as 'delicate artist', connoisseur, Stoic sage who spoke no evil of his fellow man and went into the grave still conversing.[96]

National myth played, as one may imagine, a considerable part in the elevation of a profession not necessarily destined to rise to the heights of historic greatness. Emile Duclaux, for example, in his obituary for Pasteur, his teacher and predecessor as head of the Institute, depicted his master as a 'Napoleon dying victoriously' with his benevolent spirit, even more powerful than the Emperor's, spreading its aura beyond Europe to the whole wide world.[97] Napoleon 'dying victoriously' was a quotation (or lift) taken from the first two lines of the sixth part of *L'expiation*, a piece written by Victor Hugo in 1852, and later included in the collection *Les Châtiments* (1853). The poems in the collection were familiar to tens of thousands of French people at the time.[98] National myth was the humus from which arose the figure of the scholar adorned with all the gleaming trappings of the great man. It is an easy task to draw up the long list of national icons exploited in Academy eulogies. George Weisz wrote a scathing criticism of Charles Achard's eulogy of Grancher. Then there was the delicious portrait of Pasteur Vallery-Radot as Cyrano de Bergerac, hero of Edmond Rostand's play, penned by Carlos Chagas Filho (1910-2000), a biologist, corresponding member of the Académie de medicine, for the centenary of Pasteur's grandson's birth.[99] This ideological ailment is not, needless to say, peculiar to France.[100] 'Real greatness is a mystery', said Burckhardt.[101] What historical greatness requires is not the positivist language of the norm – the only one recognised by our 'audit societies' – but the existential language of value. The romantic kitsch we have here is proof of the agonistic climate surrounding the memory and history of learned men.

The twilight of greatness

Academy biographies, with their 'unstable combination of biographical veracity and hagiographic morality',[102] sought to pass down to posterity an ideal image of the scientist. In the Age of Enlightenment, however, the tone of the eulogies had moved well away from that of epic rhapsody or tragedy. Certainly, the savant was still shown as a Plutarchian hero, embodying spiritual strength and almost religious wisdom, *fortitudo et sapientia*. He could likewise be characterised as a political reformer, capable of combining action with contemplation, or as a tireless and upright defender of truth. Other biographies described a character as simple and frugal as an Arcadian shepherd, whose asceticism was the moral counterpart of his love of science. He could also be a Stoic sage, a valiant fighter, a paragon serving the Good and the True. Academy biographies, while ensconcing Science in the seat reserved for Love in the idylls, provided 'a veritable catalogue of saintly attributes'[103] – virtue, love of truth, moral purpose – out of which the savant's life was woven. The cultural background could vary and the style and references could change, but the ideal remained inviolate.[104] In sum, the biographies nurtured a kind of charismatic expectancy.

Roland Barthes discerned in biography the danger of a history reduced to names, to a 'succession of individual men'.[105] But it was very much something else – a reflecting glass for the academies.[106] Cuvier, who, according to Sainte-Beuve, had established the 'true idea of the [epidictic] form', strongly emphasised this in prefacing the collection of his eulogies. 'The small benignly-written biographies called historical Eloges are more than tokens of affection which the learned companies believe they owe to members removed from them by death; they also offer precious examples and admonitions to the younger generation.'[107] They are the implements of a rite, a collective action.[108] This was demonstrated until quite recently by the bi-annual trek by the members of the Pasteur Institute down to the Master's mausoleum on the anniversaries of his birth and death and, as climax to the ceremony, the brief homily by the Institute's Director extolling the virtues upon which the 'House' was founded.[109] There was probably no better exemplar of this biographical approach than William Osler. Following upon Carlyle, he viewed the history of medicine as a succession of biographies. He held that evoking the great doctors of the past could imbue students with 'a sense of their profession's overarching mission'. On that account he wanted libraries to devote 'alcoves of Fame' to great men, with each country holding them up as objects of adoration for its young.[110] This pet idea was shared not only by Cuvier, as we have seen, but by all the medical biographers and all the Academicians.[111]

Science and the great man have always entertained a symbolic exchange relation. The institution's ritualised word-feast guaranteed the Academicians' renown, but it amounted only to a 'testimony of gratitude to the men who of old or of late rendered good service to that medical profession of which the Academy is together the tangible image, the consciousness and the spiritual court.'[112] 'The greatness is that of the obituarists as well as of the persons commemorated,' as Keith Thomas shrewdly remarked.[113] As most authors see it, the epidictic form seeks to depict science as an apolitical, socially neutral activity;[114] it is a matter of saving the skin of scientists and doctors in times of political turmoil. What they are forgetting is that the projected image of the scientist or doctor – as Stoic sage, Arcadian shepherd, visionary or guide – aims above all at masking the double visage of the will to know: thirst for knowledge on the one hand, jealousy and envy on the other. Jealousy and envy, sometimes ill-concealed by the rhetorical, flourishes : 'without carrying abnegation to the point of selflessness, wrote one Secretary of the Académie de medicine, he [Paul Brouardel] managed to do very useful work… he enjoyed the favour of the powerful and the prestige of fame… in a word, he was a happy man.'[115] This dissimulation is a particular mark of the 19th and 20th centuries; the Age of Enlightenment was not so squeamish.[116] Was not historical greatness the stake in a contest where victory was never certain? A diffuse sense of rivalry and competition, what we might call an agonistic situation, was valid only if it was all at once confirmed (by the tournament, the contest) and denied (by the eulogy). In the words of the poet, 'There are on earth two goddesses of discord': the bad one who stirs up war and barbarity, and the good one who leads not to battle but to the tourney. Science worships at both altars.[117] The dual nature of greatness is therefore not so surprising. Yes to glory, that is, science and philosophy; no to power, that is, politics.[118]

Greatness settles the confrontation between death and the 'great man' by arranging the persona's posthumous destiny. The myth of greatness pushes back death by several centuries.[119] Thanks to it, the persona becomes glorious; he revives his presence by crossing into a 'second life, lasting without duration'.[120] The quality of glory is to shine across the ages. The moment of glory is too fleeting not to need repetition, continual reaffirmation. This is why Burckhardt regards the recurrent (or generality) as a more important ingredient in greatness than the singular (or peculiarity).[121] The hero is the product of a running process connecting myth, permanent by definition, and 'heroic' deeds, by nature intermittent. Thanks to this process, renown weathers the erosion of time. It is exactly this perpetual recreation of the self, the foundation of greatness, which post-modernism demolishes. Post-modernism could be defined as the clinical reappropriation of society and culture. As Emile Cioran aptly phrases it, 'Devotees of the fragment and the stigma, we belong to a clinical age where all that count are cases.'[122] Can we imagine anyone eulogising a case?

Myth is not merely the guarantee of survival down the centuries. It is also an imaginary self, an identity which the subject is well-advised to construct and climb into while still in his 'preposthumous' life, to use Musil's expression.[123]

Cuvier, with the calibrated theatricality of his public appearances, the knowing exposure of certain parts of his private life and the dramatisation of his discoveries, was a virtuoso of Self-mythologising, to the point where he is his own first biographer.[124] Was he insuring himself against the risk of seeing his glory inexorably tarnished after his death? Just see how he was ill-treated by his successors.[125] This was not an isolated case. The Private Science of Louis Pasteur by Gerald Geison is not a history of Pasteurian biology. What one critic justifiably described as 'scientific biography at its best', this veritable *damnatio memoriae* tears the subject down from his pedestal.[126] The author wilfully disperses the charismatic glow ordinarily surrounding the inventor of the rabies vaccine. The Pasteurian legend cannot withstand the brutal revelation of the dark side of a scientist who would stop at practically nothing to acquire immortal fame, at least as is implied by a reading of his laboratory notebooks and a careful decoding of his writing and publication strategies. Statues also die! The pill was bitter enough to evince a public protest from a French diplomat at a scientific gathering held in Mexico City shortly after the publication of Geison's book.[127] The disillusioned reader will recognise in this story a world where the race to success, even in science, is not run without the occasional dirty trick. The historian will discover in Geison's biography the ambivalence proper to the scientific eulogy, torn between praise and blame.

Banality of the exceptional

An agonistic situation thus forbids the 'exclusiveness'[128] of genius in the sense used by Carlyle or Burckhardt. Rivalry and antagonism secure some kind of a democratic usage of biography. It was Baudelaire who said, 'The tremendous appetite we have for biographies stems from a deep sense of equality.'[129] The need satisfied by biography is the fair distribution of praise and criticism. The same duality may be responsible for today's approach to biography, which is no longer that of the almightiness of a single, indivisible personality. Modern biographies do not claim to portray everything in a life; they present a succession of discrete images, scattered signs connected with their subject's career.[130] But, whether the persona provides the angle from which the sources are viewed or whether the person's story is attacked from the reverse angle, how can the discordancy between persona and person, between biography and chronicle, be attenuated ?

How can the relative importance of the subject and his will, the contingent and the incidental, be measured without indulging in 'genre painting'? Or without committing the too frequent biographical fault of using the frame (the period) and the subject (the life) as exogenous components of what the author himself wishes to say? Or without falling into the teleological trap?[131]

Perhaps the solution lies in matching biographised 'lives' against a standard curriculum (family, studies, career, honours, writings, etc.), part biographical data and part statistics.[132] For more than fifty years now, prosopography, imported from political or religious history, has been widely used as a method in social history. A triumph of erudition, it may be described as 'collective biography' designed for compiling lists of dignitaries and militants,[133] or the numerical strength of groups and institutions. Prosopography is on the scale of such things as activism, which involves not only individuals but also groups; it is on the scale of every aristocratic, bourgeois or proletarian elite. This makes it particularly suited to the study of learned or medical societies.[134] By using a stock portrait composed from data derived from chosen sources (correspondence, diaries), 'standard deviations' can be determined and a 'complex image' created of partisans, specialists and men of good works.[135] The individual is placed in a series, beyond biography.[136] Since the idea is to rescue obscure figures from anonymity, the biography of the major personalities recedes into the background.[137] The disagreement between persona and person seems in this way to be eliminated, since they merge together in the dark, where 'all cats are grey'.[138]

Despite being disdained by 'learned' history, biography, firmly rooted in our institutions (Academy eulogies), is in fine fettle. This, even though the 'heroarchy'[139] treasured by Carlyle has long since been toppled, like the statues of Lenin after the collapse of the USSR. Biography is alive and well since it is a protection against genius; since it is opposed to the exclusiveness of genius, as we have said. It is in good shape since it is more capable than 'learned' history of praising and blaming. In doing so, it meets a very real need. Whereas the Last Judgement has dropped out of history, the Academy eulogy and biography do what they can to establish, according to merit, a strict hierarchy among personae, not persons. The agonistic situation – simultaneously manifested (competition among posthumous reputations) and denied (encomiastic rules) – extinguishes the charismatic glow which once haloed the giants.[140] At every moment, the historian oscillates between regret for the exceptional and heady freedom before the banal.

Translated from the French by Owen Leeming

---

1 As regards disdain, see the unusually acrimonious passages which Furet reserved for R. Cobb: F. Furet, *L'atelier de l'histoire* (Paris: Flammarion, 1982), 19-28. E.H. Carr took a very severe view of biography, a holdover from the past swept aside by sociology, but at least he mentioned it, E.H. Carr, *What is History?* (London: Macmillan, 1961), chap.2. Significantly, R.J. Evans, *In Defence of History* (London: Granta Books, 1997), 161-165, seeking to measure the progress made since Carr, chose to quarrel with political history, the preferred medium for an elitist historiography of 'great men', and not with biography, which he did not even mention. In November 2001, a number of historians, gathered to celebrate the fortieth anniversary of Carr's Cambridge lectures, raised questions about the development of their discipline. The subject of biography was not brought up and the word itself was not pronounced, D. Cannadine (ed.), *What is History Now?* (Basingstoke: Palgrave, 2002).

2 Bibliographie Nationale Française, publication statistics, 7 February 2007.
3 D. Porter, 'The Mission of the Social History of Medicine: A Historical View', *Soc. Hist. Med.*, 8 (1995), 345—59.
4 On the more general aspects of biography in relation to new trends in history, see E. Engelberg and H. Schleier, 'Zur Geschichte und Theorie der historischen Biographie', *Zeitschrift für Geschichtswissenschaft*, 38 (1990), 195—217; T.C.W. Blanning and D. Cannadine (eds), *History and Biography. Essays in Honour of Derek Beales* (Cambridge: Cambridge University Press, 1996); and, where France is concerned, F. Dosse, *Le pari biographique. Ecrire une vie* (Paris: La Découverte, 2005).
5 W.F. Bynum and H. Bynum, 'Introduction', in W.F. Bynum and H. Bynum (eds), *Dictionary of Medical Biography*, 1 (Westport, Conn.: Greenwood Press, 2007), XXV.
6 L. Stone, 'The Revival of the Narrative: Reflections on a New Old History', *Past & Present* (1979), 3—24.
7 Furet, *L'atelier*, 10-7.
8 For the most part, concerning practitioners deeply interested in social medicine and public health.
9 K. Thomas, 'How it strikes a contemporary', *Times Literary Supplement*, Dec 16, 2005.
10 Prof. Gilbert, preface to P. Busquet, *Les biographies médicales. Notes pour servir à l'histoire de la médecine et des grands médecins* (Paris: Baillière, undated [1927-1928]), 3.
11 M.D. Grmek, 'Introduction', M.D. Grmek (ed.), *Histoire de la pensée médicale en Occident. 1. Antiquité et Moyen Age* (Paris: Seuil, 1995), 9.
12 H.-U. Lammel, 'To Whom Does Medical History Belong?' in F. Huisman and J.H. Warner (eds), *Locating Medical History* (Baltimore: The Johns Hopkins University Press, 2004), 34—44: 37, 43-4. However, this disaffection may be fading, Engelberg and Schleier, Zur Geschichte und Theorie,' 198-200.
13 F. H. Garrison, *An Introduction to the History of Medicine: with Medical Chronology, Bibliographic Data and Test Questions* (Philadelphia : W.B. Saunders, 1913).
14 G. Daremberg, *Les grands médecins du XIXe siècle* (Paris: Masson, 1907), 3.
15 E. Ackerknecht, *Rudolf Virchow. Doctor, Statesman, Anthropologist* (Madison: The University of Wisconsin Press, 1953).
16 Grmek, 'Introduction,' 20.
17 F. Hartog, 'Plutarque entre les anciens et les modernes,' in Plutarque (ed.), *Vies parallèles* (Paris: Gallimard, 2001), 48.
18 Evans, *In Defence of History*, 189.
19 According to Droysen, Caesar or Frederick the Great could not be subjects for a biography; they belong to history. Only an adventurer, a failure, an outsider 'sind durch und durch biographische Figuren', J. G. Droysen, *Grundriss der Historik* (Berlin, 1857-8), edited by R. Hübner (Munich and Berlin, 1937), 292, quoted by A. Momigliano, *Les Origines de la biographie en Grèce ancienne* (Strasbourg: Circé, 1991), 11 (The Development of Greek Biography, Harvard, 1971).
20 G.L. Strachey, *Eminent Victorians* (New York: Putnam, 1918), Preface.
21 Momigliano, *Les origines*, 85, 135; Hartog, *Vies parallèles*, 29-30.
22 Plutarch, 'Life of Alexander', I, 2 and 3; R. Barthes, *Sade Fourier Loyola* (Paris: Seuil, 1971), 14.
23 Voltaire, 'to Nicolas-Claude Thiriot, around 15 July 1735', in J. Hellegouarc'h (ed.), *Correspondance choisie* (Paris: Le Livre de Poche, 1991), 75 (letter no.37).
24 A.-L. Thomas, 'Essai sur les éloges' (1773), quoted by M. Fumaroli, *Trois institutions littéraires* (Paris: Gallimard, 1994), 58-9.

25 Ibid., 59.
26 Ibid., 50-1.
27 M. Fumaroli, 'Les abeilles et les araignées', in A.-M. Lecoq (ed.), *La Querelle des Anciens et des Modernes XVIIe-XVIIIe siècle* (Paris: Gallimard, 2001), 183-4.
28 Fumaroli, *Trois institutions*, 69.
29 C.B. Paul, *Science and Immortality. The Éloges of the Paris Academy of Sciences (1699-1791)* (Berkeley: University of California Press, 1980), 13.
30 Ibid., 9-10.
31 C.-A. Sainte-Beuve, 'Eloges académiques de M. Pariset (4 mars 1850)', *Causeries du lundi, 1* (Paris: Garnier, undated), 393.
32 Ibid., 392-6. Etienne Pariset (1770-1847), succeeded Esquirol as chief of the lunatic asylum at the Salpêtrière in 1826.
33 M. Foucault, *L'ordre du discours* (Paris: Gallimard, 1971), 41-7. As to the 20th century, one of the most referred-to French collections of medical biographies comprises obituaries delivered to the Academy by its author: E. Rist, *Vingt-cinq portraits de médecins français, 1900-1955* (Paris: Masson, 1955).
34 Sainte-Beuve, 'Eloges académiques,', 410.
35 P. Hadot, Preface to E. Bertram, *Nietzsche. Essai de mythologie* (Paris: Editions du Félin, 1990), 18.
36 See, for example, J.R. Bartholemew, 'Japanese Nobel Candidates in the First Half of the Twentieth Century', *Osiris*, 13 (1998), 238—84.
37 Hartog, 'Plutarque', 42.
38 P.M. Haas, 'Introduction: Epistemic Communities and International Policy Coordination', *International Organization*, 46 (1992), 1—35. As regards epistemic communities and international public health, see M.D. Dubin, 'The League of Nations Health Organization', in P. Weindling (ed.), *International Health Organizations and Movements 1918-1939* (Cambridge: Cambridge University Press, 1995), 56—81.
39 E. Aujaleu, *Les Lauréats européens du Prix Léon-Bernard* (Copenhagen: WHO Regional Office for Europe, 1981), 2.
40 G. Weisz, *The Medical Mandarins. The French Academy of Medicine in the Nineteenth and Early Twentieth Centuries* (Oxford: Oxford University Press, 1995), 125.
41 Anonymous, 'Décès de M. [Paul] Brouardel', *Bulletin de l'Académie de médecine*, 56 (1906), 168—75 : 168-9 [hereafter : BAM]; R. Debré, 'Nécrologie. Louis Pasteur Vallery-Radot' (1886-1970)', *BAM*, 155 (1971), 436—48 : 448.
42 F. Nietzsche, 'La joute chez Homère', in G. Colli and M. Montinari (eds), *Oeuvres philosophiques complètes. Ecrits posthumes 1870-73* (Paris: Gallimard, 1975), 192-200.
43 Polybius, *History*, X, 21.
44 H. Mondor, *Anatomistes et chirurgiens* (Paris: Editions Fragrance, 1949), XIV.
45 P.C.-A. Louis, quoted ibid., XIV.
46 C.-A. Sainte-Beuve, 'Œuvres de François Arago (20 mars 1854)', *Causeries du lundi*, X (Paris: Garnier, undated), 9.
47 Paul, *Science and Immortality*, 10.
48 D. Outram, 'The Language of Natural Power: The Éloges of Georges Cuvier and the Public Language of Nineteenth Century Science', *History of Science*, 16 (1978), 153-178: 154.
49 E. Littré, *Sur la mort d'A. Comte* (Paris, 1857), quoted by E. Renan, 'Vie de Jésus' (preface 13th edition), *Histoire et parole*. Œuvres diverses (Paris: Laffont, 1984), 362.
50 J.-P. Sartre, *L'idiot de la famille. Gustave Flaubert de 1821 à 1857* (Paris: Gallimard, 1972), 263-4.

51 L.G. Neumann, *Biographies vétérinaires* (Paris: Asselin et Houzeau, 1896), VII. Neumann was professor at the School of Veterinary Medicine in Toulouse.
52 Cuvier, *Éloge de J. Darcet (1725-1801),* read on 15 Nivôse, Year X (5 April 1802), quoted by Mondor, op. cit. (note 45) , XV.
53 Sainte-Beuve, 'Eloges académiques', 407.
54 M.D. Grmek, 'Life and Achievements of Andrija Stampar, Fighter for the Promotion of Public Health', in M.D. Grmek (ed.), *Serving the Cause of Public Health. Selected Papers of Andrija Stampar,* Monograph Series No.3 (Zagreb: Andrija Stampar School of Public Health, 1966), 14-5.
55 P. Mercier, 'L'œuvre scientifique de Robert Debré', *BAM*, 166 (1982), 1285—94 : 1294. On Ciceronian eloquence as bel canto, see P. Veyne, 'Préface' to Seneca, *Entretiens et Lettres à Lucilius* (Paris: Laffont, 1993), V.
56 'Tardieu taught for eighteen years and left a potent reputation when he died. Brouardel showed himself to be very different from his two predecessors [Orfila and Tardieu], but he was not inferior to either one': L.H. Thoinot, 'Paul Brouardel', *Mémoires de l'Académie de médecine,* 42 (1911), 1—18: 5.
57 'Décès de M . [Joseph] Grancher', *BAM*, 58 (1907), 69—71 : 71. Jacques-Joseph Grancher (1843-1907), a paediatrician, performed the first vaccination against rabies on behalf of Pasteur on the 5 July 1885.
58 Fumaroli, *Trois institutions* , 58.
59 C.-A. Sainte-Beuve, 'Fontenelle par M. Flourens (27 janvier 1851)', *Causeries du lundi,* 3 (Paris: Garnier, undated), 335. Times obituaries, for their part, separated 'distinguished or remarkable persons' from 'persons of less importance', Thomas, op. cit. (note 9)', 6.
60 E. Pariset, *Membres de l'Académie royale de médecine, ou recueil des éloges lus dans les séances publiques* (Paris: Baillière, 1850), vol.2, 316, translated and quoted by Weisz, op. cit. (note 40) , 125.
61 E. Pariset, Membres de l'Académie royale de médecine, BAM, 1 (1837), 387, translated and quoted by Weisz, *The Medical Mandarins*, 127.
62 For example, the three pages devoted to the Pasteurian, bacteriologist, Etienne Burnet (1873-1960) by Gaston Ramon in 1961 were no more than a dry succession of facts and dates, with nothing said about the man. In fine, the Pasteurian motto: Work, salvation, peace. G. Ramon, 'Nécrologie. Etienne Burnet (1873-1960)', *BAM*, 145 (1961), 189—91.
63 Neumann, *Biographies vétérinaires*, VII.
64 See, for example, C. Achard, 'Eloge de Joseph Grancher', *BAM*, 90 (1923), 533—46: 533; and F. Bezançon, 'Centenaire de Grancher. Grancher phtisiologue', *BAM,* 127 (1943), 406—14: 407: '... my task before you is to demarcate between what has enriched our medical heritage for all time and what should be discarded.'
65 E. Cassirer, *The Myth of the State* (New Haven: Yale University Press, 1979 [1946]), 191.
66 B. Groethuysen, *Mythes et portraits* (Paris: Gallimard, 1947), 103-4.
67 J. Burckhardt, *Considérations sur l'histoire universelle* (Paris: Payot, 1971), 240-3, 245, 274 (*Weltgeschichtliche Betrachtungen*, 1905).
68 *Les Lauréats européens*, 61.
69 D.P. Verene (ed.), *Symbol, Myth, and Culture. Essays and Lectures of Ernst Cassirer (1935-1945)* (New Haven: Yale University Press, 1979), 191.
70 Sainte-Beuve, 'Eloges académiques', 410.
71 Ibid., 406.

72 H. Wölfflin, *Principes fondamentaux de l'histoire de l'art* (Paris: Gallimard, 1952), 15 (*Kunstgeschichtliche Grundbegriffe: das Problem der Stilentwicklung in der neueren Kunst*, 1915).

73 H.E. Sigerist, 'William Harveys Stellung in der europäischen Geistesgeschichte', *Arch. Kulturg.*, 19 (1928), 158—68, quoted by O. Temkin, *The Double Face of Janus and Other Essays in the History of Medicine* (Baltimore: The Johns Hopkins Press, 1977), 115-6.

74 A rarity is the physical portrait of Joseph Grancher offered by J. Renault in 1943. J. Renault, 'Centenaire de Grancher. Grancher pédiatre', *BAM*, 127 (1943), 401—6: 406. In general, all one gets is a vague sketch: 'He was of average height, and sturdy-looking.' R. Dujarric de la Rivière, 'Nécrologie de Georges Brouardel (1869-1959)', *BAM*, 143 (1959), 624—30: 629. One later exception: M. Druon, 'Louis Pasteur Vallery-Radot ou le génie de l'amitié', *BAM*, 170 (1986), 613—34 : 621, but the author was a novelist.

75 R. Piédelièvre, 'Notice nécrologique sur M. Balthazard', *BAM*, 135 (1951), 249—53 : 252.

76 Examples of friendship are so numerous that we need not quote them. There is, however, Robert Debré's eulogy of Pasteur Vallery-Radot in 1971, a fine meditation on friendship in the Stoic and Péguy sense. (Debré had studied philosophy before taking up medicine.) Debré, 'Nécrologie', 442.

77 J. Marie, 'Robert Debré (1882-1978). L'homme, le médecin, le professeur', *BAM*, 166 (1982), 1257—64 : 1259. Robert Debré was the father of Michel Debré, Prime Minister of France from 1959 to 1962. See M. Debré, 'Robert Debré, réformateur', *BAM*, 166 (1982), 1295—1303. (Died in 1978, Debré held the Paris Chair of Pediatrics since 1933 and instigated in the early 1960s a reform in medical studies and hospital practice.)

78 Thomas, 'How it strikes)'.

79 Sainte-Beuve, 'Œuvres de François Arago', 13.

80 For a more recent example, in addition to the eulogy of Grancher by Charles Achard (1860-1944) in 1923 and that delivered by F. Bezançon (1868-1948) twenty years later, already mentioned, see Mercier, 'L'œuvre scientifique', 1285—94.

81 J. Marie devotes only three pages out of thirteen to Robert Debré's scientific work. J. Marie, 'Eloge de Robert Debré (1882-1978)', *BAM*, 162 (1978), 607—19.

82 L. Bernard, 'Nécrologie. La vie et l'œuvre d'Albert Calmette', *BAM*, 110 (1933), 426—38 : 431. See also R. Dujarric de la Rivière, 'Eloge de Charles-Albert Calmette (1863-1933)', *BAM*, 148 (1964), 648—55 : 652.

83 Sainte-Beuve, 'Œuvres de François Arago', 11, 13.

84 Weisz, *The Medical Mandarins*, 129.

85 L. Jordanova, *History in Practice* (London: Arnold, 2000), 101.

86 P.A. Lawrence, 'The Politics of Publication', *Nature*, 422 (20 March 2003), 259—61: 260.

87 D. Outram, 'Scientific Biography and the Case of Georges Cuvier: with a Critical Bibliography', *History of Science*, 14 (1976), 101—137: 102.

88 Dujarric de la Rivière, 'Eloge de Charles-Albert Calmette', 654.

89 J. Burckhardt, *La Civilisation de la Renaissance en Italie* (Paris: Le Livre de Poche, 1958), Vol.2, 252-4, 247.

90 The role allotted to wives was symmetrically obverse. Emile Roux saw in Madame Pasteur 'the model scholar's wife, devoted to the point of renunciation, and the most useful of helpers'. Quoted by P. Lépine, 'Le petit-fils de Pasteur', *BAM*, 170 (1986), 625—28 : 625. Convention weighs heavily here. See A. Dufour, 'Eloge de Xavier Leclainche

(1899-1984)', *BAM*, 168 (1984), 717—25: 724 (endnote ' ma chère Eva'). It is clear that a wife was measured, not against her husbands' person, but against his persona, which was not very sporting.

91 Veyne, 'Préface', III.

92 P. Milliez, 'Le médecin et l'homme', *BAM*, 170 (1986), 617—19 : 617; Debré, 'Nécrologie,', 446. The RPF (Rassemblement du peuple français) was founded by General de Gaulle in April 1947. Pasteur Vallery-Radot, elected under the party's standard in 1951, resigned his seat in the following year.

93 Lépine, 'Le petit-fils,' 628. Grancher also is shown in his role as acquaintance of anyone who was anybody in medicine, science, literature, the arts and politics; Renault, 'Centenaire de Grancher', 406.

94 Marie, 'Eloge de Robert Debré', 617, 619; Mercier, 'L'œuvre scientifique,' 1285.

95 J. Bernard, 'Robert Debré: L'humanisme et les académies', *BAM*, 166 (1982), 1281—84 : 1283.

96 'Décès de Fernand Bezançon', *BAM*, 132 (1948), 430; P. Pruvost, 'Fernand Bezançon (1868-1948)', *BAM*, 133 (1949), 3—13: 11, 3.

97 Quoted by G.L. Geison, *The Private Science of Louis Pasteur* (Princeton NJ: Princeton University Press, 1995), 272.

98 'Enfin, mort triomphant, il vit sa délivrance / Et l'océan rendit son cercueil à la France.' ('At last, triumphant dead, he saw his deliverance / And the ocean returned his casket to France.') Regarding the extreme popularity of Les Châtiments among the French during the century 1850-1950, see T. Zeldin, *France 1848-1945,* Vol.1: Ambition, Love and Politics (Oxford: Clarendon Press, 1973), 746; and P. Pia, *Romanciers, poètes et essayistes du XIXe siècle* (Paris: Denoël, 1971), 94-5.

99 C. Chagas, 'Pasteur Vallery-Radot et le rayonnement de la France', *BAM,* 170 (1986), 629—33 : 633.

100 K.F. Quinn, 'Banting and his Biographers: Maker of Miracles, Makers of Myth', *Queen's Quarterly*, 89 (1982), 243—59.

101 Burckhardt, *Considérations* , 237.

102 Paul, *Science and Immortality*, 12.

103 Ibid., 102.

104 See the eulogy written by H. Cumming, in the name of the U.S. Public Health Service, when Joseph Goldberger died in January 1929, quoted by A.M. Kraut, *Goldberger's War. The Life and Work of a Public Health Crusader* (New York: Hill & Wang, 2003), 243.

105 R. Barthes, *Sur Racine* (Paris: Seuil, 1963), 138.

106 Outram, 'The Language,' 160.

107 Sainte-Beuve, 'Eloges académiques', 406; also Mondor, *Anatomistes et chirurgiens*, XV.

108 This aspect of biographical practice was noted by Outram, op. cit. (note 48), 154 and by Weisz, *The Medical Mandarins*, 125.

109 F. Jacob, The Statue Within: an Autobiography (New York: Basic Books, 1988), 244-7, quoted by Geison, *The Private Science* , 263-4.

110 E. Fee and T.M. Brown, 'Using Medical History to Shape a Profession', F. Huisman and J.H. Warner (eds), Locating Medical History(Baltimore: The Johns Hopkins University Press, 2004), 139—64: 140-4. On Carlyle and history as a succession of biographies, see Cassirer, *The Myth of the State*, 191.

111 Pr. Gilbert, preface to Busquet, *Les biographies médicales*, 4; J. Hamburger, 'Introduction à la séance consacrée à la commémoration du centenaire de la naissance de Pasteur Vallery-Radot (1886-1970)', *BAM*, 170 (1986), 613—34: 615.

112 G. Duhamel, surgeon and author, on 24 May 1938, proposing the inclusion of Justin Godart in the short-list of candidates to fill a vacancy in the Academy's free member section, X. Leclainche, 'Eloge de Justin Godart (1871-1956)', *BAM*, 156 (1972), 943—52: 952.
113 Thomas, 'How it strikes a contemporary", 6.
114 Paul, *Science and Immortality*, 87; Weisz, *The Medical Mandarins*, 231.
115 Anonymous, 'Décès de M. [Paul] Brouardel', 175 ; Paul Brouardel (1837-1906), holder of the chair of forensic medicine of the Faculty of Paris and dean of the Faculty, he was commissaire du gouvernement at the turn of the century, when the parliament elaborated the law of public health. Or see the barely hidden spite vented at the celebration of the centenary of Pasteur Vallery-Radot's birth by Paul Milliez (1912-1994), another of his friends and a member of the Academie de médecine, against Robert Debré (by then dead), author of the eulogy of the deceased in 1971, Milliez, 'Le médecin et l'homme', 617.
116 Weisz *The Medical Mandarins*, 225.
117 Outram, 'The Language of Natural Power,' 155.
118 Debré, 'Robert Debré, réformateur', 1299.
119 Burckhardt, *Considérations*, 254.
120 M. Blanchot, *L'Entretien infini* (Paris: Gallimard, 1969), 544.
121 J. Burckhardt, *Griechische Kulturgeschichte*, quoted by E. Cassirer, *'Political History and the History of Civilization: Burckhardt', The Problem of Knowledge. Philosophy, Science, and History since Hegel* (New Haven: Yale University Press, 1978 [1950]), 277.
122 E. Cioran, *Syllogismes de l'amertume* (Paris: Gallimard, 1952), 1.
123 R. Musil, *Nachlass zu Lebzeiten* (Zürich: Humanitas, 1936).
124 Outram, 'Scientific Biography', 101-2.
125 Outram, 'Scientific Biography', 105-7.
126 Geison, *The Private Science* , 277-8; the critic quoted on the book jacket is R. Olby.
127 Personal message from Dr A.-M. Moulin.
128 Nietzsche, 'La joute chez Homère', 197.
129. C. Baudelaire, *'Pierre Dupont (1851)', Œuvres complètes*, vol. II (Paris: Pléiade-Gallimard, 1976), 28.
130 M.-L. Desclos (ed.), *Biographie des hommes, biographie des dieux, Recherches sur la philosophie et le langage*. Cahier 21 (Paris: Vrin, 2000); see the review by F. Gherchanoc, *Annales*, 57 (2002), No.3, 697--9. On this important point, see Barthes, *Sade Fourier Loyola*, 14.
131 Furet, *L'atelier de l'histoire*, 19.
132 R. Bange, 'Base de données pour une étude prosopographique: les auditeurs du cours de Lamarck au Muséum national d'histoire naturelle (1795-1823)', *Annales historiques de la Révolution française*, No.320 (2006), http://ahrf.revues.org/document167.html, consulted on 6 March 2007, 3.
133 P. Brown, *La vie de Saint Augustin* (Paris: Seuil, 2001), 627 (Augustine of Hippo. A Biography, 2000). We should point to the extreme recentness of the vogue in prosopography outside of the fairly small circle of specialists in early century Roman or Christian ruling classes. The controversy which raged in Great Britain in the 1930s when L. Namier embarked on a prosopography of British 18th century parliamentary elites had little effect on biographical methods, Engelberg and Schleier, 'Zur Geschichte und Theorie der historischen Biographie', 202.
134 Jordanova, *History in Practice*, 179.

135 M. Brejon de Lavergnée, 'La Société de Saint-Vincent-de-Paul à Paris au XIXe siècle (1833-1871)', *Revue d'histoire du XIXe siècle* (posted on the Internet on 9 January 2007), http://rh19.revues.org/document1186.html, consulted on 6 March 2007.

136 C. Nicolet, 'Prosopographie et histoire sociale: Rome et l'Italie à l'époque républicaine', *Annales ESC*, 25 (1970), 1216.

137 Bange, 'Base de données', 2.

138 The aesthetics of banality were pushed to their limits by A. Corbin, *Le monde retrouvé de Louis-François Pinagot: sur les traces d'un inconnu 1798-1876* (Paris: Flammarion, 1998). Without making much of a stir at the time, a biography of the 'nameless' had been proposed for the first time by Austrian literary historian R.M. Werner, 'Biographie der Namenlosen', *Biographische Blätter*, 1 (1895), quoted in Engelberg and Schleier, 'Zur Geschichte und Theorie der historischen Biographie', 201.

139 Cassirer, *The Myth of the State*, 192.

140 S. Mazzarino, *Trattato di storia romana*, vol.II (Rome: Tumminelli, 1956), 416, quoted by Brown, *La vie de Saint Augustin*, 665.

Notes on Contributors

Iris Borowy is adjunct lecturer at the University of Rostock. Her research interests focus on twentieth century international relations and on the politics of international health. She has published on various aspects of interwar health, including 'International Social Medicine Between the Wars. Positioning a Volatile Concept,' *Hygiea Internationalis*, 6, 2 (2007), 13–35, and 'Die internationale Gesundheitspolitik des Völkerbundes zwischen globalem Denken und europäischem Führungsanspruch', *Zeitschrift für Geschichtswissenschaft*, 54:10 (2006), 864-875. Together with Wolf D. Gruner she is co-editor of *Facing Illness in Troubled Times. Health in Europe in the Interwar Years, 1918 - 1939,* (Berlin: Peter Lang Verlag, 2005). She is currently finishing *Coming to Terms with World Health. The League of Nations Health Organisation,* expected to be published in 2009.

Zeljko Dugac is senior researcher of the Croatian Academy of Sciences and Arts, Institute for the History and Philosophy of Science, Division for the History of Medicine. His research forcuses on the history of public health and health promotion between the World Wars, on the history of Rockefeller philanthropy and on the work of Andrija Štampar as an expert of the League of Nation Health Organization as well as the Rockefeller Foundation. He also explores a history of folk medicine in Croatia. Recent publications include 'Mothers Care about Children's Health, «Seljacka Sloga» Campaign for Medical Education, 1939-1941', *Casopis za suvremenu povijest* 38:3 (2006), 983-1005; *Opposing diseases and ignorance: The Rockefeller Foundation in the Interwar Yugoslavia* (Zagreb: Srednja Europa, 2005); 'Popular Health Education and Venereal Diseases in Croatia between Two World Wars', *Croatian Medical Journal*, 45:4 (2004), 490-498.

Anne Hardy was educated at Oxford, and joined the staff of the Wellcome Institute in 1990 after a period of research funding. Her research interests are in the modern period, more especially in the history of disease, environment and nutrition. She is the author of *The Epidemic Streets: Infectious disease and the rise of preventive medicine, 1856-1900* (Oxford, 1993), *Health and Medicine in Britain since 1860* (London, 2001), co-author of *Prevention and Cure: A history of the London School of Hygiene and Tropical Medicine* (London, 2001), and co-editor of two volumes of collected essays. She has published numerous articles in academic journals. Her on-going research project is on the history of the salmonellas and salmonellosis since 1880. She is currently Professor of the History of Modern Medicine and Deputy Director of the Wellcome Trust Centre for the History of Medicine at UCL.

Erik Ingebrigtsen is a post doctoral fellow at the Department of History, Norwegian University of Science and Technology, in Trondheim, Norway. He is affiliated with the *Program on East European Cultures and Societies* (PEECS), where he is a participant in the project *Imagining the West - Perceptions of the Western Other in Modern and Contemporary Eastern Europe and Turkey*. In 2007, Ingebrigtsen defended his PhD thesis, *The Continuation of Revisionism with other Means: Rockefeller Foundation and Public Health in Hungary, 1920-1940* (title translated from the Norwegian). Forthcoming is a paper titled *Privileged Origins: 'National Models' and Reforms of Public Health in Interwar Hungary*. (in anthology, Slavica Publishers)

Socrates Litsios worked with WHO for 30 years (1967-97). His writings include articles and books on the history of malaria, control of infectious diseases, WHO, and the life of Selskar Gunn. His most recent works include the official history of WHO's 3rd decade (1968-77), which is expected to be published in the fall of 2008; 'Selskar Gunn and Paul Russell of the Rockefeller Foundation: A Contrast in Styles,' in Benjamin B. Page and David A. Valone (eds.), *Philanthropic Foundations and the Globalization of Scientific Medicine and Public Health* (Lanham, Maryland: University Press of America, 2007); and 'The Health, Poverty, and Development Merry-Go-Round: The Tribulations of WHO,' in S. William Gunn et al. (eds.), *Understanding the Global Dimensions of Health*, (Springer: 2005). He is currently working on a sequel to *Plague Legends: From the Miasmas of Hippocrates to the Microbes of Pasteur* (Chesterfield: Science & Humanities Press, 2001) entitled *Plague Legends II: In Search of Public Health 1830-1940*.

Esteban Rodriguez-Ocaña is Professor of History of Science at the University of Granada. His fields of research include the social history of diseases and the history of public health and occupational and environmental health. Among his recent publications are *La acción médico-social contra el paludismo en la España metropolitana y colonial del siglo XX* (Madrid: CSIC, 2003, together with Rosa Ballester; Enrique Perdiguero; Rosa Mª. Medina and Jorge Molero), *Salud Pública en España: Ciencia, profesión, política, siglos XVIII-XX* (Granada: Editorial Universidad de Granada, 2005). With Patrick Zylberman he is co-editor of the dossier 'Improving Public Health Amidst Crises: the Interwar Years in Europe' in *Dynamis*, 2008; vol. 28. Currently he is finishing a book on the relationship between the Rockefeller Foundation and Spain, 1911-1941.

Zoe C. Sprigings was a Coombs Scholar at Somerville College, Oxford and graduated in Modern History in 2007. Her undergraduate thesis *LNHO to WHO:*

From the Last of the League to the First of the United Nations focused on the epistemic community which moved between these two organisations, and was the History Faculty nominee for the best History of Science essay. She is currently a civil servant in the UK Department for Environment, Food and Rural Affairs.

Patrick Zylberman is senior researcher at the Centre de Recherche Médecine, Sciences, Santé et Société (CNRS, Paris). Among his publications are: 'Fewer Parallels than Antitheses : René Sand and Andrija Stampar on Social Medicine, 1919-1955,' *Social History of Medicine*, 17, 1 (2004); and *L'Hygiène dans la République, la santé publique en France ou l'utopie contrariée, 1870-1918* (Fayard, 1996, co-authored with Lion Murard). He co-edited with Susan Gross Solomon (University of Toronto) and Lion Murard (CERMES, Paris) *Shifting Boundaries of Public Health: Europe in the Twentieth Century* (University of Rochester Press, 2008) and with Esteban Rodríguez-Ocaña a special dossier 'Improving Public Health Amidst Crises: the Interwar Years in Europe' in *Dynamis* 2008, vol. 28. He is currently working on bioterror and anti-pandemic scenarios, which impose new images of microbial threats that might affect the management of epidemic crises.

Nicolaas A. Rupke (ed.)

Eminent Lives in Twentieth-Century Science and Religion

Frankfurt am Main, Berlin, Bern, Bruxelles, New York, Oxford, Wien, 2007.
255 pp.
ISBN 978-3-631-56803-3 · pb. € 40.10*

Can science and religion coexist peacefully, even symbiotically? Or is conflict inevitable and are the enterprises mutually exclusive? In this volume an international team of distinguished scholars address these enduring yet urgent questions by examining the lives of eminent twentieth-century biologists, chemists and physicists whose careers were marked by the interaction of science and religion: Charles Coulson, Theodosius Dobzhansky, R.A. Fisher, Julian Huxley, Pascual Jordan, Ivan Pavlov, Michael Pupin, and E.O. Wilson. The team's rich empirical studies show a diversity of creative engagements between science and religion that defy efforts to set the two at odds.

Contents: Nicolaas A. Rupke: *Introduction: Telling Lives in Science and Religion* · Arie Leegwater: *Charles Alfred Coulson: Mixing Methodism and Quantum Chemistry* · Jitse M. van der Meer: *Theodosius Dobzhansky: Nothing in Evolution Makes Sense Except in the Light of Religion* · James Moore: *Ronald Aylmer Fisher: A Faith Fit for Eugenics* · Peter J. Bowler: *Julian Huxley: Religion without Revelation* · Richard H. Beyler: *Pascual Jordan: Freedom vs Materialism* · Torsten Rüting: *Ivan Petrovich Pavlov: From Russian Orthodox Monastery to Big Science Laboratory* · Edward B. Davis: *Michael Idvorsky Pupin: Cosmic Beauty, Created Order, and the Divine Word* · Mark Stoll: *Edward Osborne Wilson: The Gospel According to Sociobiology* · Ronald L. Numbers: *Epilogue: Science, Secularization, and Privatization*

www.ingramcontent.com/pod-product-compliance
Ingram Content Group UK Ltd.
Pitfield, Milton Keynes, MK11 3LW, UK
UKHW020121290926
15471UKWH00003B/207

9 783631 580448